Essential Concepts of Electrophysiology through Case Studies: Intracardiac EGMs

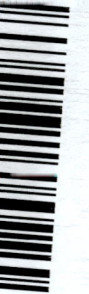

ESSENTIAL CONCEPTS OF ELECTROPHYSIOLOGY THROUGH CASE STUDIES: INTRACARDIAC EGMs

EDITED BY

Kenneth A. Ellenbogen, MD

CONTRIBUTORS

Roderick Tung, MD

David S. Frankel, MD

Prabal K. Guha, MD

Reginald T. Ho, MD

cardiotext®

PUBLISHING

Minneapolis, Minnesota

© 2015 Kenneth A. Ellenbogen, Roderick Tung, David S. Frankel, Prabal K. Guha, Reginald T. Ho

Cardiotext Publishing, LLC

750 2nd St NE Suite 102

Hopkins, MN 55343

USA

www.cardiotextpublishing.com

Any updates to this book may be found at: www.cardiotextpublishing.com/essential-concepts-of-electrophysiology-through-case-studies-intracardiac-egms Comments, inquiries, and requests for bulk sales can be directed to the publisher at: info@cardiotextpublishing.com.

This book is intended for educational purposes and to further general scientific and medical knowledge, research, and understanding of the conditions and associated treatments discussed herein. This book is not intended to serve as and should not be relied upon as recommending or promoting any specific diagnosis or method of treatment for a particular condition or a particular patient. It is the reader's responsibility to determine the proper steps for diagnosis and the proper course of treatment for any condition or patient, including suitable and appropriate tests, medications, or medical devices to be used for or in conjunction with any diagnosis or treatment. Due to ongoing research; discoveries; modifications to medicines, equipment, and de vices; and changes in government regulations, the information contained in this book may not reflect the latest standards, developments, guidelines, regulations, p roducts, or devices in the field. Re aders are responsible for keeping up to date with the latest developments and are urged to review the latest instructions and warnings for any medicine, equipment, or medical device. Readers should consult with a specialist or contact the vendor of any medicine or medical device where appropriate.

Except for the publisher's website associated with this work, the publisher is not affiliated with and does not sponsor or endorse any websites, organizations, or other sources of information referred to herein.

The publisher and the authors specifically disclaim any damage, liability, or loss incurred, directly or indirectly, from the use or application of any of the contents of this book.

Unless otherwise stated, all figures and tables in this book are used courtesy of the authors.

Library of Congress Control Number: 2015935642

ISBN: 978-1-935395-33-1

6 7 8

Dedication

To my wife and family, Phyllis, Michael, Amy, and Bethany, whose support and love sustain my intellectual journey.

—Kenneth A. Ellenbogen, MD

To my parents, who have supported me in every way possible and shown me the value of education, perseverance, and passion. I am an exceptionally fortunate product of their American dream.

To my parents, Patricia and Theodore, and my sister, Candice, for always showing me the road ahead. To Mark Josephson and Kalyanam Shivkumar, who have been instrumental in my training and development as a young physician.

—Roderick Tung, MD

To my wife and son for their love. To my mother and father for teaching me the right way. And to my brothers and sister, lifelong partners in crime.

—David S. Frankel, MD

To my parents; my wife, Simi; and my sons, Etash and Ayan, for their love and support, which made this endeavor possible.

—Prabal K. Guha, MD

To my wife, Maromi; sons, Ethan and Jeremy; and my parents, whose love and support are always enduring.

—Reginald T. Ho, MD

Contents

About the Contributors

Editor:

Kenneth A. Ellenbogen, MD, FACC, FHRS, is Kontos Professor of Cardiology and Chairman of the Pauley Heart Center at the Virginia Commonwealth University School of Medicine, Richmond, Virginia

Contributors:

Roderick Tung, MD, FACC, FHRS, is Assistant Professor of Medicine and Director of the Specialized Program for Ventricular Tachycardia at the UCLA Cardiac Arrhythmia Center, UCLA Ronald Reagan Medical Center, Los Angeles, California

David S. Frankel, MD, FACC, FHRS, is Assistant Professor of Medicine and Associate Director of the Cardiac Electrophysiology Fellowship Program, Perelman School of Medicine at the University of Pennsylvania, Philadelphia, Pennsylvania

Prabal K. Guha MD, FACC, is Assistant Professor of Internal Medicine at the University of South Carolina School of Medicine, Columbia; Electrophysiologist at McLeod Regional Medical Center, Florence, South Carolina; Director of the Electrophysiology Laboratory at Carolinas Hospital, Florence, South Carolina

Reginald T. Ho, MD, FACC, FHRS, is Associate Professor of Medicine, Division of Cardiology/Electrophysiology at Thomas Jefferson University Hospital, Philadelphia, Pennsylvania

Preface

One of the most essential skills in electrophysiology is the ability to analyze and decipher electrophysiologic recordings, using all the data that can be gained from a careful review of every aspect of the tracing. This second volume of tracings builds on our first volume, utilizing formal analysis of the surface ECG to complex intracardiac tracings.

We hope these tracings prove challenging and lead to review of the relevant literature. We have tried to focus on critical and important concepts.

We hope you enjoy reading and studying this manual as much as we enjoyed selecting and annotating the cases. We anticipate it will provide a valuable review for a wide variety of professionals (physicians, associated professionals, nurses, and technicians) preparing for certification and recertification examinations in electrophysiology.

—Kenneth A. Ellenbogen, MD
Richmond, Virginia

Roderick Tung, MD
Los Angeles, California

David S. Frankel, MD
Philadelphia, Pennsylvania

Prabal K. Guha, MD
Florence, South Carolina

Reginald T. Ho, MD
Philadelphia, Pennsylvania

Abbreviations

AF	atrial fibrillation
AIVR	accelerated idioventricular rhythm
ARVC	arrhythmogenic right ventricular cardiomyopathy
AV	atrioventricular
AVNRT	atrioventricular nodal reentrant tachycardia
AVRT	AV reentrant tachycardia
BBR	bundle branch reentry
BBRT	bundle branch reentrant tachycardia
CHF	congestive heart failure
CL	cycle length
CS	coronary sinus
ECG	electrocardiogram
EF	ejection fraction
EGM	electrogram
ICD	implantable cardiac defibrillator
ILR	implantable loop recorder
JT	junctional tachycardia
LAA	left atrial appendage
LBBB	left bundle branch block
LCC	left coronary cusp
LSPV	left superior pulmonary vein
LV	left ventricle or left ventricular
MI	myocardial infarction
NICM	nonischemic cardiomyopathy
ORT	orthodromic reentrant tachycardia
PAC	premature atrial contraction
PPI	postpacing interval
PV	pulmonary vein
PVC	premature ventricular contraction
RBBB	right bundle branch block
RCC	right coronary cusp
RV	right ventricle or right ventricular
SVT	supraventricular tachycardia
TCL	tachycardia cycle length
VA	ventriculoatrial
VF	ventricular fibrillation
VP	ventricular pacing
VT	ventricular tachycardia
WCT	wide complex tachycardia

PART 1

Electrophysiologic Concepts

Question

The maneuver proves:

A) Absence of retrogradely conducting bypass tract

B) Absence of septal bypass tract

C) Presence of retrogradely conducting bypass tract

D) Presence of septal bypass tract

Figure 1.A.1

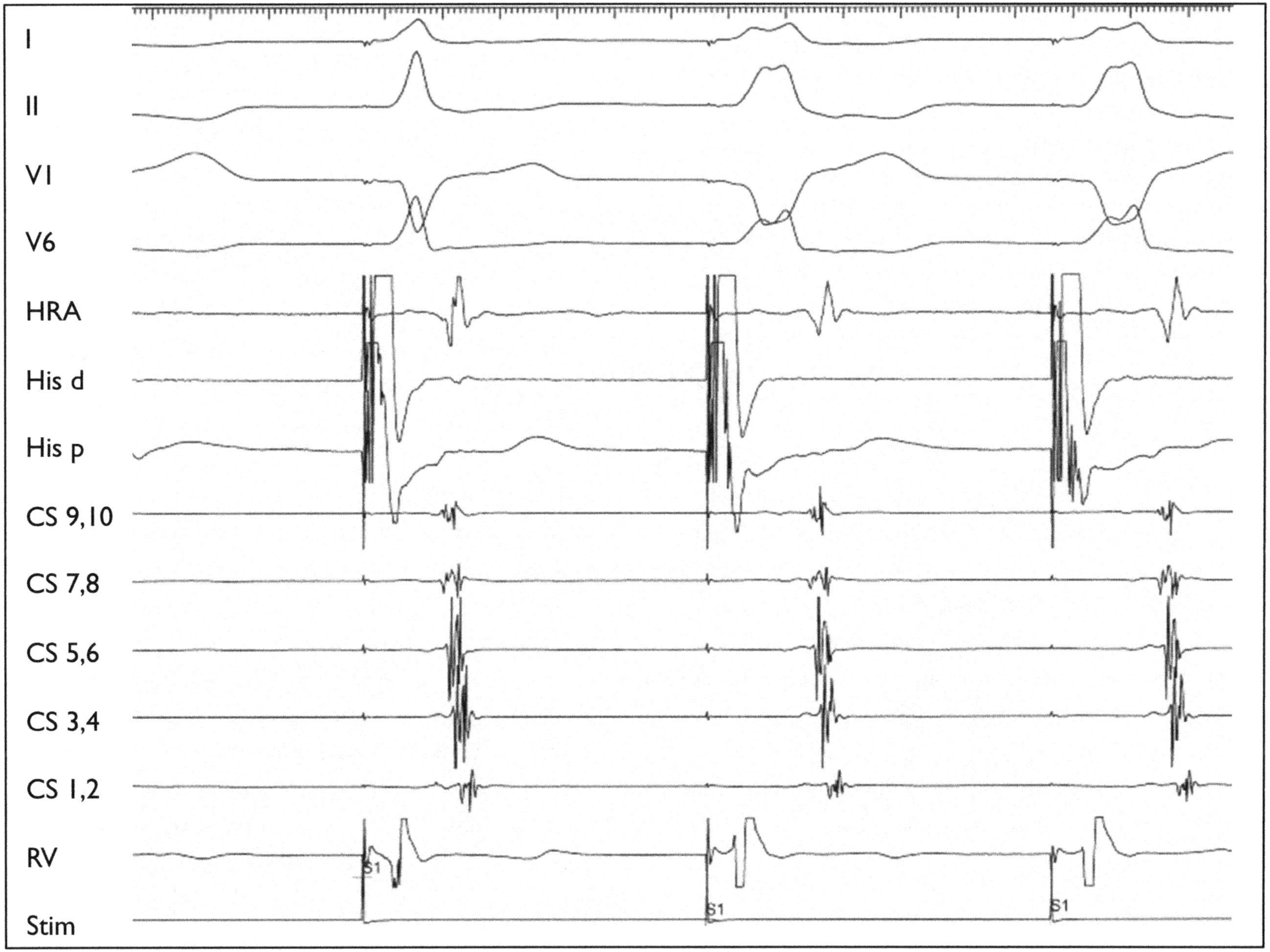

*A*nswer

The correct answer is B. Parahisian pacing technique is used to determine the presence of retrograde atrial activation over a bypass tract. Pacing is carried out near the His bundle with varying output. Capture of His and right bundle results in a narrow QRS. Decrease in output results in loss of His capture, and only RV is captured (His bundle is well insulated and needs high output for capture). The changes in stimulus to atrial activation timing, atrial activation pattern, and His-to-A timing can indicate retrograde conduction over a septal pathway, AV node, or both. Readers are referred to the excellent papers referenced for a detailed description of the patterns and interpretation.

With His + RB capture (narrower QRS) the SA (135 ms) is shorter by 35 ms as compared to RV-only capture (wide QRS) (170 ms). There is no significant change in atrial activation. This indicates that the activation was conducted only over the AV node.

However, if the insertion of the bypass tract is away from the septum, changes in the atrial activation may not be apparent unless atrial activation is recorded near the site of insertion of the accessory pathway, in which case it may show fusion. Based on the findings shown in this tracing only, a septal pathway can be ruled out. In fact, a careful analysis of this tracing should lead one to suspect the possible presence of a right-sided accessory pathway. This can be discerned by the observation of the near simultaneous activation of the high right atrial electrogram with a far-field His atrial electrogram on the first and subsequent beats.

In this case, a right lateral bypass tract was present. Postablation, repeat Parahisian pacing shows changes consistent with conduction over the AV node; however, SA time was increased as compared to baseline (HB + RB capture: 133 ms, and RV capture only: 190 ms). This indicates there was fused conduction over AV node and pathway during the baseline tracing.

It should be noted that, although a rapidly conducting septal AP is excluded, a slowly conducting, decremental AP (as seen with PJRT) is not. In such a case, rapid retrograde AVN conduction could preempt slow retrograde AP conduction during both His/RV and RV-only capture.

References

1. Takatsuki S, Mitamura H, Tanimoto K, et al. Clinical implications of "pure" Hisian pacing in addition to para-Hisian pacing for the diagnosis of supraventricular tachycardia. *Heart Rhythm*. 2006;3:1412–1418.

2. Hirao K, Otomo K, Wang X, et al. Para-Hisian pacing. A new method for differentiating retrograde conduction over an accessory AV pathway from conduction over the AV node. *Circulation*. 1996;94:1027–1035.

3. Nakagawa H, Jackman WM. Para-Hisian pacing: useful clinical technique to differentiate retrograde conduction between accessory atrioventricular pathways and atrioventricular nodal pathways. *Heart Rhythm*. 2005;2:667–672.

4. Sheldon SH, Li HK, Asirvatham SJ, McLeod CJ. Parahisian pacing: technique, utility, and pitfalls. *J Interv Card Electrophysiol*. 2014;40:105–116.

Figure 1.A.2

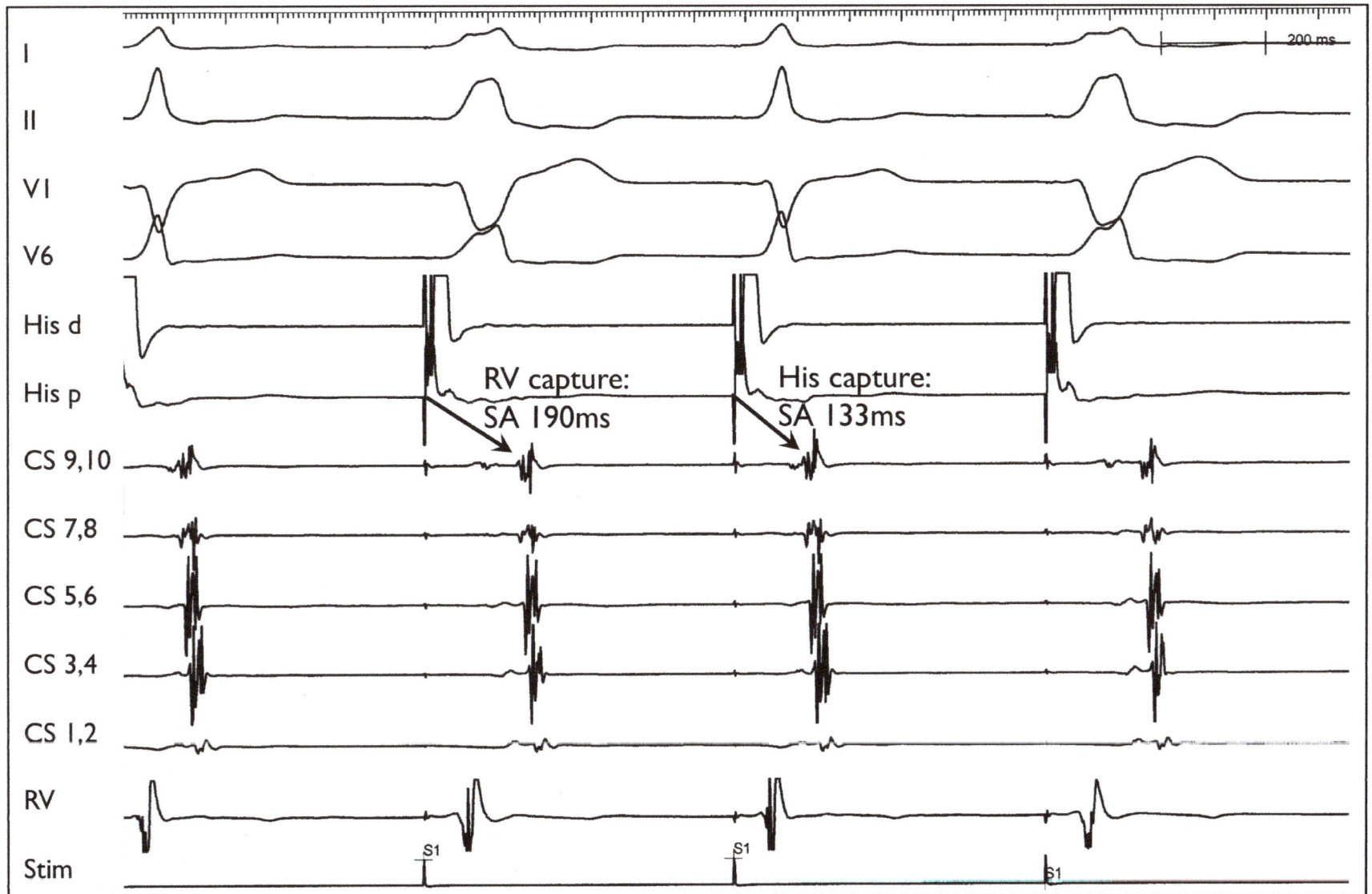

Question

An electrophysiological study was performed in a 70-year-old woman with presyncope.

This study demonstrates conduction system disease in the:

A) AV node

B) His bundle

C) Infrahisian system

D) B and C

E) All of the above

Figure 1.B.1

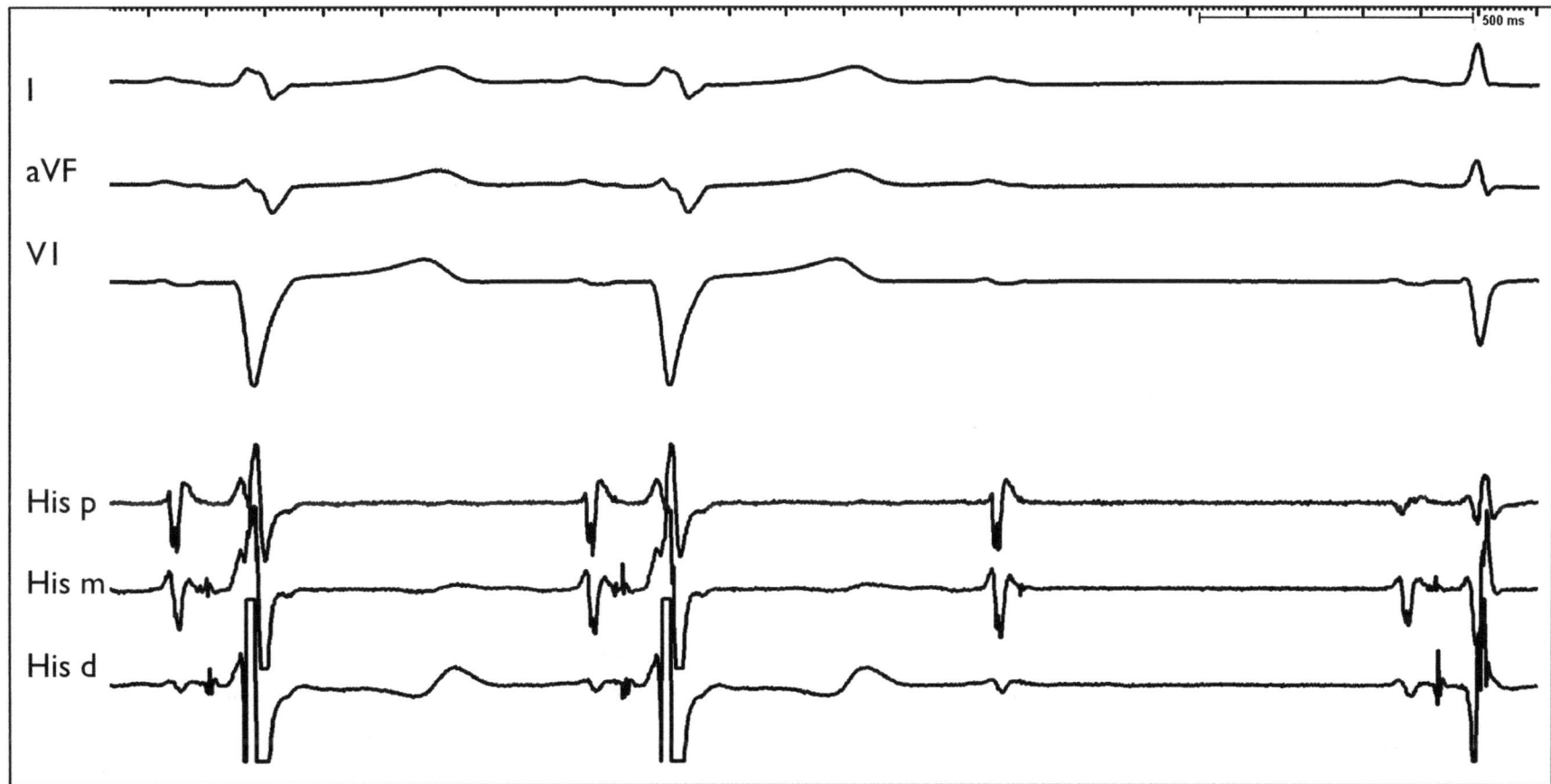

*A*nswer

The correct answer is **D**. Intrahisian block is seen, with evidence of infrahisian conduction disease in the left bundle.

AV block is seen with 3:2 conduction without evidence of PR prolongation or Wenckebach behavior. The presence of a left bundle branch block with a normal PR interval increases the pretest probability that the block is infrahisian. During block, a His bundle electrogram is seen, which is supportive of this diagnosis. However, closer inspection demonstrates a split His bundle potential with block between the proximal (H1) and distal (H2) His. Note the complete absence of the H2 on the distal His electrode during block. Left bundle branch block is alleviated due to diastolic recovery from the resultant pause, and a conducted narrow QRS complex with the same HV interval (60 ms) as the conducted wide complex beat is seen. AV block in the setting of normal PR interval and narrow complex QRS is suggestive of intrahisian block.

References

1. Iesaka Y, Rozanski JJ, Pinakatt T, Gosselin AJ, Lister JW. Intrahisian functional bundle branch block. *Pacing Clin Electrophysiol.* 1982;5(5):667–674.
2. McAnulty JH, Murphy E, Rahimtoola SH. Prospective evaluation of intrahisian conduction delay. *Circulation.* 1979;59(5):1035–1039.

Figure 1.B.2

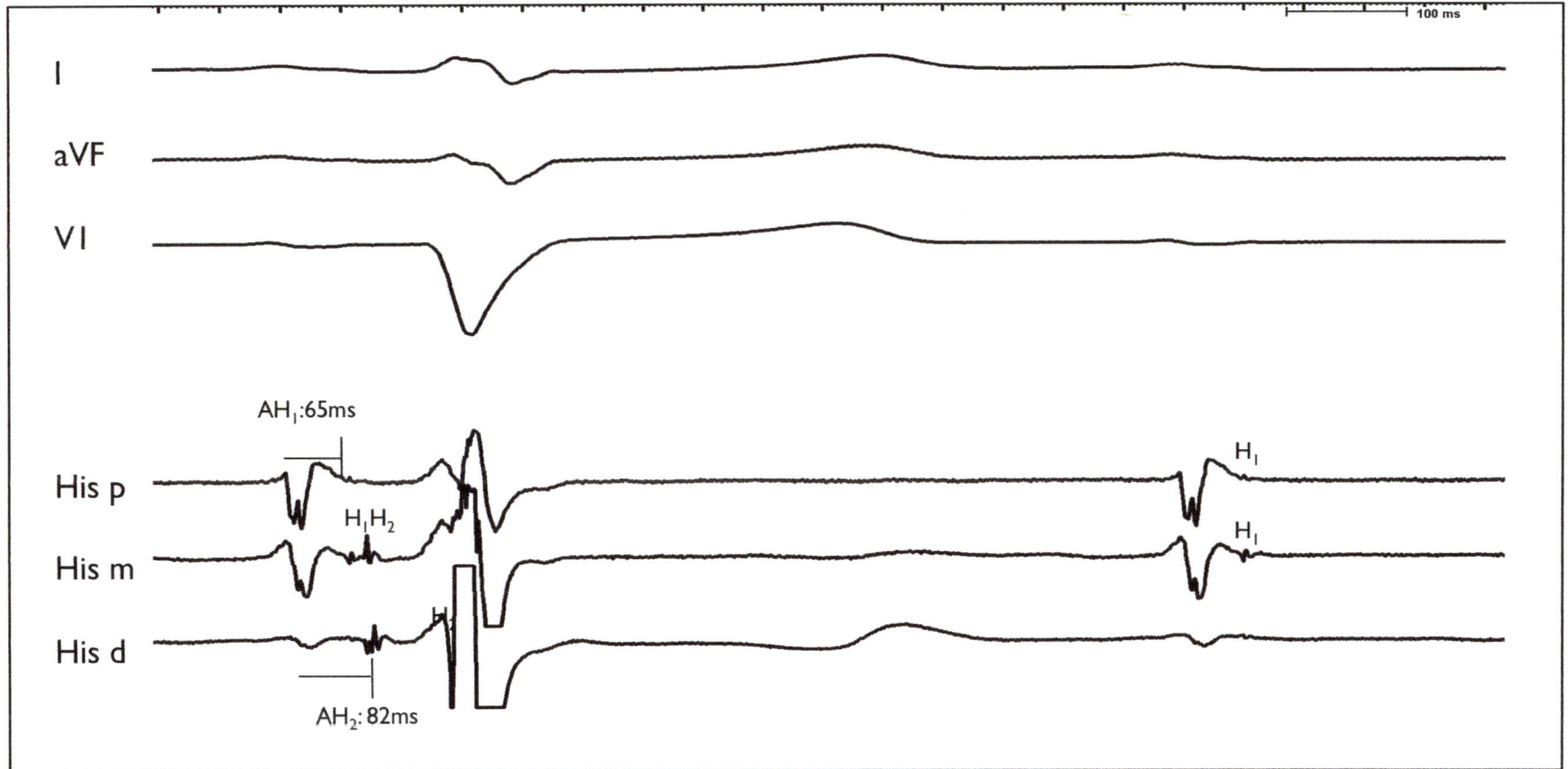

Question

What is the best explanation for the widening of the QRS complex observed during this tracing?

A) Accelerated idioventricular rhythm

B) Intermittent left bundle branch block

C) Intermittent preexcitation over a right free wall atrioventricular accessory pathway

D) Intermittent preexcitation over an atriofascicular accessory pathway

Figure 1.C.1

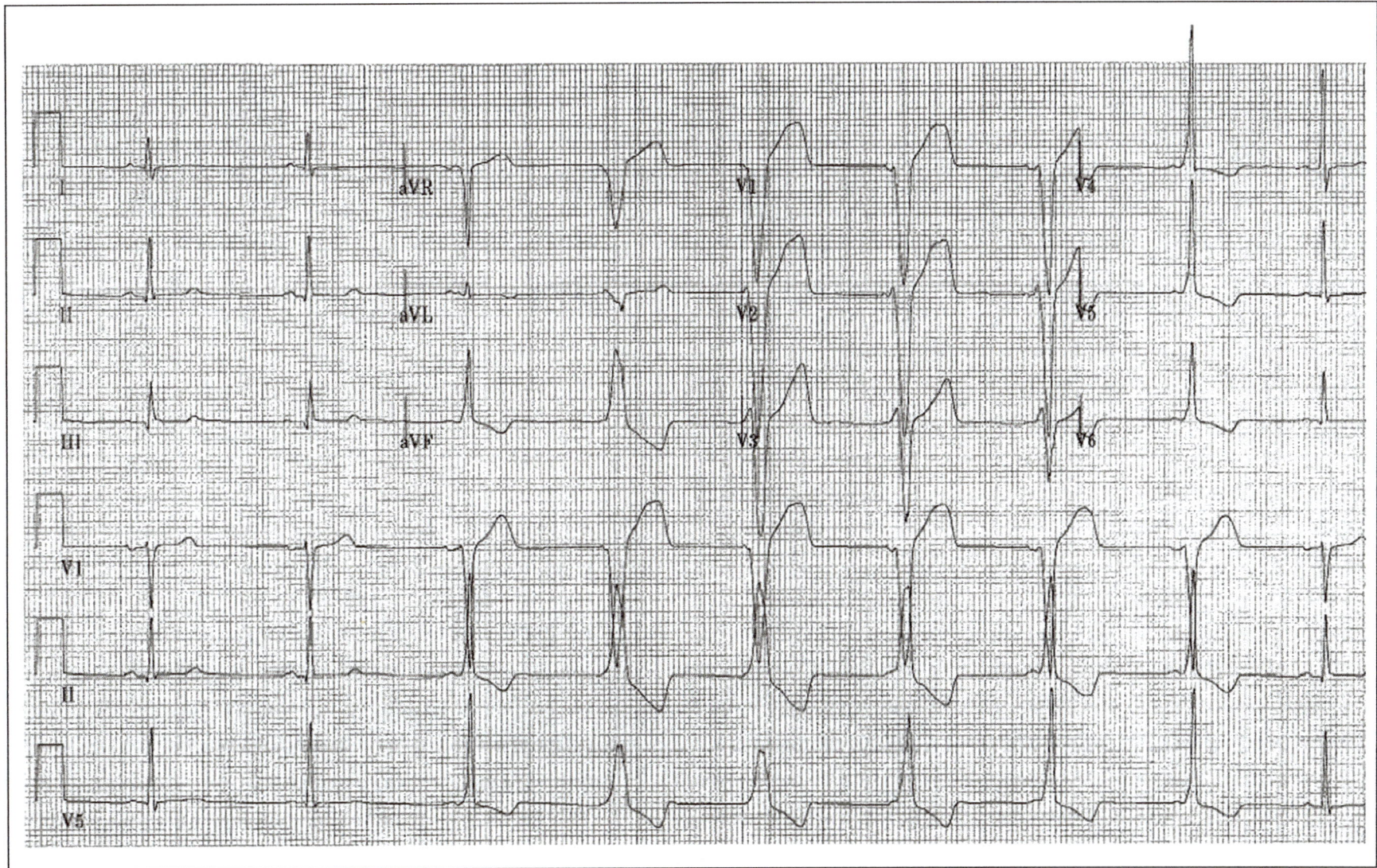

Answer

The correct answer is **A**. The third through eighth beats on the tracing are **accelerated idioventricular rhythm (AIVR)**, nearly isorhythmic to the sinus rate. The third, sixth, seventh, and eighth QRS complexes (identified by stars in the second image) are marked by varying degrees of fusion between AIVR and native conduction. Importantly, the PR interval and QRS morphology vary from beat to beat. With intermittent preexcitation, the PR interval and QRS morphology tend to be constant during all preexcited beats. Further, the PR interval on the fifth and sixth beats is 40 ms, far too short for an atrial impulse to reach the ventricle. The AIVR morphology is right ventricular outflow tract, with left bundle configuration in lead V_1, precordial transition at V_4, and inferior axis.

Figure 1.C.2

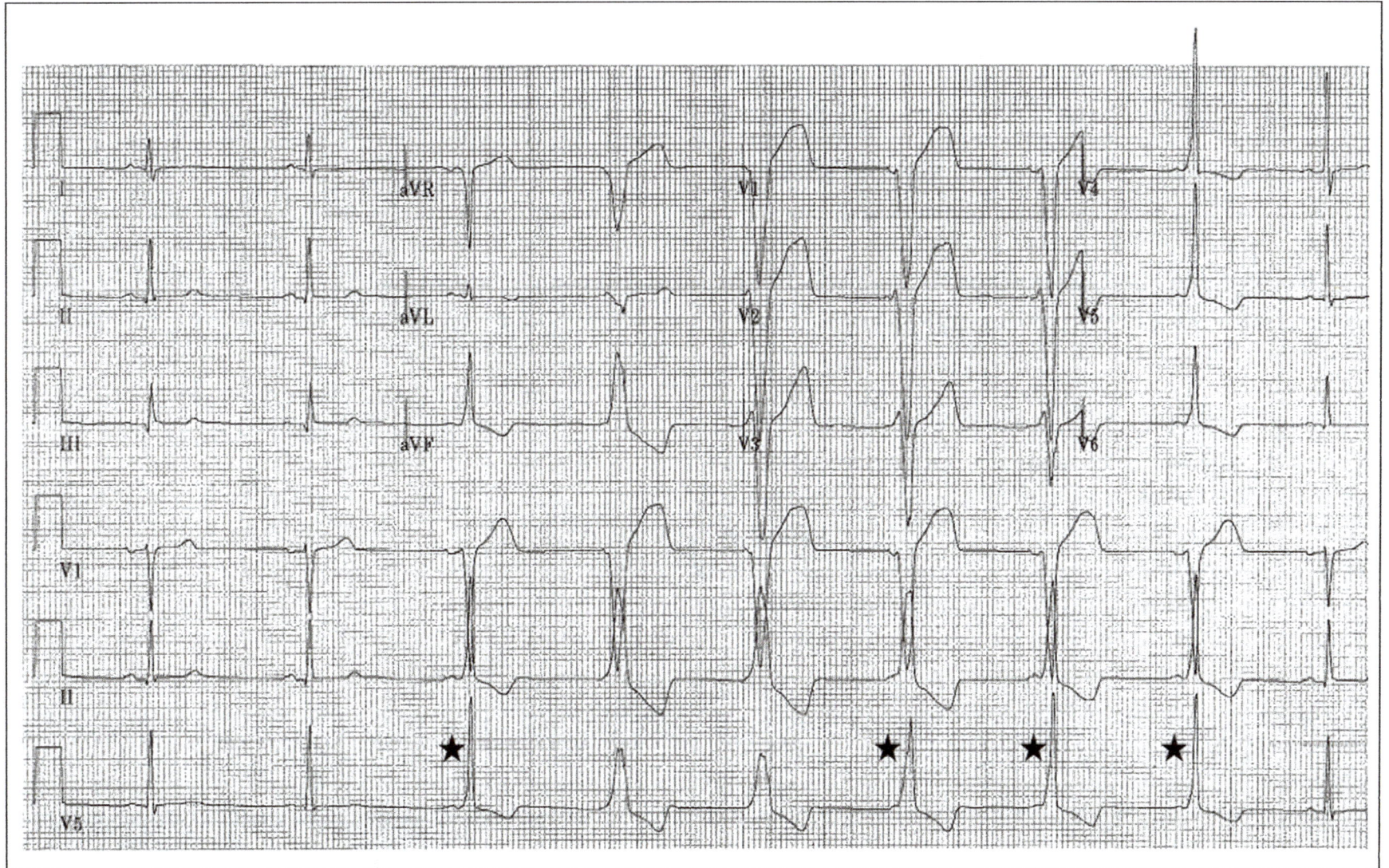

Question

A 71-year-old man with first-degree AV block and left bundle branch block presented with syncope. The following was observed during EP study.

What is the most likely explanation for the left bundle branch block morphology of the first QRS complex?

A) Premature ventricular contraction with concealed conduction into the His-Purkinje system

B) Conduction over an atriofascicular pathway

C) Block in the left bundle branch

D) Slowed conduction through the left bundle branch

Figure 1.D.1

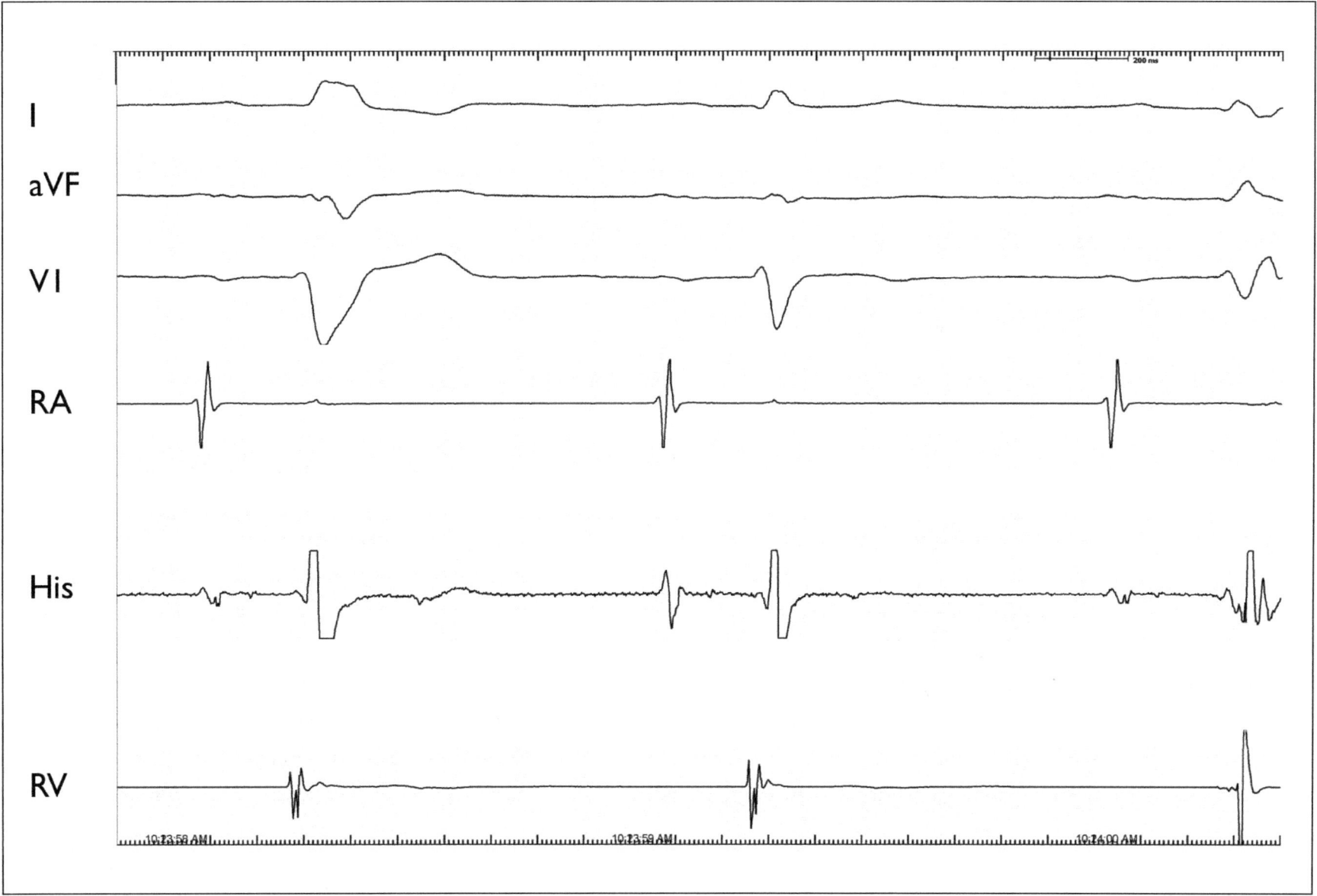

*A*nswer

The correct answer is **D**. On the first beat, conduction occurs over the right bundle branch, resulting in a left bundle branch block morphology. On the second beat, conduction occurs over both bundle branches, resulting in a narrow QRS complex. Equal delay in the right bundle branch is not a possible mechanism for narrowing of the second QRS complex, since the HV interval remains 80 ms. Rather, spontaneous recovery of conduction over the left bundle branch is the most likely explanation. On the third beat, conduction either blocks or slows severely in the right bundle branch, resulting in prolongation of the HV interval to 120 ms and right bundle branch block morphology. If the left bundle branch were actually blocked, then concurrent block in the right bundle branch would have resulted in AV block. **Based on the prolongation of the HV interval and change in QRS morphologies from the 1st to 3rd complexes, we can conclude that left bundle branch conduction is delayed rather than blocked in the 1st complex.**

Neither a premature ventricular contraction nor preexcitation over an atriofascicular pathway would result in a long HV interval.

Figure 1.D.2

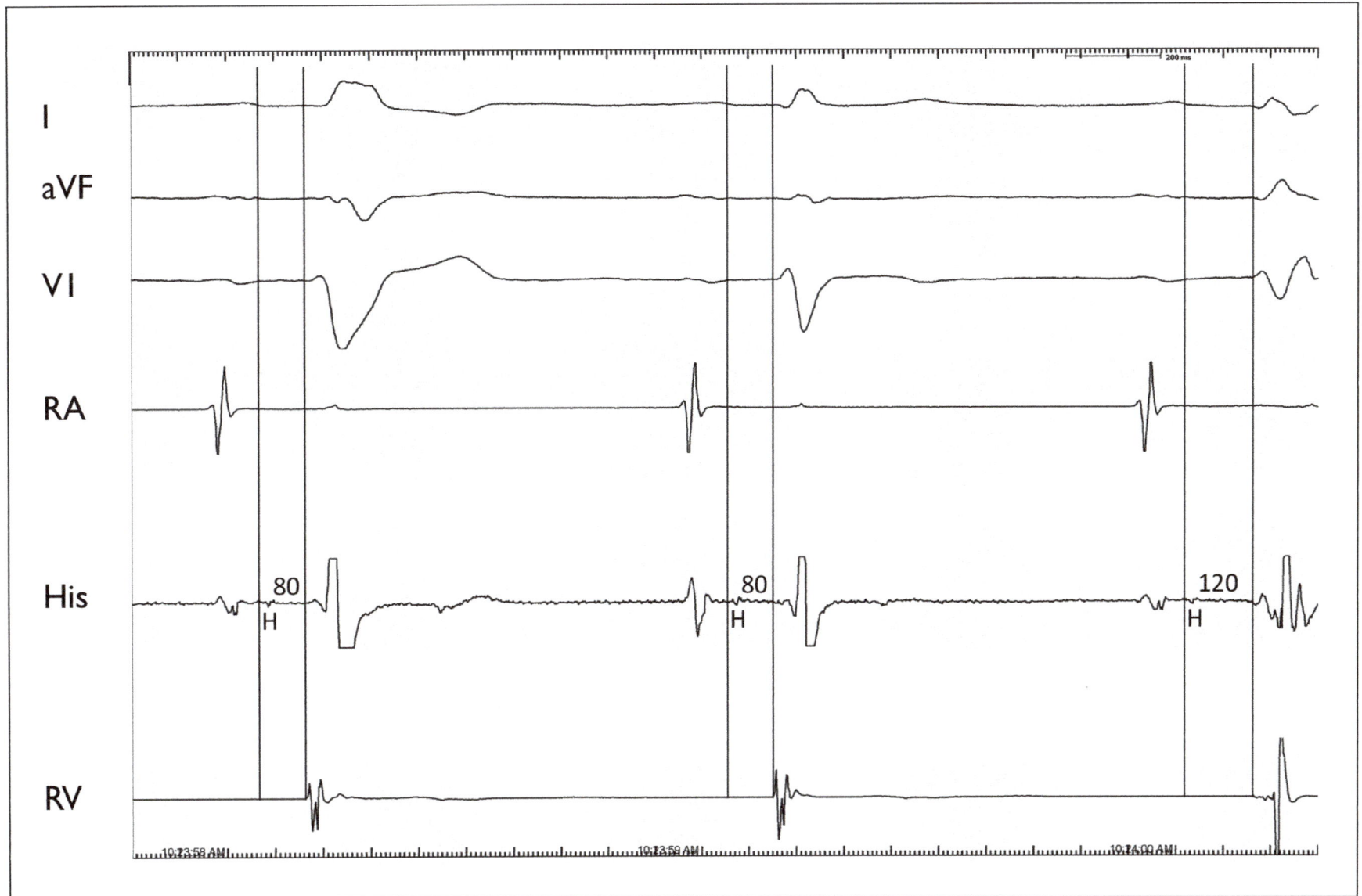

Figure 1.D.2

Reference

1. Josephson ME. *Clinical Cardiac Electrophysiology: Techniques and Interpretations*, 4th ed. Philadelphia: Lippincott Williams & Wilkins; 2008:114–144.

Question

A 55-year-old man with prior CABG/AVR (ejection fraction = 45%) was admitted with syncope.

What single best answer explains the findings on the figure?

A) Dual antegrade responses, AVNRT with phase 3 LBBB

B) Pathologic infrahisian block, phase 4 LBBB, and BBRT

C) Physiologic intranodal block, phase 4 LBBB, and BBRT

D) Phase 4 LBBB with antidromic nodofascicular reentrant tachycardia

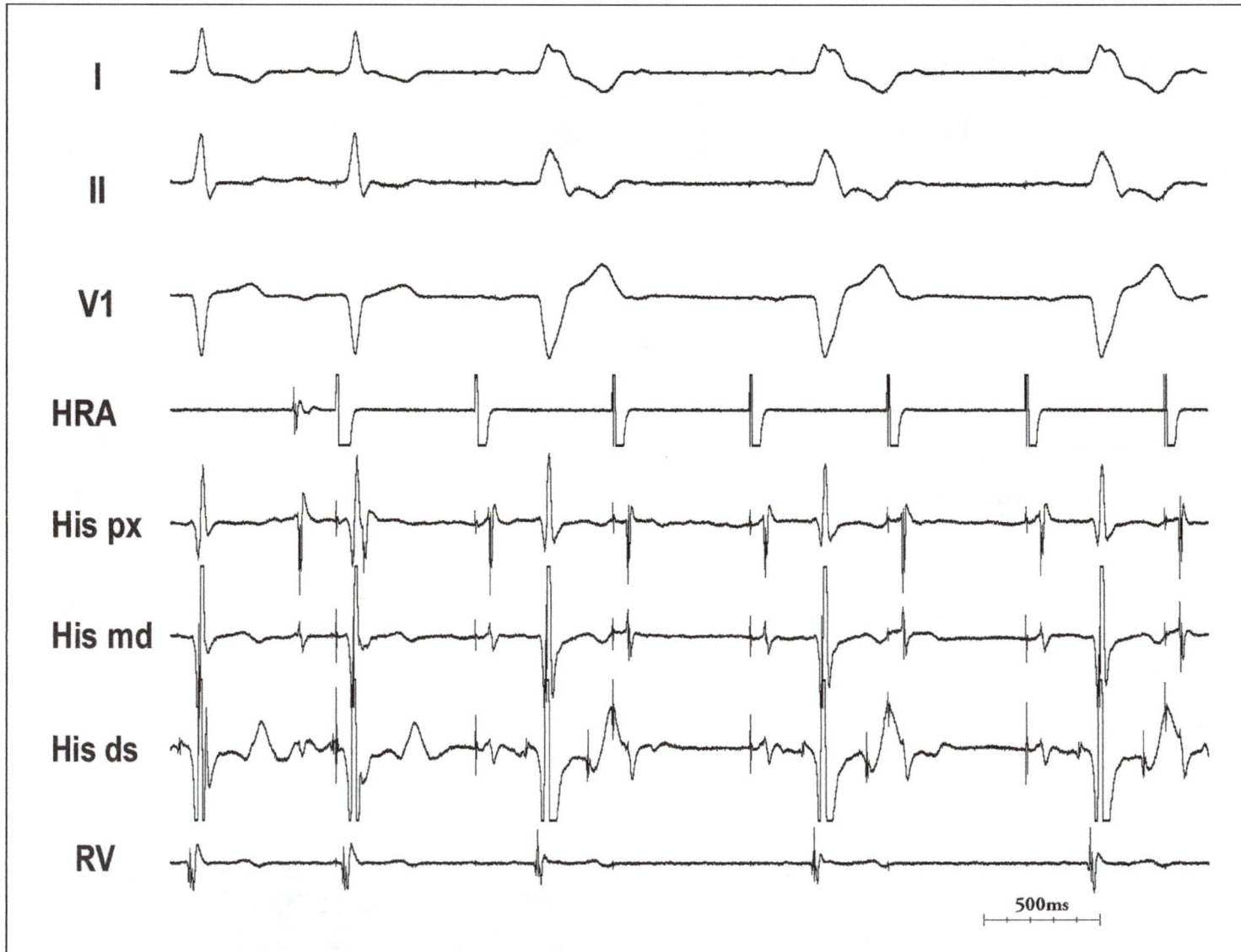

Figure 1.E.1A

Figure 1.E.1B

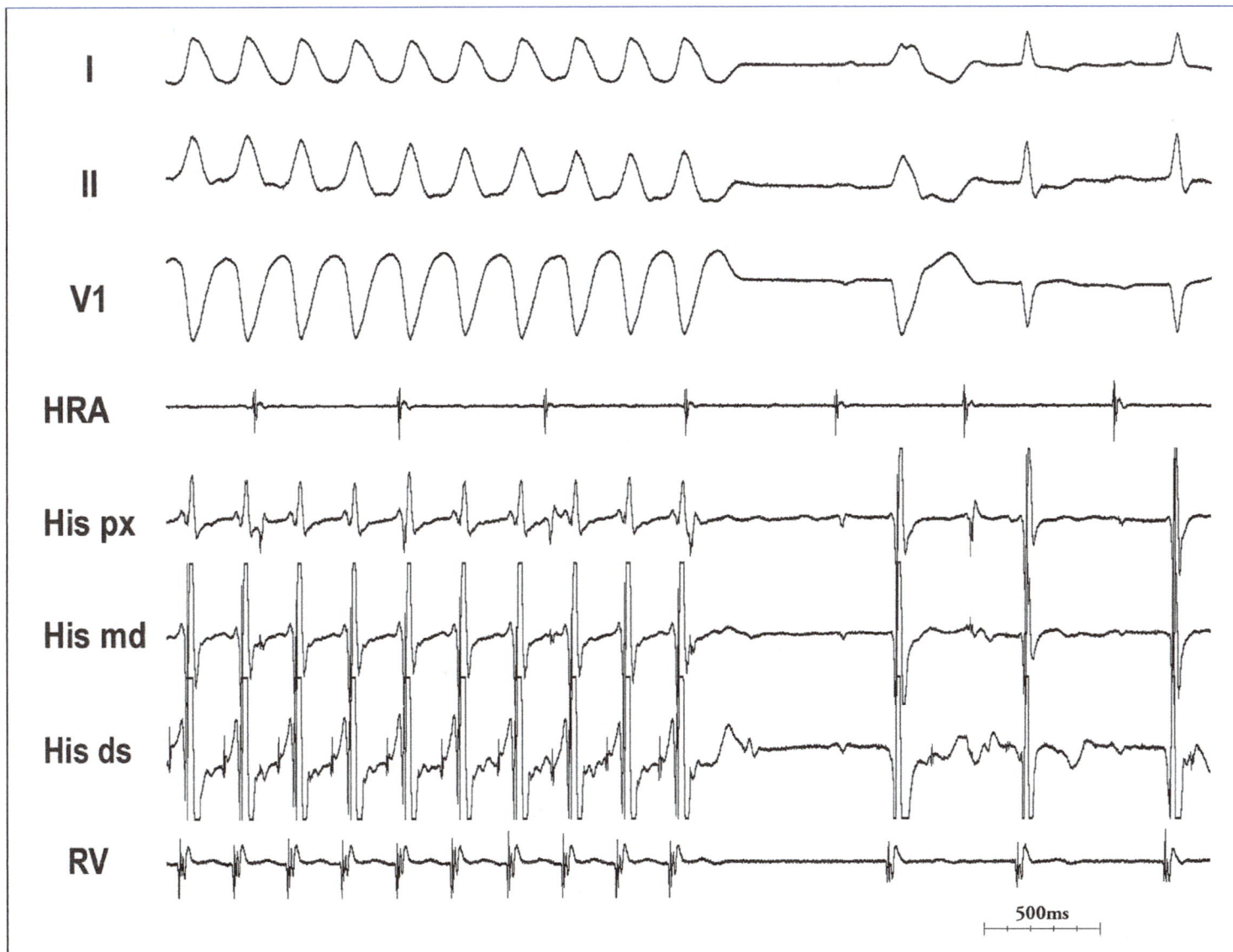

Answer

The correct answer is **C**. During HRA pacing, the first stimulus captures the atrium but fails to conduct over the AV node. The ensuing pauses cause phase 4 block (pause or bradycardia-dependent block) in the left bundle so that the second stimulus captures the atrium, conducts over the AV node–His–RB axis, and crosses the septum to retrogradely activate the LB and His bundle (rH) and retrogradely conceal into the AV node. Functional refractoriness in the RB after the pause prevents recurrent antegrade RB conduction. The third pacing stimulus finds the recently depolarized AV node refractory and fails to conduct to the ventricle, which with continued pacing promotes a self-perpetuating cycle of physiologic intranodal block, causing phase 4 LBBB and vice versa. This is the ideal substrate for BBRT (bottom), which was induced by a single ventricular extrastimulus (not shown). His bundle potentials precede LBBB QRS complexes with mildly prolonged

HV intervals. Tachycardia terminates with retrograde block in the left bundle, causing a pause that again induces phase 4 LBBB. Bundle branch reentrant tachycardia is not reinitiated because of functional antegrade RB refractoriness following the pause. The second-to-last sinus complex finds the AV node relatively refractory and conducts to the ventricle. While dual antegrade responses can explain two His bundle electrograms for a single atrial complex, it fails to explain its occurrence with only LBBB complexes; moreover, observing both phase 3 and 4 LBBB in the same patient would be unusual. Despite LBBB, AV block during HRA pacing is functional and intranodal rather than pathologic and infrahisian. While antidromic nodo-fascicular tachycardia can produce a LBBB tachycardia with AV dissociation, His bundle potentials would occur slightly after rather than before QRS onset.

Figure 1.E.2A

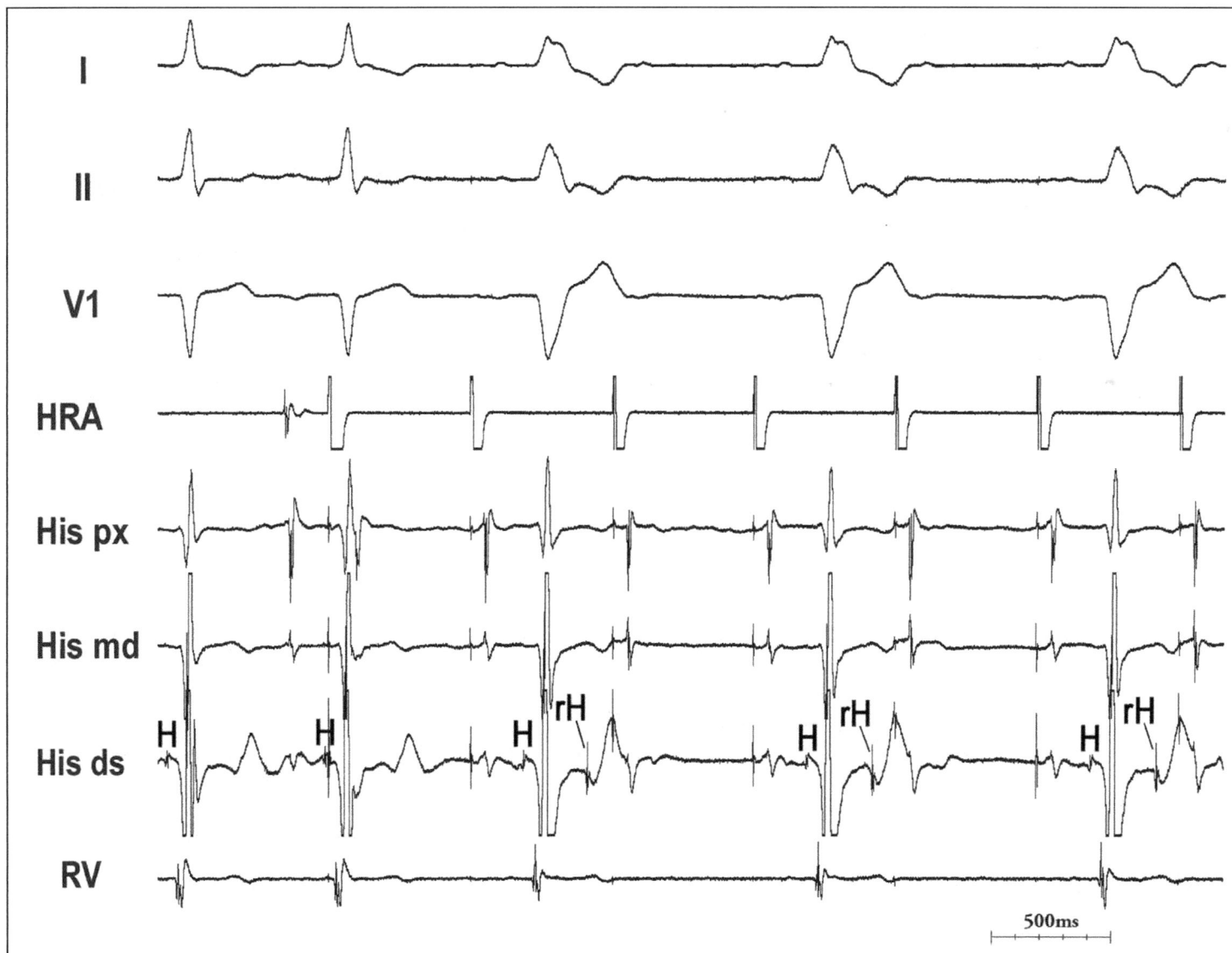

Figure 1.E.2B

References

1. Massumi R. Bradycardia-dependent bundle branch block: a critique and proposed criteria. *Circulation*. 1968;38:1066–1073.

2. Fisch C, Miles W. Deceleration-dependent left bundle branch block: a spectrum of bundle branch conduction delay. *Circulation*. 1982;65:1029–1032.

3. Akhtar M, Damato A, Batsford W, Ruskin J, Ogunkelu B, Vargas G. Demonstration of reentry within the His-Purkinje system in man. *Circulation*. 1974;50:1150–1162.

4. Caceres J, Jazayeri M, McKinnie J, Avitall B, Denker S, Tchou P, Akhtar M. Sustained bundle branch reentry as a mechanism of clinical tachycardia. *Circulation*. 1989;79:256-270.

Question

A 35-year-old man with GERD and nephrolithiasis underwent electrophysiologic evaluation because of rapid palpitations that occurred while the patient was power lifting.

What is the most likely diagnosis?

A) Antidromic tachycardia

B) AVNRT with a bystander preexcitation

C) Septal atrial tachycardia with RBBB aberration

D) Ventricular tachycardia

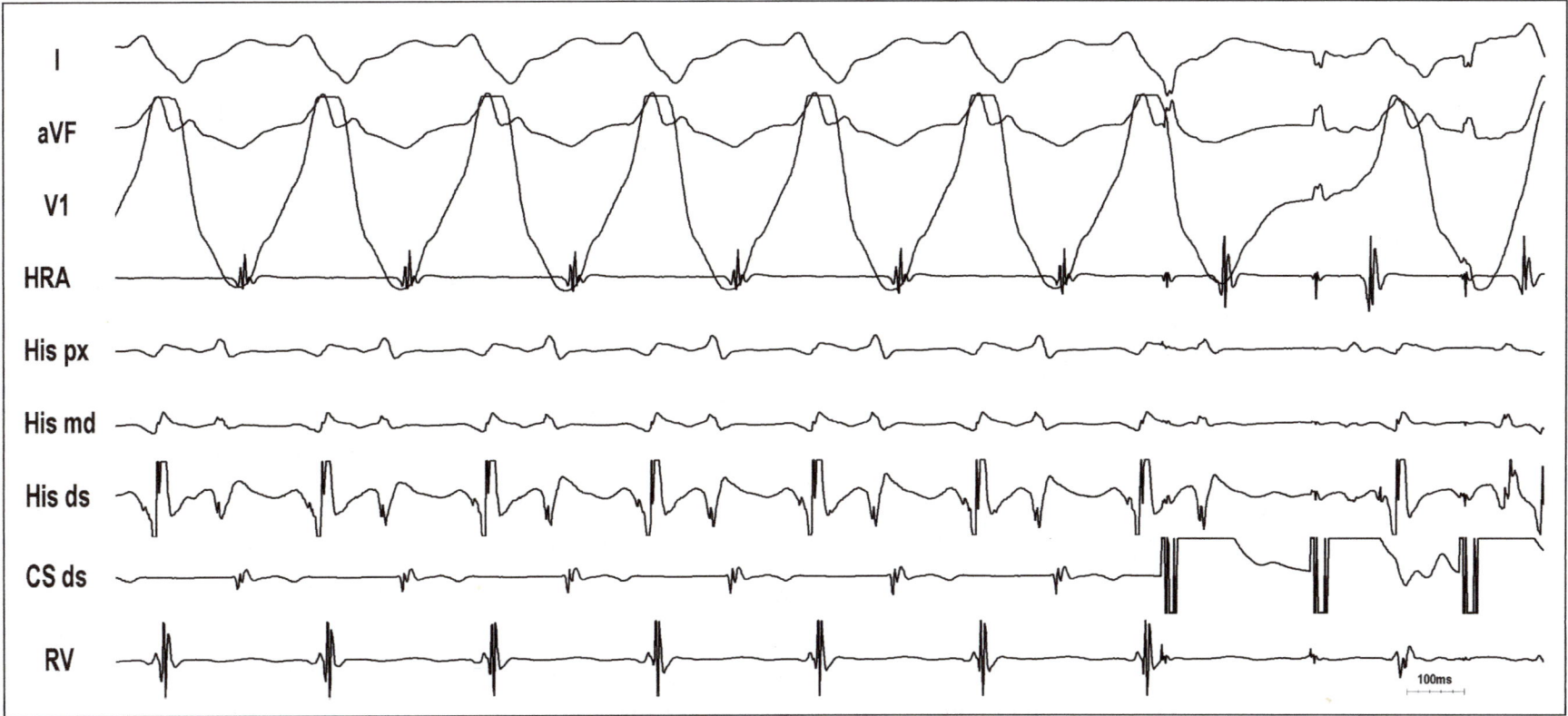

100ms

*A*nswer

The correct answer is **A**. The figure shows a regular wide complex tachycardia with right bundle branch block morphology. Its morphology is consistent with a ventricular origin, and the absence of His bundle potentials preceding each QRS excludes SVT with aberration.

Rapid pacing stimuli delivered from the distal CS capture the atrium—the first of which terminates tachycardia without reaching the ventricle. The ability of an APD equivalent to terminate a wide complex tachycardia with AV block excludes VT. Furthermore, the first pacing stimulus terminates tachycardia without affecting the septal atrium. Such an AV J-refractory APD would not be able to terminate AVNRT (nor an AT that had already depolarized the septum), and therefore its ability to terminate tachycardia with AV block is diagnostic of antidromic tachycardia. In this case, antegrade conduction occurred over a left free wall AP and retrograde conduction over the AV node. Note the retrograde His bundle potentials at the onset of the ventricular

electrogram ("short VH tachycardia") resulting from retrograde conduction over the left bundle (ipsilateral to the AP). Upon tachycardia termination, pacing stimuli conduct with ventricular preexcitation and a negative HV interval.

References

1. Kuck KH, Brugada P, Wellens HJ. Observations on the antidromic type of circus movement tachycardia in the Wolff-Parkinson-White syndrome. *J Am Coll Cardiol.* 1983;2:1003–1010.
2. Atie J, Brugada P, Brugada J, Smeets J, Cruz F, Peres A, Roukens MP, Wellens HJ. Clinical and electrophysiologic characteristics of patients with antidromic circus movement tachycardia in the Wolff-Parkinson-White syndrome. *Am J Cardiol.* 1990;66:1082–1091.
3. Packer DL, Gallagher JJ, Prystowsky EN. Physiological substrate for antidromic reciprocating tachycardia—prerequisite characteristics of the accessory pathway and atrioventricular conduction system. *Circulation.* 1992;85:574–588.

Figure 1.F.2

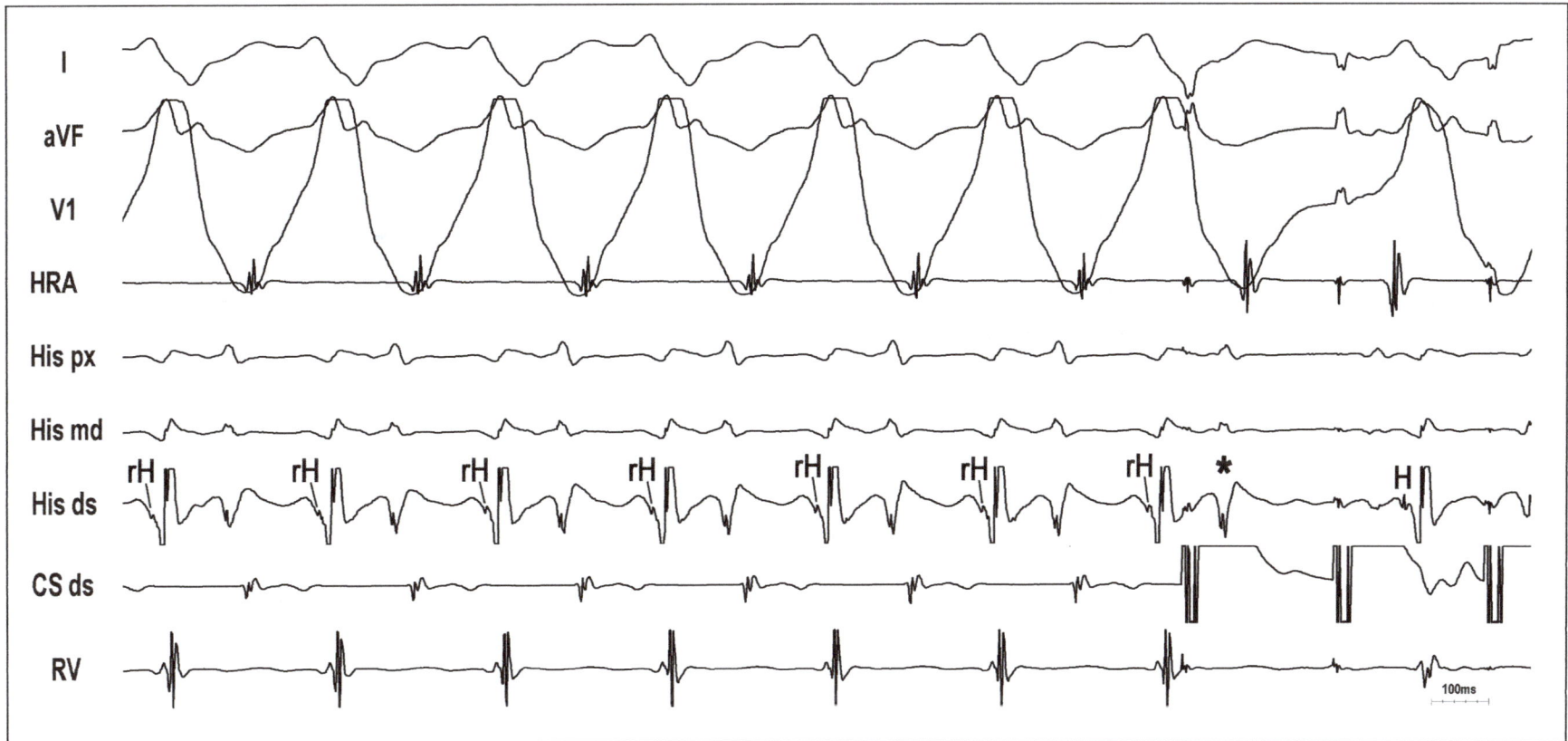

Question

A 55-year-old man with pulmonary sarcoidosis presents with 2 weeks of fatigue.

Which of the following answers is the least likely to explain the findings in the figure?

A) Infrahisian AV block in the setting of RBBB/ LAFB with premature ventricular complexes arising from the left anterior fascicle

B) Infrahisian AV block in the setting of RBBB/ LPFB with ventricular escape complexes arising from the left posterior fascicle

C) Infrahisian AV block in the setting of RBBB/ LAFB with conduction during the supernormal period of the left anterior fascicle

D) Infrahisian AV block in the setting of RBBB/ LAFB with gap conduction over the left anterior fascicle

Figure 1.G.1

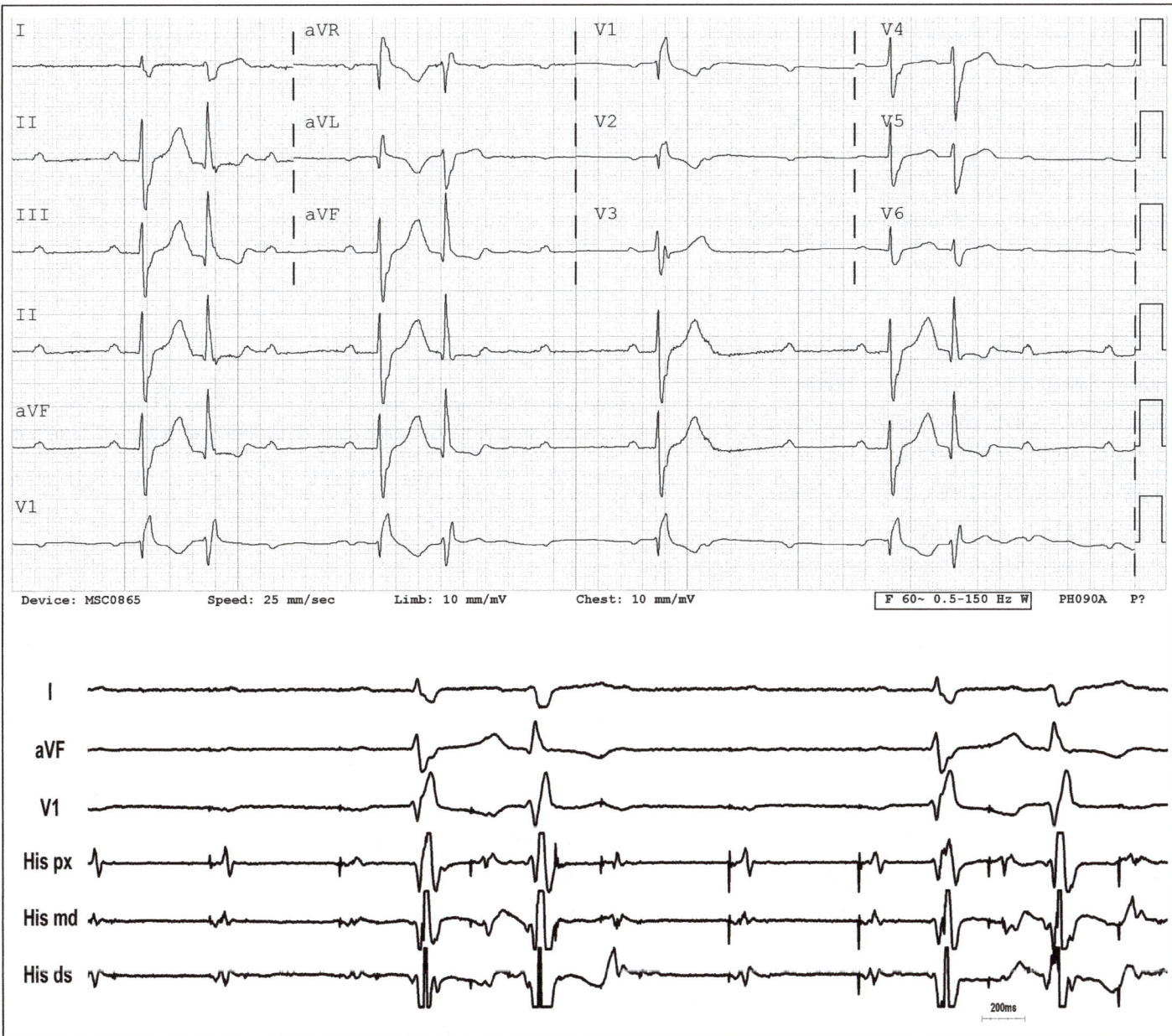

Device: MSC0865   Speed: 25 mm/sec   Limb: 10 mm/mV   Chest: 10 mm/mV   F 60~ 0.5-150 Hz W   PH090A   P?

Answer

The correct answer is **D**. The 12-lead ECG shows sinus rhythm, high-grade AV block, and bigeminal cycles of RBBB with alternating LAFB/LPFB. His bundle recordings demonstrate block below the His bundle, but the second QRS complex (RBBB/LPFB) is preceded by a paradoxical shortening of the HV interval. One explanation is that the second QRS complex of each cycle is a PVC arising from the LAF, resulting in a foreshortened "HV" interval. Alternatively, it is possible that the first QRS complex (RBBB/LAFB) is actually a ventricular escape complex arising from the LPF, giving the appearance of a long HV interval. By concealing into the LAF and "peeling back refractoriness" or Wedensky facilitation, the escape facilitates subsequent LAF conduction. A third explanation is that the second P wave of each cycle falls into the supernormal period of the LAF, creating RBBB/LPFB complexes with shorter HV intervals. Evidence supporting supernormality is the observation that a nonconducted P wave (★) has a different RP relationship than conducted P waves because it falls outside the supernormal window. While gap conduction could explain unexpected LAF conduction, there is no visible conduction delay proximal to the LAF (AH and His bundle durations are constant) and the gap phenomenon would not account for the sizeable (71 ms) paradoxical shortening of the HV interval.

References

1. Rosenbaum MB, Elizari MV, Lazzari J, Nau GJ, Levi RJ, Halpern MS. Intraventricular trifascicular blocks. Review of the literature and classification. *Am Heart J*. 1969;78:306–317.

2. Massumi RA, Amsterdam EZ, Mason DT. Phenomenon of supernormality in the human heart. *Circulation*. 1972;46:264–275.

3. Schamroth L. "Supernormal" phase in hemiblock conduction. *J Electrocardiol*. 1989;22:257–261.

Figure 1.G.2

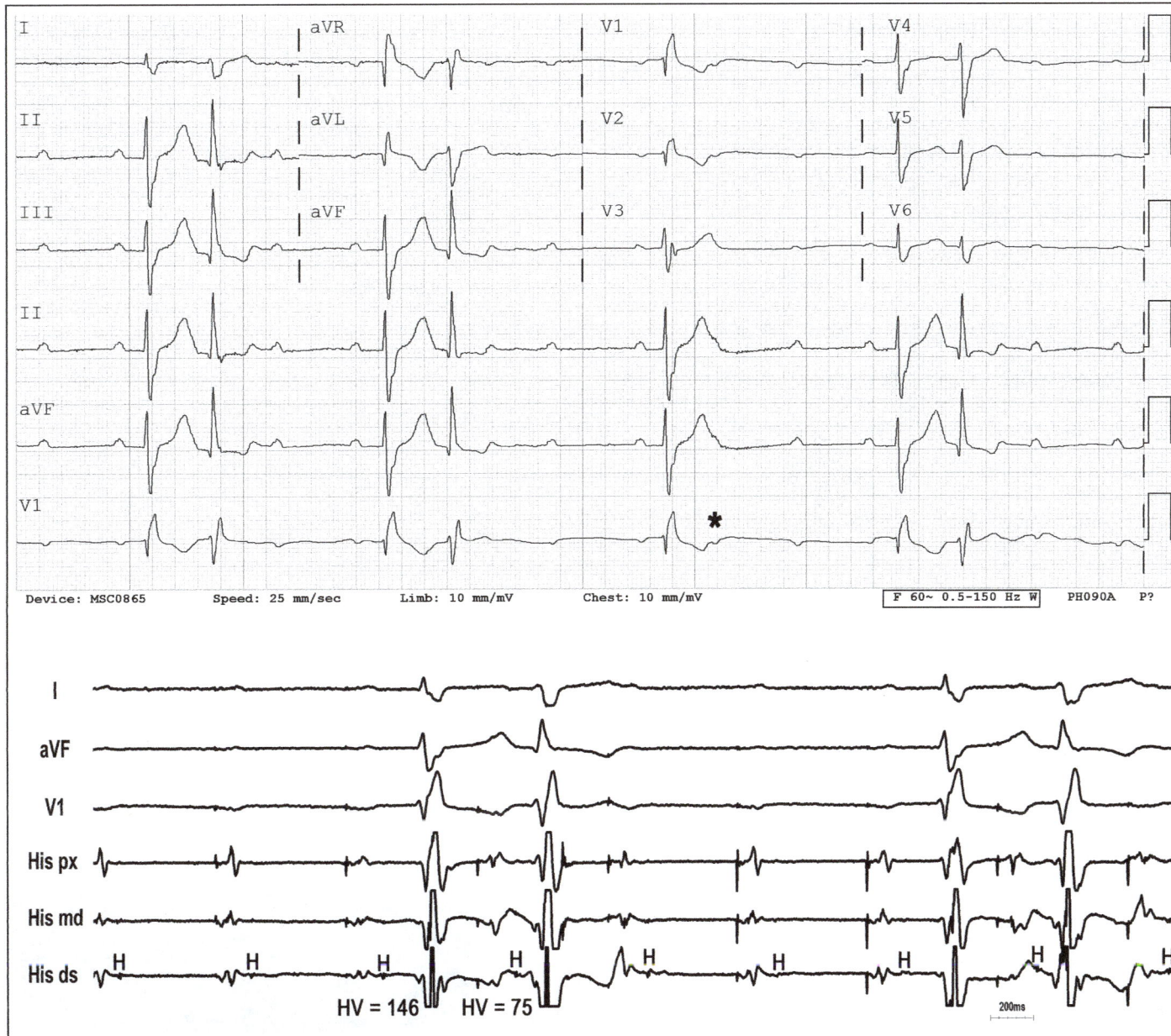

Device: MSC0865   Speed: 25 mm/sec   Limb: 10 mm/mV   Chest: 10 mm/mV   F 60~ 0.5-150 Hz W   PH090A   P?

Question

The following tracings were obtained prior to ablation of atrial flutter. A multipolar catheter is placed with its tip lateral to the right atrial isthmus. Pacing is performed from the lateral edge of the cavotricuspid isthmus. The pacing maneuver shown in this tracing demonstrates the following:

A) Pacing does not capture the circuit

B) Pacing from the exit of the circuit

C) Pacing from the central part of the circuit

D) Pacing from a bystander part of the circuit

Figure 1.H.1

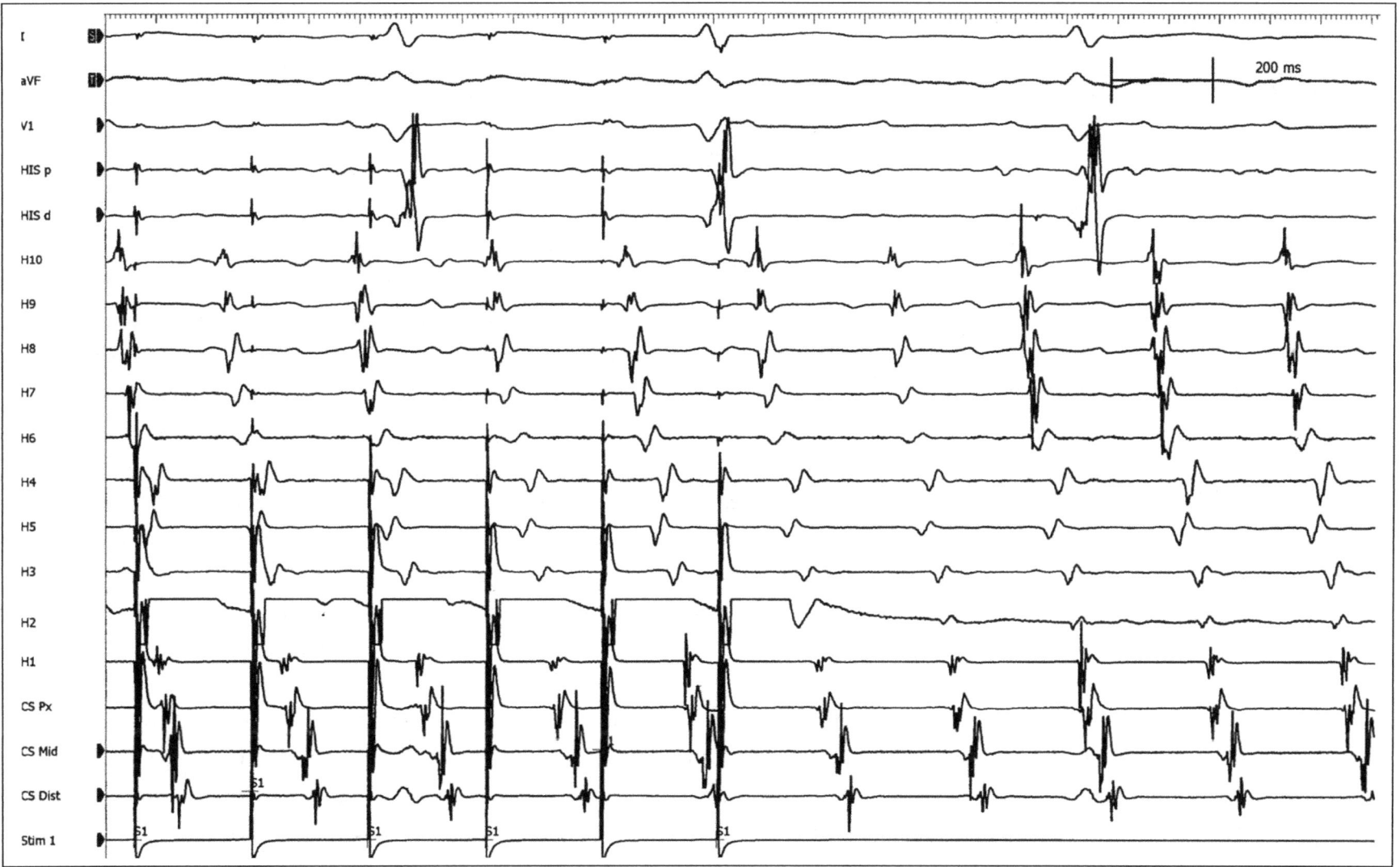

Answer

The correct answer is **A**. Pacing is performed during tachycardia to determine the mechanism of the tachycardia and to determine the proximity of the ablation catheter to the tachycardia circuit.

During evaluation of atrial flutter, entrainment is carried out from the proximal and distal coronary sinus (CS) and the cavotricuspid isthmus (CTI) to broadly differentiate between a left atrial versus right atrial tachycardia. The observation that most of the tachycardia cycle length (TCL) is encompassed by the catheters shown in the figure argues strongly for a reentrant circuit (140 ms out of 189 ms). ECG morphology also suggests counterclockwise CTI-dependent atrial flutter, confirmed by the "halo" activation pattern and proximal to distal CS activation.

The proximity of the circuit to the pacing catheter is estimated by measuring the postpacing interval (PPI), which is the difference between the timing of the electrogram that is the last captured electrogram from the pacing catheter to the first subsequent electrogram on that pacing catheter after the tachycardia resumes. In general, particularly for atrial arrhythmias, it is desirable to have a PPI-TCL less than 20 ms. Pacing or entrainment (once it is shown that the tachycardia is reentrant) is then carried out from different parts of the CTI and the right atrium to determine the nature of the circuit.

Several parameters should be checked:

1. Was the tachycardia entrained? Did the tachycardia accelerate to the pacing cycle length?
2. Did the tachycardia resume at the initial cycle length and the same activation pattern/sequence?
3. Is concealed entrainment present?

In the tracing on the previous page, the tachycardia is not accelerated and there is no evidence of atrial capture; hence, the maneuver should be repeated after repositioning the catheter or pacing at a higher output.

The following image shows the outcome of repeat pacing at a higher output with better catheter contact. During this maneuver, the tachycardia is clearly accelerated to the pacing cycle length. The flutter wave morphology in lead V_1 is unchanged and the atrial electrogram morphology and sequence are unchanged indicating concealed entrainment and the tachycardia continues after cessation of pacing.

The postpacing interval is 2 ms greater than the tachycardia cycle length; PPI-TCL < 20 ms indicates site of pacing is within the circuit.

The stimulus to flutter wave timing is same as the electrogram to flutter wave and is about half of the TCL. This means that the site of pacing is in the middle of the area of slow conduction (in this case, the cavotricuspid isthmus).

References

1. Cosio FG, Lopez Gil M, Arribas F, Goicolea A. Radiofrequency catheter ablation for the treatment of human type 1 atrial flutter. *Circulation*. 1993;88:804–805.
2. Cosio FG, Lopez-Gil M, Goicolea A, Arribas F, Barroso JL. Radiofrequency ablation of the inferior vena cava-tricuspid valve isthmus in common atrial flutter. *Am J Cardiol*. 1993;71:705–709.
3. Stevenson WG, Sager PT, Friedman PL. Entrainment techniques for mapping atrial and ventricular tachycardias. *J Cardiovasc Electrophysiol*. 1995;6:201–216.

Figure 1.H.2

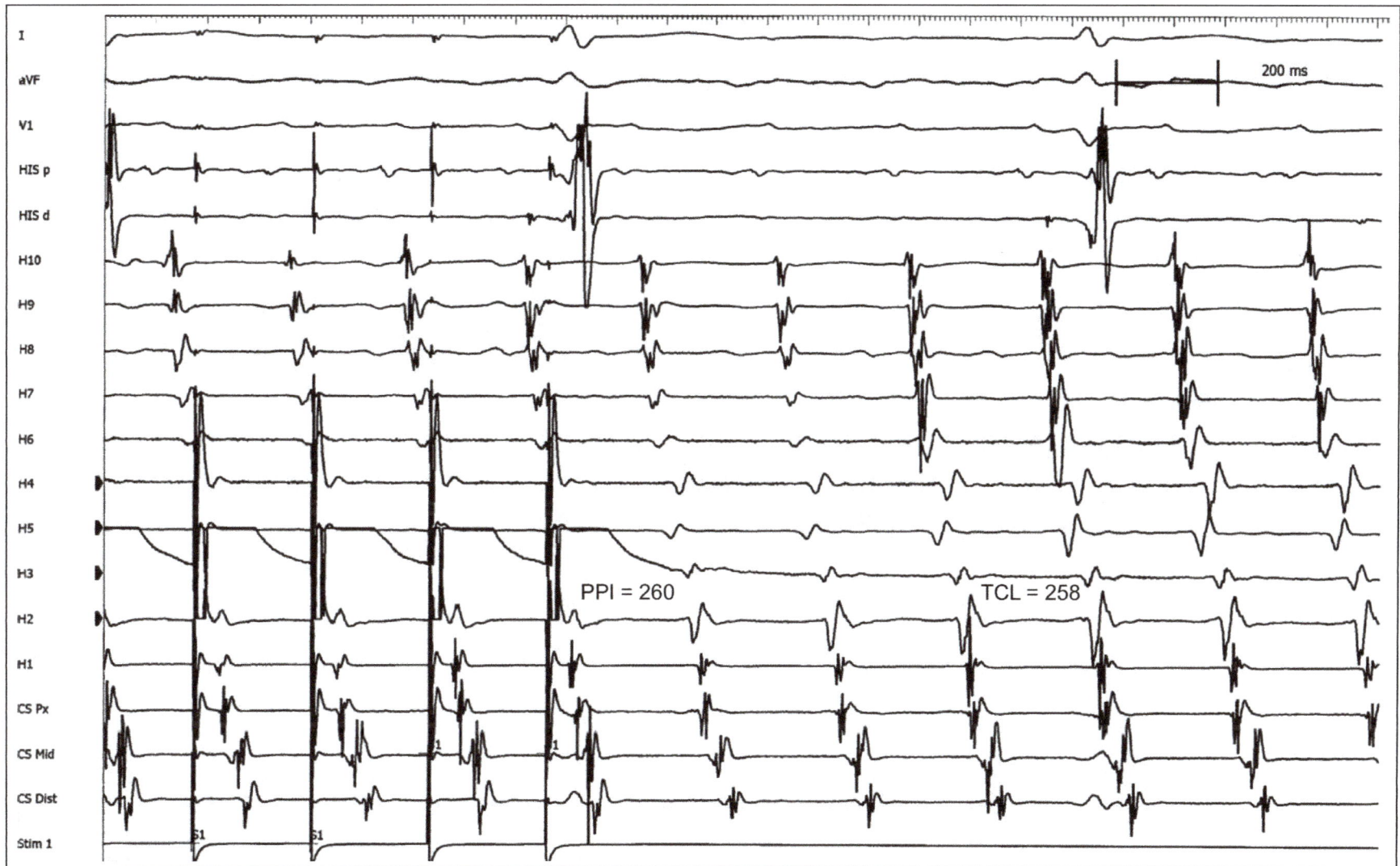

Question

Based on the following pacing maneuver, the most likely diagnosis in this patient with recurrent wide complex tachycardia is:

A) AVNRT with a bystander accessory pathway

B) Antidromic tachycardia

C) Atriofascicular antidromic tachycardia

D) Fascicular VT

Figure 1.I.1

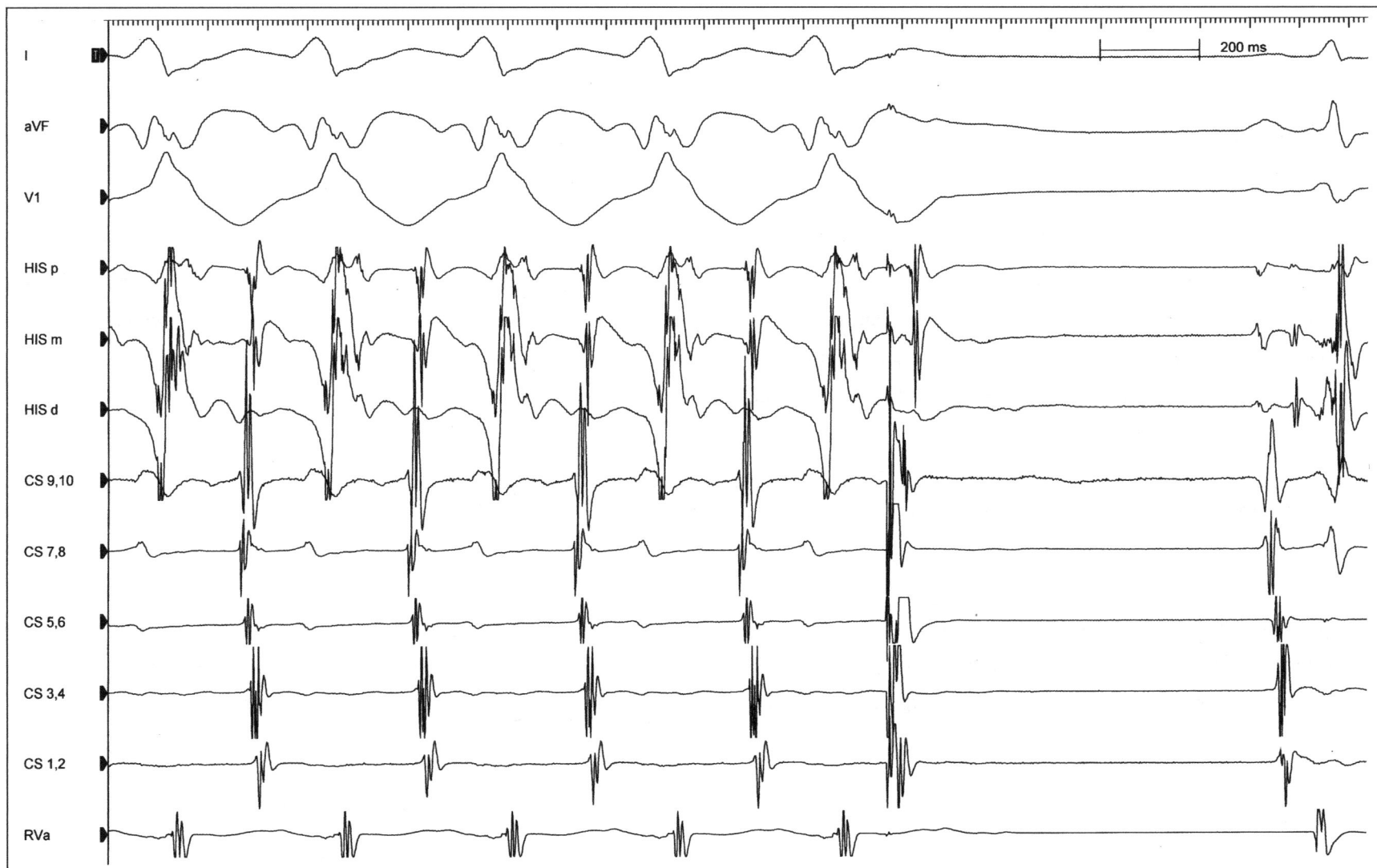

Answer

The correct answer is **B**. This tracing shows a wide complex tachycardia (WCT). The differential diagnosis has been previously discussed, but can be separated into ventricular tachycardia and preexcited tachycardia. This tracing shows a wide complex tachycardia with 1:1 VA relationship. The septal VA interval measured from the onset of QRS to the A electrogram on the His or proximal CS channel is ~240 ms. Septal VA interval, which is significantly greater than 70 ms, makes AVNRT with a bystander accessory pathway unlikely. (While typical AVNRT shows VA < 70 ms, other "atypical" forms of AVNRT can show septal VA intervals > 70 ms. Furthermore, while the septal VA < 70 ms or > 70 ms pertains to narrow complex tachycardias, it may not be so for preexcited tachycardias, where ventricular activation starts early over the AP compared to the HPS, resulting in a relatively longer VA interval in patients with AVNRT and a bystander pathway).

Fascicular VT has a short or negative HV interval. The His potential usually follows the QRS by 5 to 30 ms. There may be 1:1 VA conduction. Atriofascicular pathways insert into the right ventricle near the right bundle branch and produce a left bundle branch morphology.

To differentiate between these possibilities, an atrial extrastimulus is delivered when the His A (septal A) is refractory. If the late PAC advances the next ventricular activation, a bypass tract is present. If the tachycardia is reset, then the bypass tract is integral to the tachycardia. In this case, the PAC is delivered within 50 ms of septal activation (atrial electrogram in His and proximal CS channel). The septal A on the His and proximal CS are on time, hence the septum was refractory. The tachycardia terminates, which means the PAC led to concealment in the bypass tract, which forms the antegrade limb of the tachycardia. Furthermore, please note that the PAC was delivered near the site of the accessory pathway, namely from the left atrium in this patient with a left-sided accessory pathway. An atrial premature beat introduced when the His A was refractory (not perturbed or on time) that terminates a WCT with AV block excludes preexcited AVNRT (and preexcited AT) and VT.

Reference

1. Bardy GH, Packer DL, German LD, Gallagher JJ. Preexcited recipro-cating tachycardia in patients with Wolff-Parkinson-White syndrome: incidence and mechanisms. *Circulation*. 1984;70:377–391.

Question

An 83-year-old woman with preserved left ventricular function undergoes electrophysiologic study because of recurrent syncope.

What is the single best explanation for the figure?

A) Concealed His bundle extrasystoles causing decremental conduction within the His bundle

B) Wenckebach block within the AV node

C) Wenckebach block within the His bundle

D) Wenckebach block within the right bundle

Figure 1.J.1

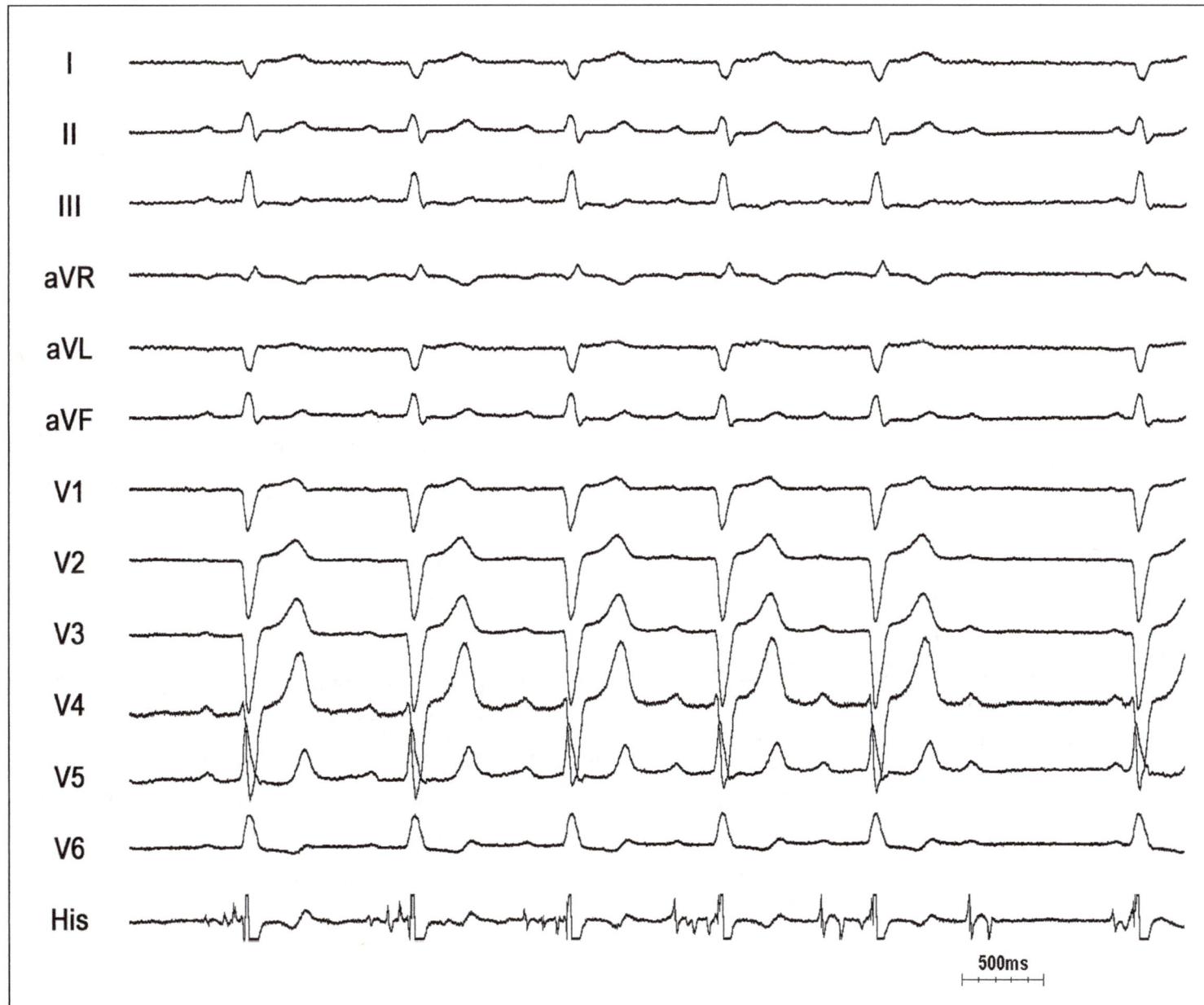

*A*nswer

The correct answer is **C**. The figure shows second–degree AV block (Wenckebach) in the setting of LBBB. His bundle recording shows split His bundle potentials that progressively widen and account for the PR prolongation while AV nodal (AH_1) and right bundle (H_2V) conduction remains constant. Conduction block occurs within the His bundle (H_1 only) followed by a distal His bundle escape complex of the same QRS morphology (H_2 simultaneous with A electrogram). While the vast majority of AV Wenckebach occurs within the AV node, severely diseased His–Purkinje tissue can demonstrate decremental conduction and manifest intra– and infrahisian Wenckebach block. While nonpropagated His bundle discharges can cause "pseudo–AV block," none are seen on the tracing.

References

1. Bharati S, Lev M, Wu D, Denes P, Dhingra R, Rosen KM. Pathophysiologic correlations in two cases of split His bundle potentials. *Circulation*. 1974;49:615–623.

2. Amat-Y-Leon F, Dhingra R, Denes P, Wu D, Wyndham C, Chuquimia R, Rosen KM. The clinical spectrum of chronic His bundle block. *Chest*. 1976;70:747–754.

3. Gupta PK, Lichstein E, Chadda KD. Chronic His bundle block: clinical, electrocardiographic, electrophysiological, and follow-up studies in 16 patients. *Br Heart J*. 1976;38:1343–1349.

Figure 1.J.2

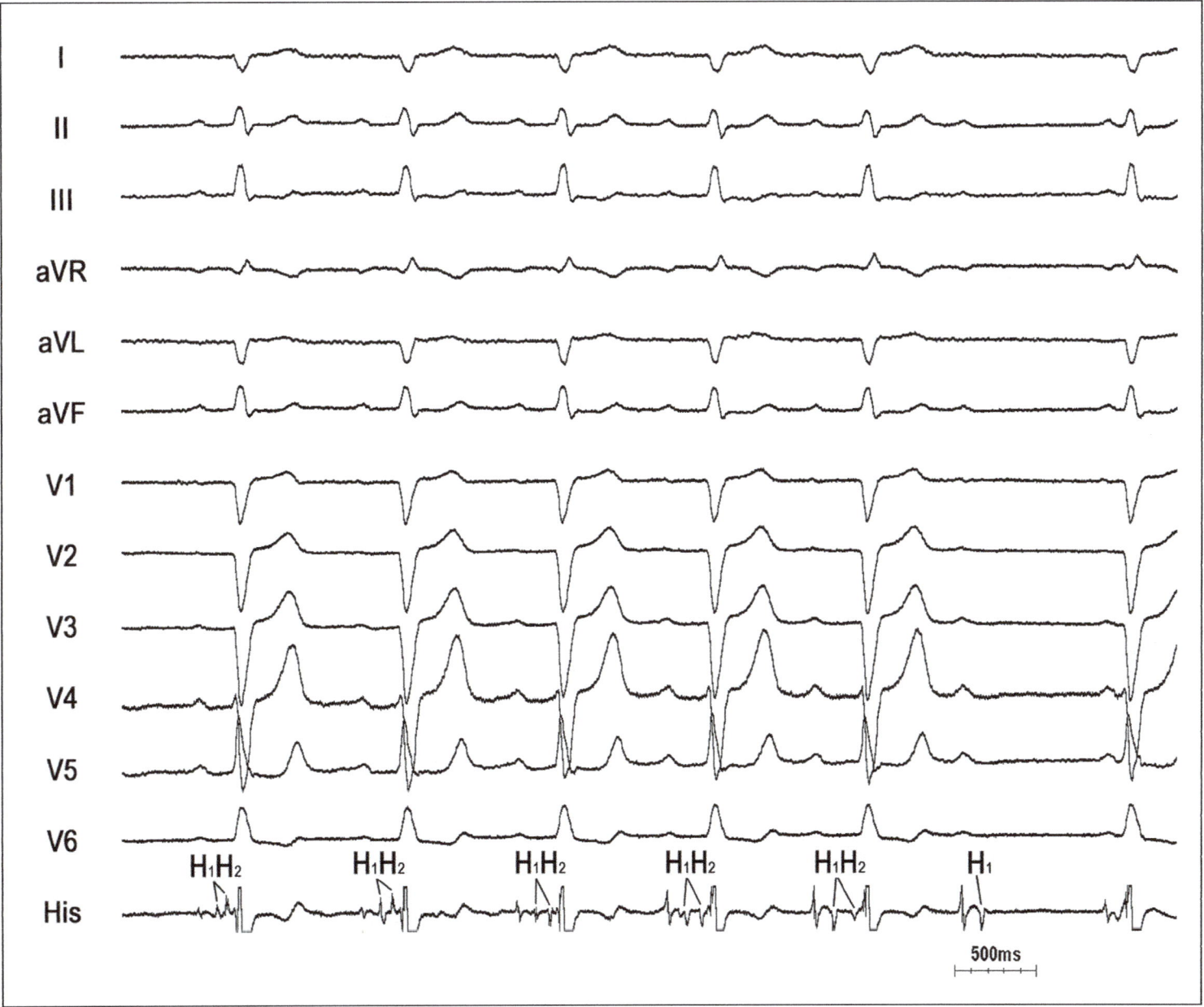

Question

A 54-year-old man with hypertension presents with fatigue and lightheadedness.

Which of the following reflect what is observed in the following figure?

A) Sinus rhythm with APCs, intranodal AV block, and competing ventricular/junctional escape rhythm

B) Sinus rhythm with APCs, intranodal AV block, and intermittent ventricular preexcitation

C) Sinus rhythm with intranodal AV block, 2:1 ventricular preexcitation, and junctional escape rhythm with retrograde AP conduction

D) Sinus rhythm with infrahisian AV block, 2:1 ventricular preexcitation, and junctional escape rhythm

Figure 1.K.1

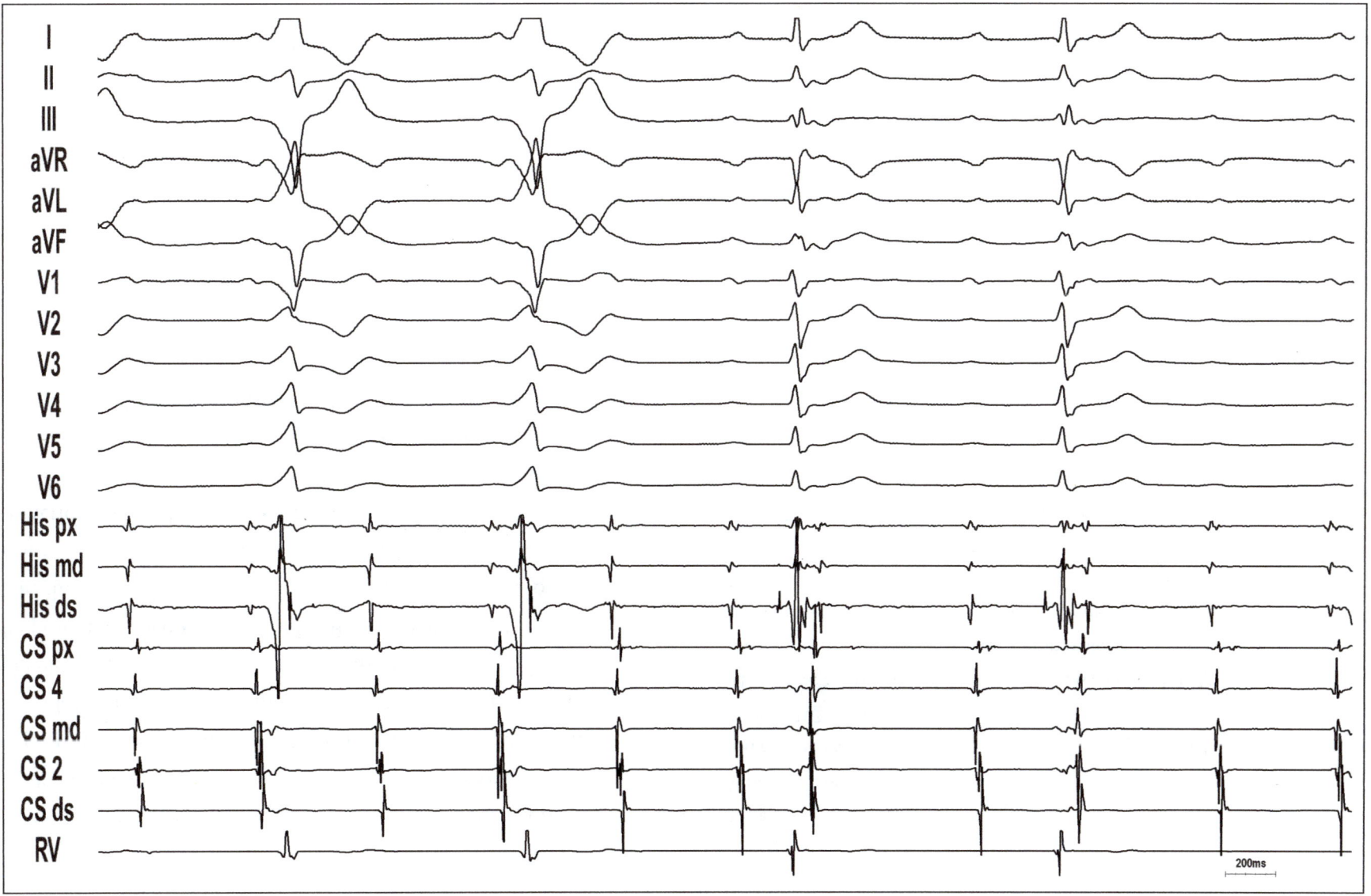

Answer

The correct answer is **C**. The figure shows sinus rhythm with intranodal AV block interrupted by 2:1 manifest preexcitation over a posteroseptal AP. Short but fixed PR intervals argue against a ventricular escape rhythm (unless the escape rate happens to be completely isorhythmic with half the sinus rate). Retrograde His bundle potentials follow preexcited QRS complexes, but retrograde block in the AV node prevents antidromic reentry. Abrupt loss of preexcitation reveals an underlying junctional escape rhythm with each junctional complex associated with retrograde AP conduction. The fixed relationship of AP conduction to junctional and not sinus complexes excludes APCs, and its failure to conduct antegradely over the AV node prevents orthodromic reentry.

References

1. Wolff L, Parkinson J, White PD. Bundle-branch block with short P-R interval in healthy young people prone to paroxysmal tachycardia. *Am Heart J*. 1930;6:685–704.

2. Milstein S, Sharma AD, Guiraudon GM, Klein GJ. An algorithm for the electrocardiographic localization of accessory pathways in the Wolff-Parkinson-White syndrome. *Pacing Clin Electrocardiol*. 1987;10:555–563.

3. Wellens H, Durrer D. Patterns of ventriculo-atrial conduction in the Wolff-Parkinson-White syndrome. *Circulation*. 1974;49:22–31.

Figure 1.K.2

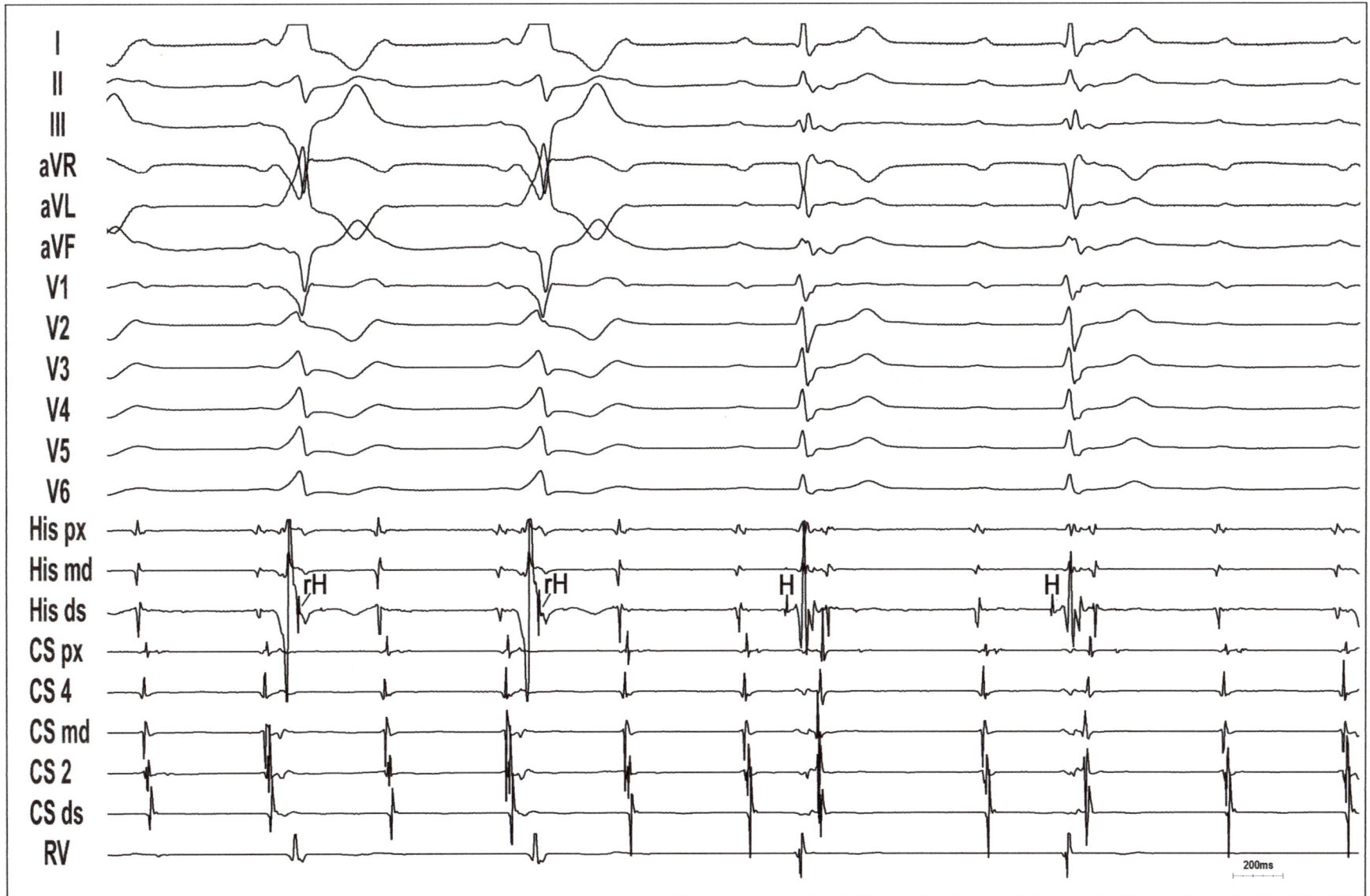

Question

A 35-year-old man undergoes electrophysiologic study because of palpitations and a wide QRS complex tachycardia. Tachycardia reproducibly terminates following delivery of a single VPD.

Which is the most likely diagnosis?

A) Atrioventricular nodal reentrant tachycardia with RBBB aberration

B) Septal atrial tachycardia with bystander preexcitation

C) Antidromic tachycardia

D) Focal ventricular tachycardia arising from the basal posterolateral left ventricle

Figure 1.L.1

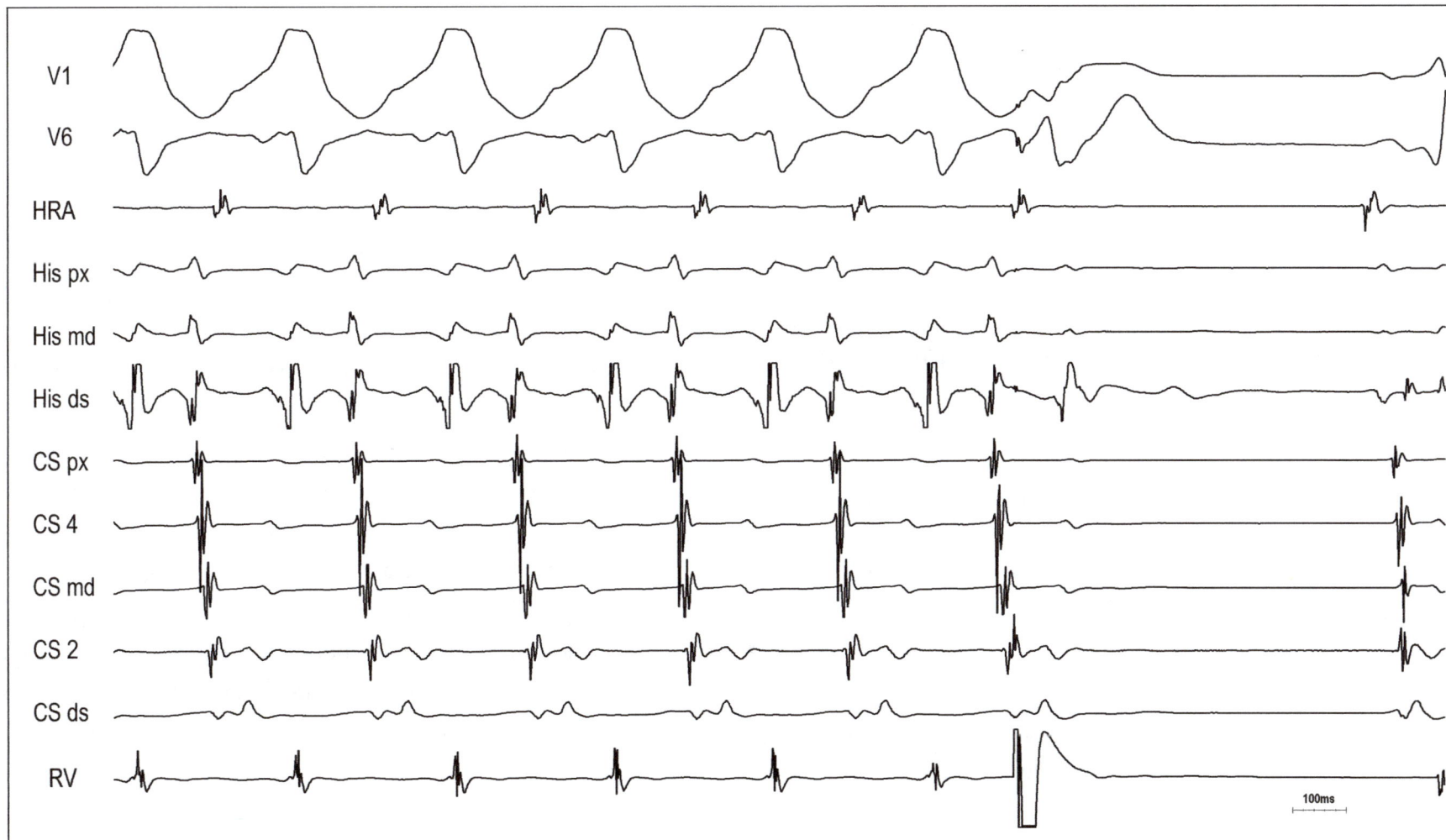

Answer

The correct answer is **C**. The tracing demonstrates a RBBB morphology tachycardia with a 1:1 AV relationship and midline atrial activation pattern. The monophasic R wave in V_1 and absence of His bundle electrograms preceding each QRS complex excludes SVT with RBBB aberration. Tachycardia terminates by a VPD delivered from the right ventricular apex that fails to reach the atrium. Such a finding argues against an atrial tachycardia. Note that the VPD is a fused complex resulting from both pacing-induced right ventricular and tachycardia-mediated left ventricular activation. While the ventricular electrograms on the His bundle catheter are advanced by the pacing stimulus, none of them (arrows) on the coronary sinus are affected. Such a VPD arising from the right ventricle would not be able to terminate a focal tachycardia arising from the basal posterolateral left ventricle without also being able to depolarize the tachycardia site of origin.

The correct answer is, therefore, an antidromic tachycardia using a left free wall accessory pathway terminated by an early VPD that failed to conduct retrogradely to the atrium (VA block).

References

1. Kuck KH, Brugada P, Wellens HJ. Observations on the antidromic type of circus movement tachycardia in the Wolff-Parkinson-White syndrome. *J Am Coll Cardiol.* 1983;2:1003–1010.
2. Atie J, Brugada P, Brugada J, Smeets J, Cruz F, Peres A, Roukens MP, Wellens HJ. Clinical and electrophysiologic characteristics of patients with antidromic circus movement tachycardia in the Wolff-Parkinson-White syndrome. *Am J Cardiol.* 1990;66:1082–1091.
3. Packer DL, Gallagher JJ, Prystowsky EN. Physiological substrate for antidromic reciprocating tachycardia—prerequisite characteristics of the accessory pathway and atrioventricular conduction system. *Circulation.* 1992;85:574–588.

Figure 1.L.2

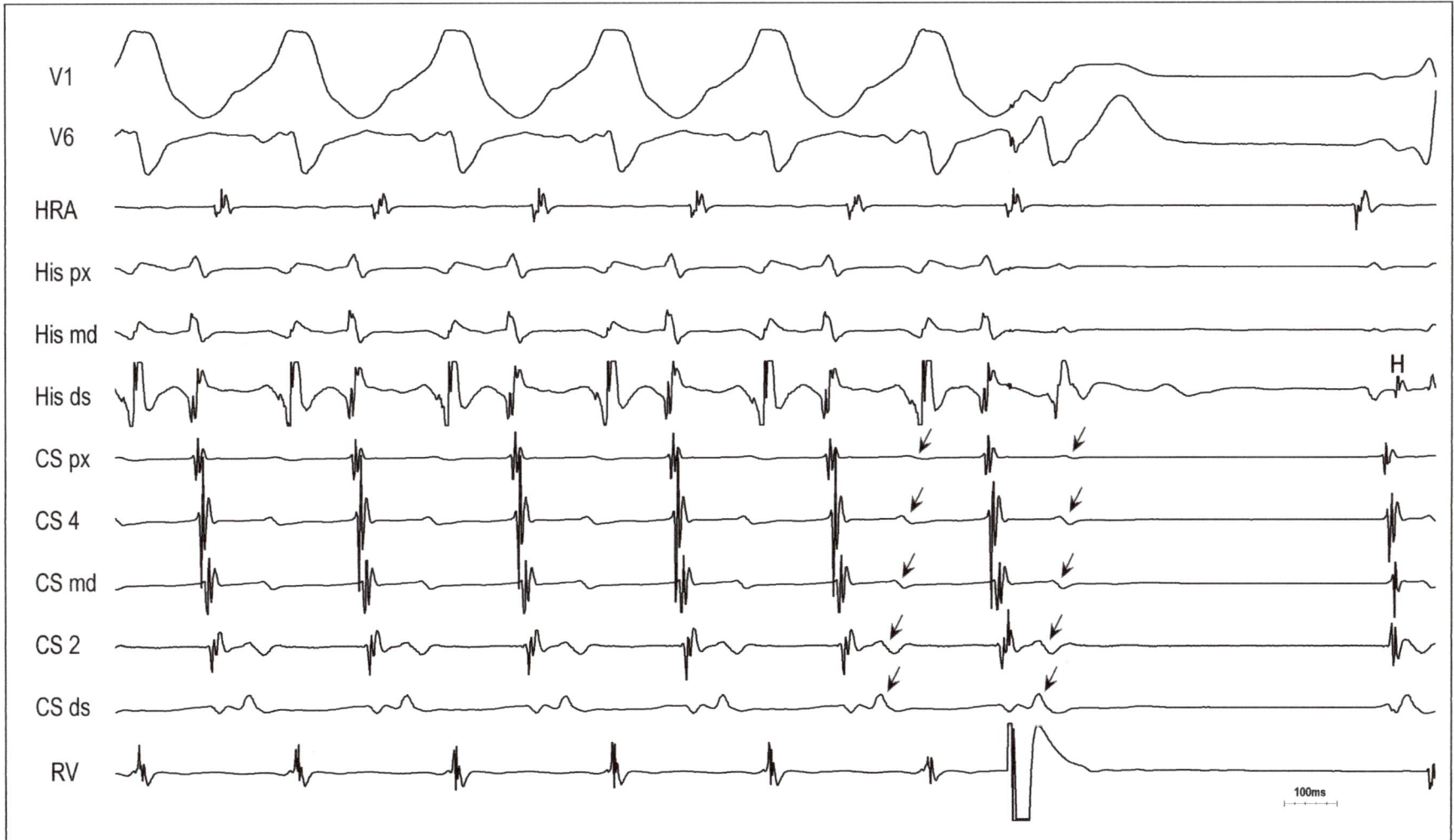

Question

A 60-year-old female with recurrent palpitations under-goes electrophysiology study. The following was recorded during the study.

What is the most likely explanation for the findings shown in this recording?

A) Two beats of ventricular tachycardia

B) Two beats of atrial tachycardia

C) Two AV nodal echo beats

D) Bundle branch reentrant beat followed by an AV nodal echo beat

Figure 1.M.1

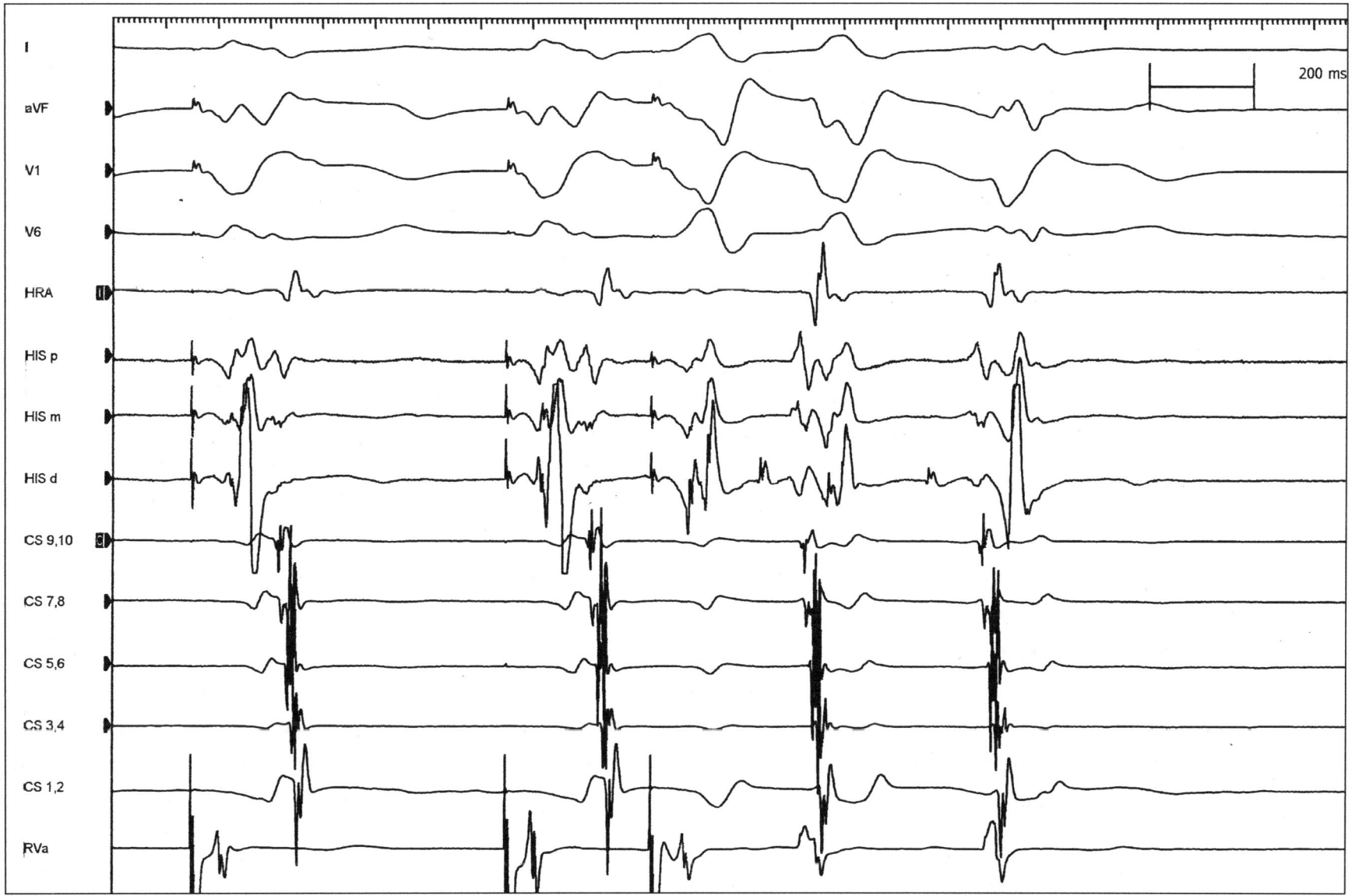

Answer

The correct answer is **D.** The tracing shows ventricular pacing with an extrastimulus being introduced. During ventricular pacing from the RV apex, activation proceeds retrogradely over the right bundle to the His bundle and may activate the atrium (depending on the refractoriness of the AV node). A retrograde His is seen on the first two beats of right ventricular pacing. After the extrastimulus at this critical coupling interval (see +), there is retrograde right bundle branch block resulting in delay; therefore, transseptal conduction proceeds retrogradely over the left bundle branch. The resultant delay from the transseptal conduction promotes a bundle branch reentrant beat (morphology similar to a right ventricular paced beat). Retrograde activation occurs over the AV node and results in atrial activation. The ventricle is activated via the right bundle with a left bundle branch block morphology.

This is sometimes described as the V_3 phenomenon (beat marked by a "+"). The next beat has a narrower QRS. The ventricle is activated anterogradely via the slow pathway. The long AH allows retrograde conduction to the atrium over the fast pathway, resulting in an AV nodal reentrant echo beat. The increase in VA interval between the ventricular drive train and extrastimulus occurs at the expense of an increase in the VH interval (HA intervals appear constant) indicating that retrograde atrial activation is linked to retrograde His bundle activation and confirms that retrograde conduction occurs over the fast pathway of the AV node.

References

1. Reddy CP, Khorasanchian A. Intraventricular reentry with narrow QRS complex. *Circulation*. 1980;61:641–647.

2. Kapa S, Henz BD, Dib C, et al. Utilization of retrograde right bundle branch block to differentiate atrioventricular nodal from accessory pathway conduction. *J Cardiovasc Electrophysiol*. 2009;20:751–758.

3. Akhtar M, Damato AN, Batsford WP, Ruskin JN, Ogunkelu JB, Vargas G. Demonstration of re-entry within the His-Purkinje system in man. *Circulation*. 1974;50:1150–1162.

Figure 1.M.2

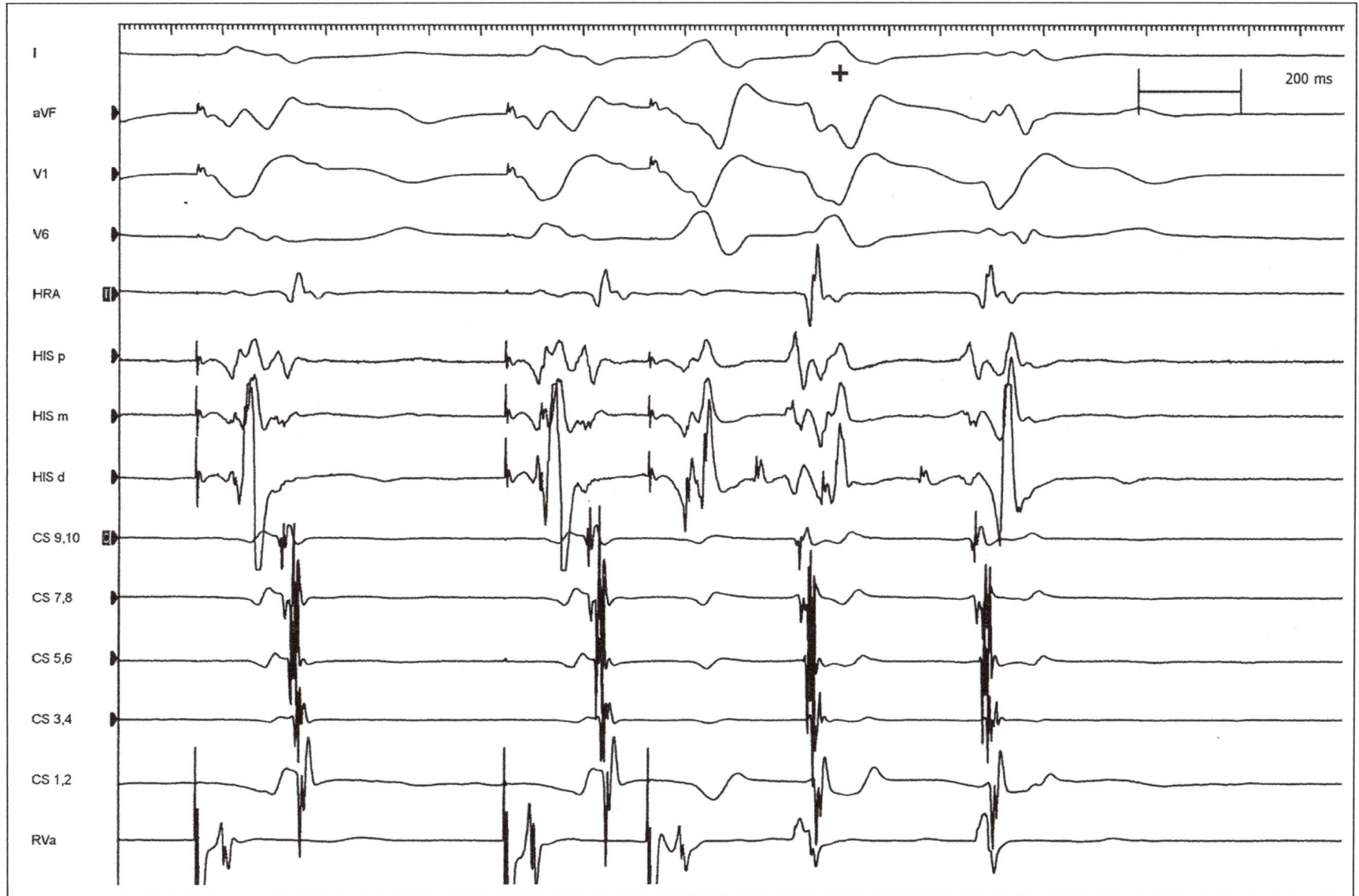

Figure 1.M.3

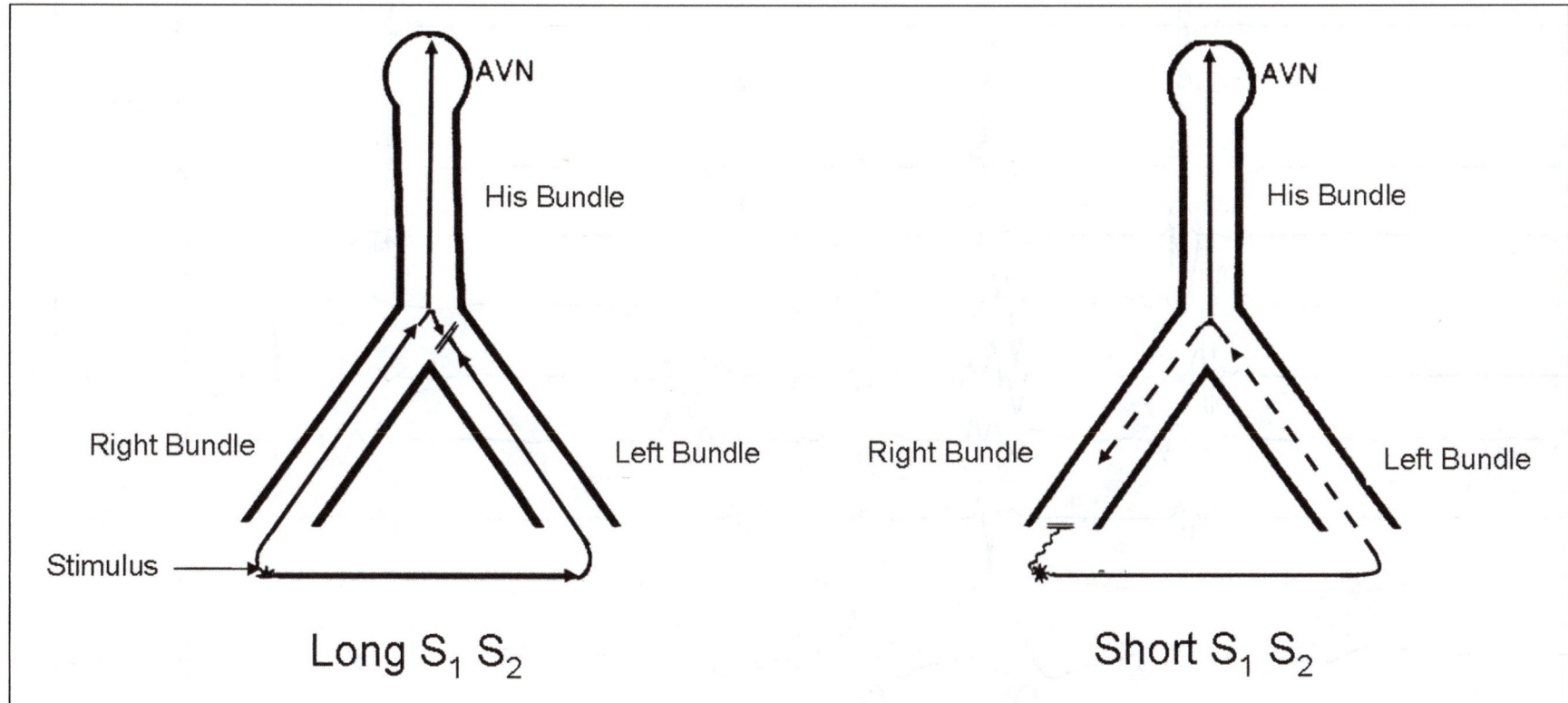

Long $S_1 S_2$

Short $S_1 S_2$

PART

2

Supraventricular Tachycardia (SVT)

Question

What is the most likely mechanism for narrowing of the final QRS complex?

A) Gap phenomenon

B) PVC peels back refractoriness

C) Supernormal conduction

D) Fusion of the conducted complex with a PVC

Figure 2.A.1

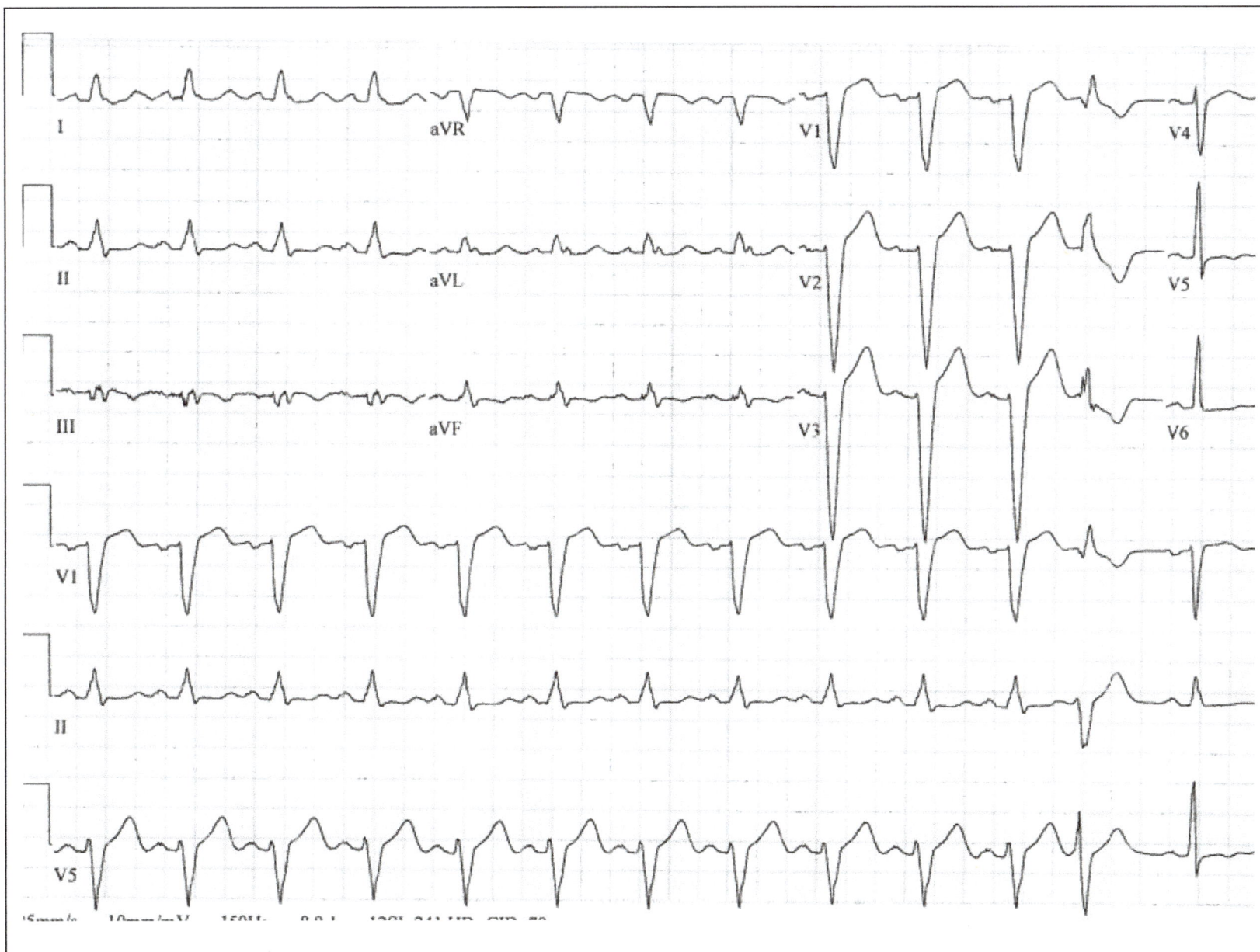

*A*nswer

The correct answer is **B**. Left bundle branch block is present at baseline. A PVC occurs (arrow) and the following P wave conducts without aberration (★). During the first 11 beats, conduction occurs over the right bundle branch. The wavefront of activation then crosses the ventricular septum and conceals into the left bundle branch, causing it to be refractory when the next wavefront arrives from the His bundle, thereby perpetuating the left bundle branch block. The PVC breaks this cycle by depolarizing both bundle branches. This results in a short–long sequence. The short interval decreases the refractory period of the bundle branches. The subsequent long interval allows plenty of time for excitability to recover throughout the His-Purkinje system.

Gap phenomenon is when a premature impulse fails to conduct, but a more premature impulse conducts. This occurs when greater degrees of prematurity result in even longer delays in conduction proximal to the site of block. Supernormal conduction is that which occurs either more rapidly than expected or when block is anticipated. If the last conducted beat were fused with a PVC, the PR interval would be shorter.

References

1. Moe GK, Childers RW, Merideth J, et al. An appraisal of supernormal AV conduction. *Circulation*. 1968;38:5–28.
2. Josephson ME. *Clinical Cardiac Electrophysiology: Techniques and Interpretations*, 4th ed. Philadelphia: Lippincott Williams & Wilkins, 2008.

Figure 2.A.2

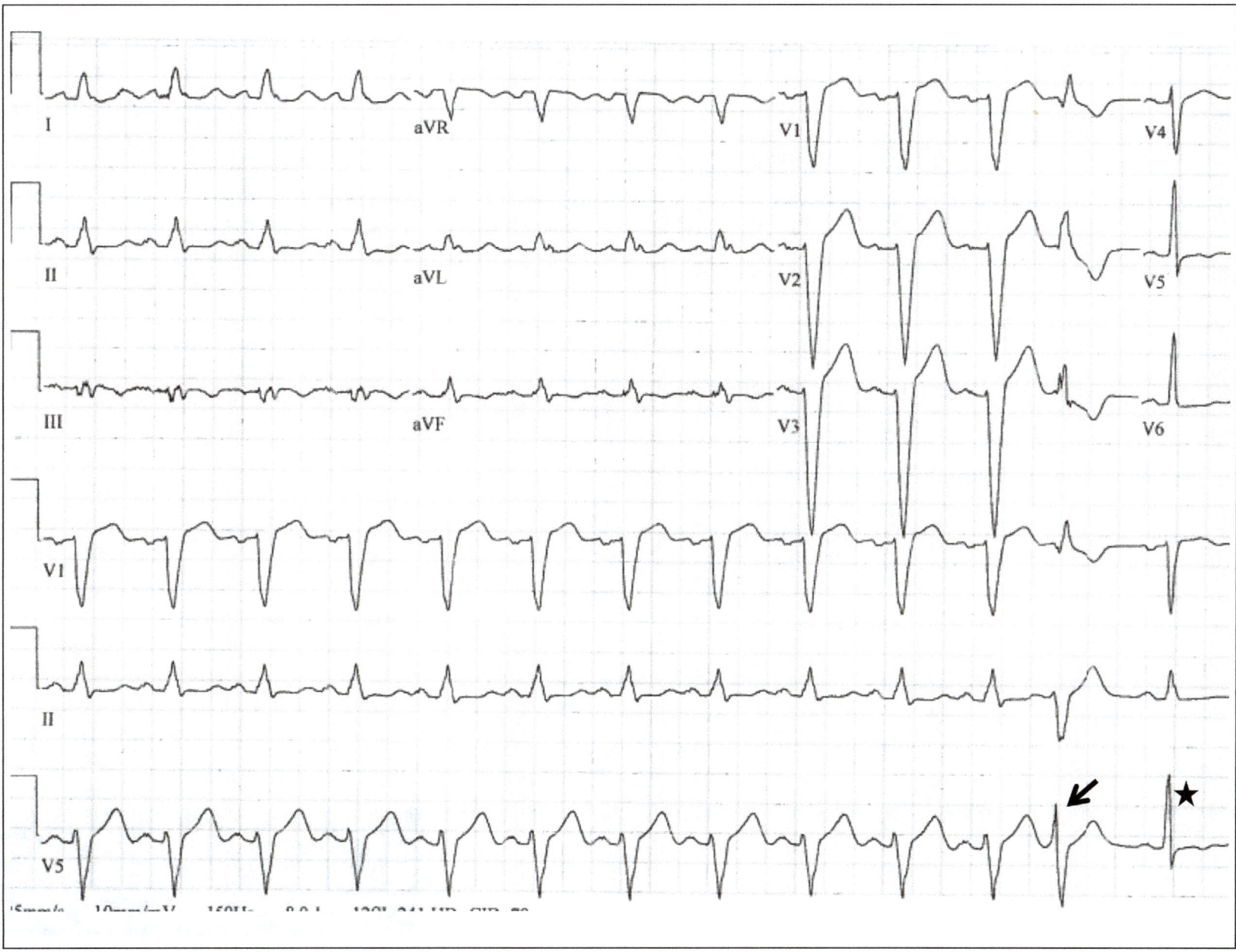

Question

What mechanism of tachycardia is demonstrated by this pacing maneuver in a 40-year-old man after slow pathway modification was performed?

A) AVNRT

B) Atrial tachycardia

C) Junctional tachycardia

D) Cannot be determined

Figure 2.B.1

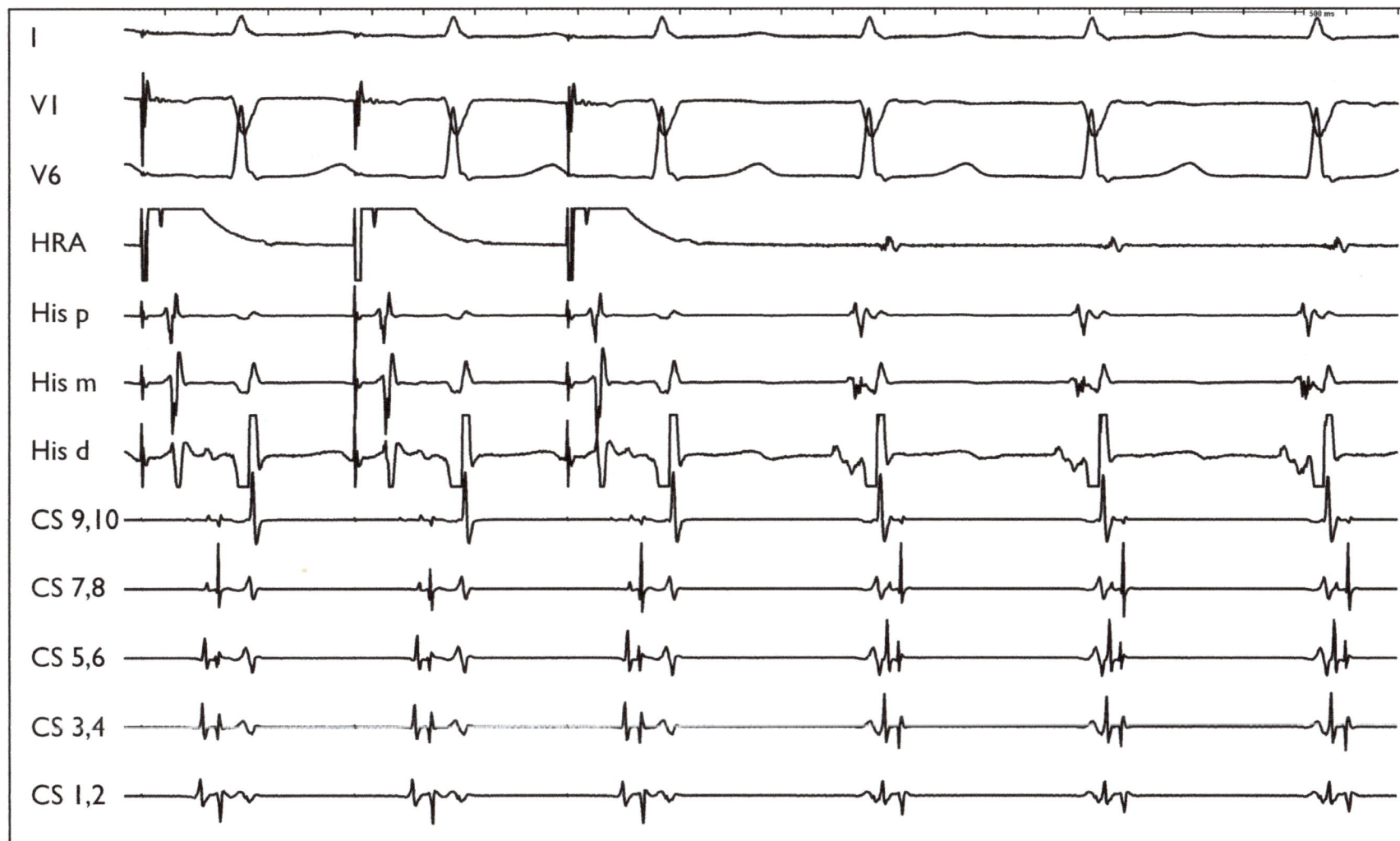

*A*nswer

The correct answer is **A**. AV node reentry is demonstrated with atrial overdrive pacing.

Differentiation between JT and AVNRT is critical to determine whether further ablation is necessary. Atrial overdrive pacing is performed 20 ms faster than the tachycardia cycle length and consistent atrial capture is seen (590 ms). With this pacing maneuver, an A-H-A response after the last paced beat is diagnostic of AVNRT, as entrainment of the His down the antegrade slow pathway occurs. Junctional tachycardia exhibits an A-H-H-A response, as entrainment with atrial overdrive pacing occurs down the fast pathway, and the reinitiation of tachycardia occurs within the His.

In this case, the conducted AH interval during atrial overdrive pacing is longer than the pacing cycle length. As a result, a "pseudo-A-H-H-A" response is seen. Measurement of the RR interval after pacing confirms that the second QRS after pacing follows the paced cycle length of 590 ms. Atrial tachycardia is excluded, as the septal VA time is <70 ms and should not reinitiate with a His electrogram. A 1:2 response with antegrade double-fire down fast and slow pathways cannot be completely excluded, although termination of AVNRT would likely be seen at the initiation of pacing if antegrade conduction switches from the slow to fast pathway during typical AVNRT.

Reference

1. Fan R, Tardos JG, Almasry I, Barbera S, Rashba EJ, Iwai S. Novel use of atrial overdrive pacing to rapidly differentiate junctional tachycardia from atrioventricular nodal reentrant tachycardia. *Heart Rhythm.* 2011;8(6):840–844.

Figure 2.B.2

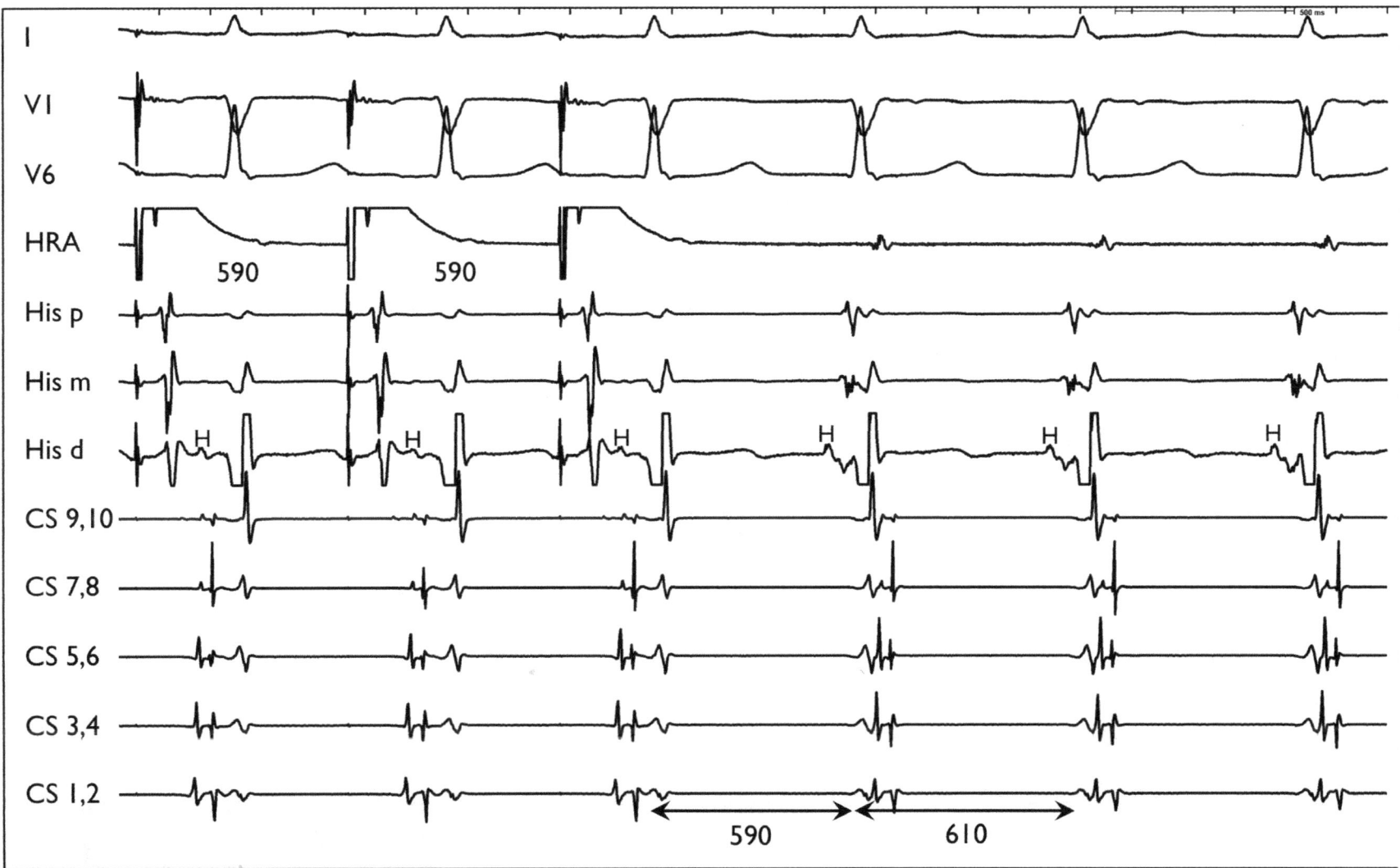

Question

A 25-year-old man presented with recurrent palpitations and documented narrow complex tachycardia on Holter monitor. The following phenomenon (Figure 2.C.1) was reproducibly noted during his EP study.

Which of the following is the most likely mechanism of tachycardia?

A) Atypical AVNRT

B) Atrial tachycardia

C) AVRT

D) No conclusions can be made, since the PVC is early

Figure 2.C.1

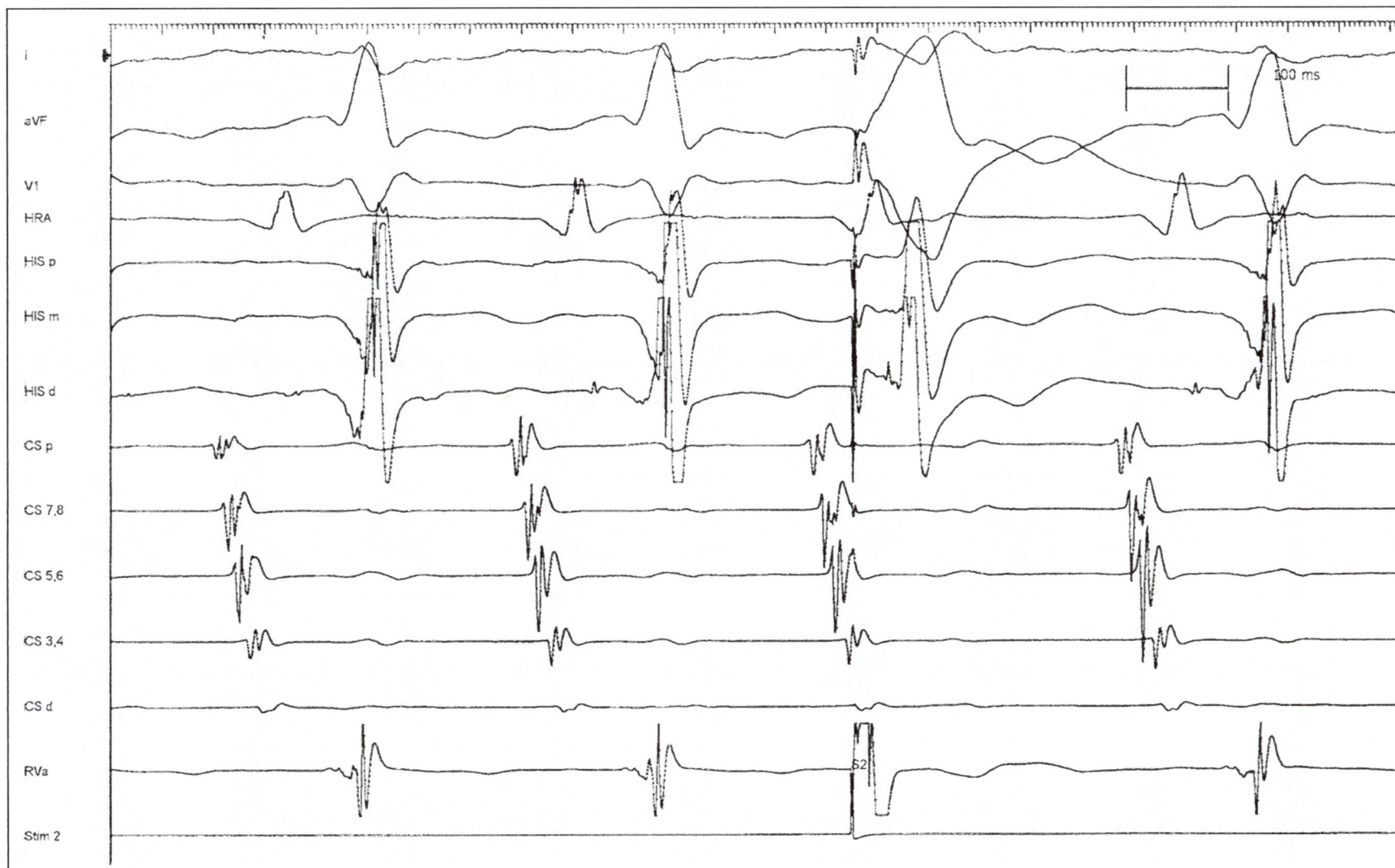

Answer

The correct answer is **C**. His-synchronous PVCs are commonly used to define the mechanism of tachycardia. The effect on the subsequent atrial activation and the tachycardia by a PVC delivered at the time or within 50 ms of the anticipated His depolarization helps in defining the mechanism. This is based on the assumption that the His bundle is refractory during its inscription. Classically, 50 ms prior to the inscription of the His deflection is used as an acceptable limit. If the PVC preexcites the atria, a retrogradely conducting accessory pathway is present. If the tachycardia is reset (e.g., atrial activation is advanced) to the same degree, then the pathway is part of the circuit. If the atrial activation is delayed (postexcitation), the involvement of the pathway in the tachycardia is likely.

Termination of the tachycardia by a His-synchronous PVC without conducting to the atria rules out atrial tachycardia and confirms the diagnosis of AVRT.

If the PVC is earlier than 50 ms of the anticipated His activation, the timing of the His inscription should be measured. If the His is advanced, then it is likely that the conduction occurred over the His. If the A is advanced by the same amount as the His, then the conduction was over the AV node. However, if the A is pulled in (e.g., advanced) more than the His, the presence of a retrograde accessory pathway is likely; although, a more definitive conclusion cannot be made about the involvement of the pathway in the tachycardia circuit.

In this case, the PVC is within 50 ms of the His activation, and the His activation is precisely on time. Additionally, another important clue to look for is the morphology of the His. In this case, the His on the PVC beat looks very similar to the His in the tachycardia, arguing for this being an anterograde His. The PVC did not affect the His activation. The atrial activity is delayed by 10 ms. The atrial activation is the same as the tachycardia beats. Postexcitation of the atrial activity by a His-synchronous PVC indicates the presence of a retrogradely conducting accessory pathway involved in the tachycardia, which confirms the diagnosis of AVRT.

One final caveat: this discussion assumes that the tachycardia cycle length is "spot on" regular with no wobble; otherwise, this maneuver and any conclusions with respect to it are invalid.

References

1. Ho RT, Kenia AS, Chhabra SK. Resetting and termination of a short RP tachycardia: what is the mechanism? *Heart Rhythm.* 2013;10:1927–1929.

2. Veenhuyzen GD, Quinn FR, Wilton SB, Clegg R, Mitchell LB. Diagnostic pacing maneuvers for supraventricular tachycardia: part 1. *Pacing Clin Electrophysiol.* 2011;34:767–782.

3. Veenhuyzen GD, Quinn FR, Wilton SB, Clegg R, Mitchell LB. Diagnostic pacing maneuvers for supraventricular tachycardias: part 2. *Pacing Clin Electrophysiol.* 2012;35:757–769.

Figure 2.C.2

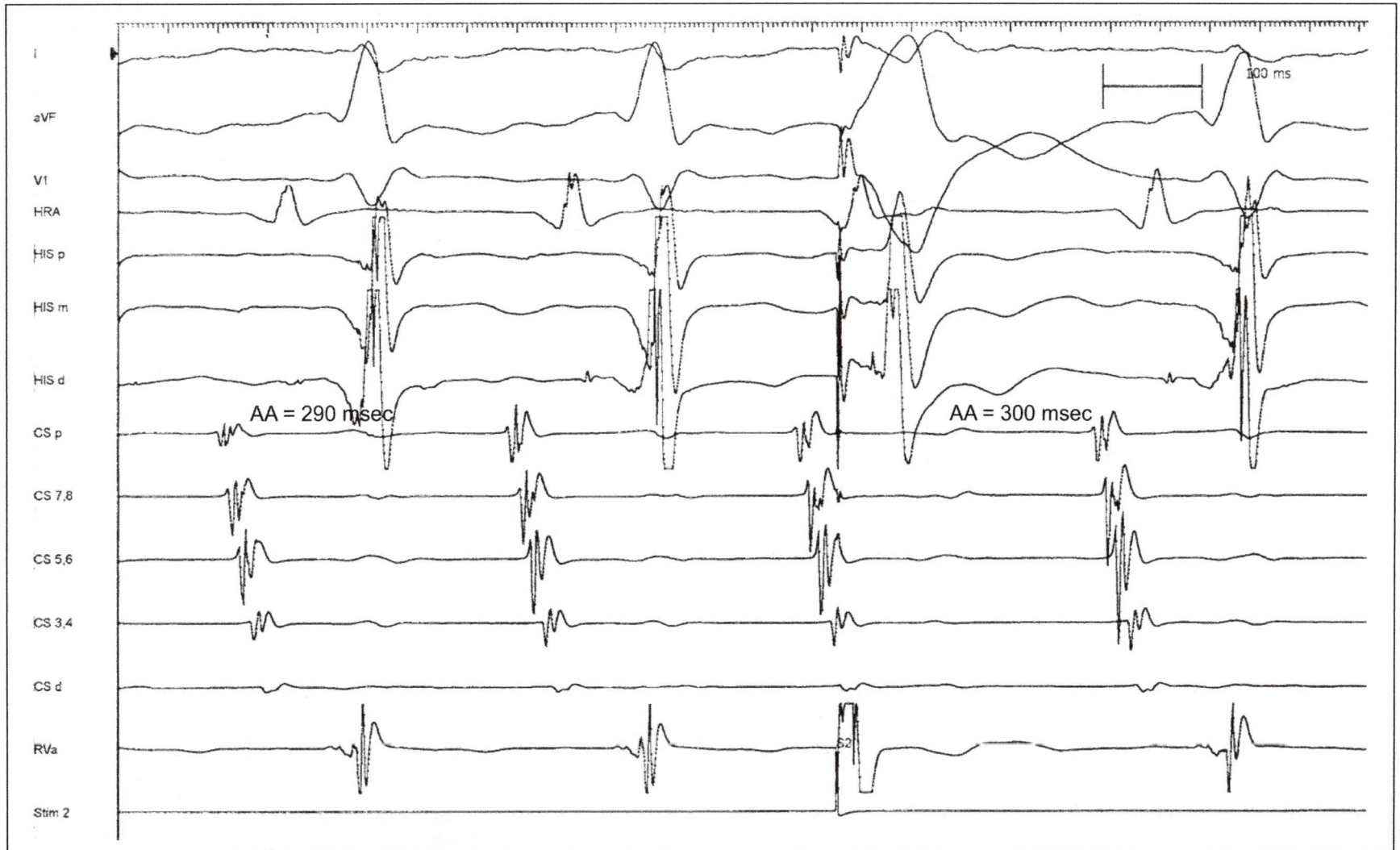

Question

A 22-year-old patient presented with SVT. The following tracing was recorded during the EP study.

Based on the findings, which of the following options is most likely?

A) AVRT and typical AVNRT

B) AVRT and atypical AVNRT

C) Atypical and typical AVNRT

D) AT and typical AVNRT

Figure 2.D.1

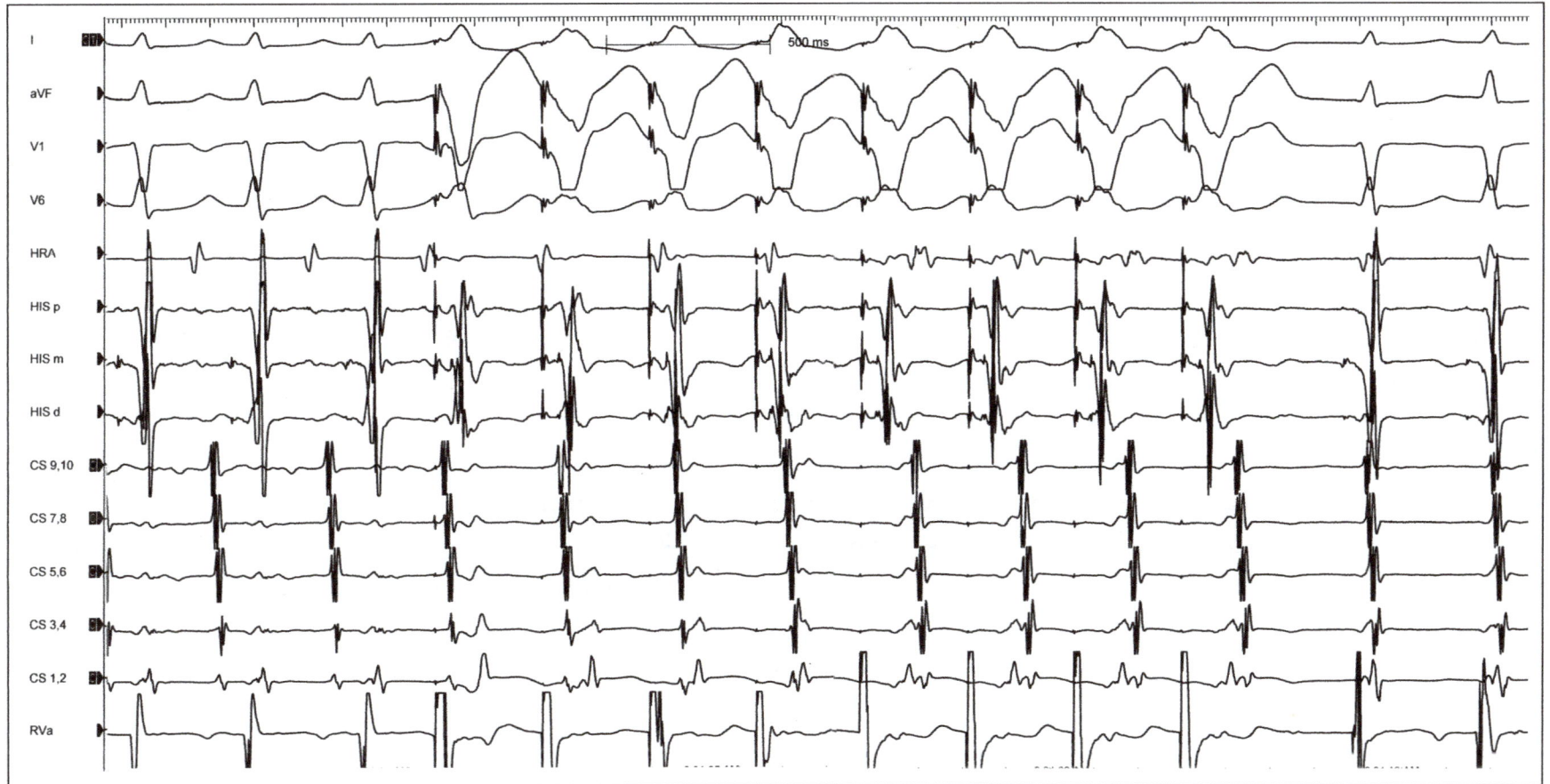

Answer

The correct answer is **D.** The initial three beats show a narrow complex long RP tachycardia. Ventricular overdrive pacing is performed to entrain the tachycardia from the right ventricle.

In the first three beats, atrial activation is high to low, i.e., high right atrium (HRA) activation is the earliest. This finding is inconsistent with AVNRT. With onset of ventricular pacing, the atrial activation and rate remain unchanged until the sixth ventricular paced beat. Absence of atrial entrainment despite complete ventricular capture and dissociation of ventricle from the atrium rules out AVRT. The initial tachycardia is an atrial tachycardia, with the earliest activation in the HRA. Also, with right ventricular pacing, one should be able to entrain conduction over a right-sided accessory pathway in all cases within two beats.

Ventricular pacing captures the atrium at the sixth beat (marked by ⋆) associated with a change in atrial activation. The short VA time during the atrial capture with earliest activation at the His catheter is consistent with retrograde conduction over a fast pathway. There is partial concealment in the slow pathway, resulting in increased refractoriness of the slow pathway, which results in antegrade conduction with long AH (342 ms as compared to 114 ms in the initial tachycardia). The prolongation of the AH allows fast pathway to recover, resulting in a second tachycardia with a septal VA ~25 ms. Tachycardia with septal VA time <60 ms and onset with AH prolongation is consistent with typical AVNRT.

Figure 2.D.2

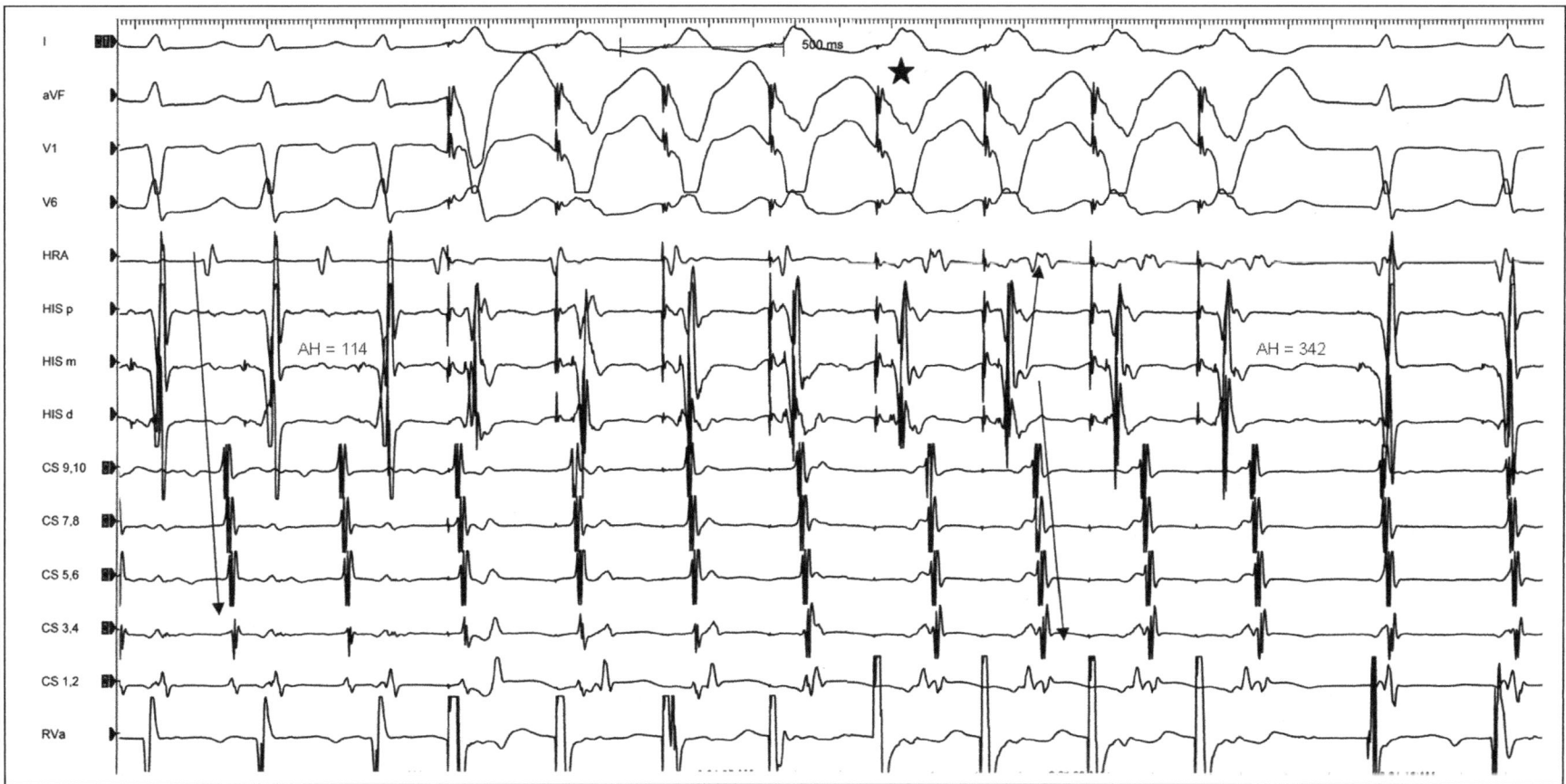

References

1. AlMahameed ST, Buxton AE, Michaud GF. New criteria during right ventricular pacing to determine the mechanism of supraventricular tachycardia. *Circ Arrhythm Electrophysiol.* 2010;3:578–584.

2. Benditt DG, Pritchett EL, Smith WM, Gallagher JJ. Ventriculoatrial intervals: diagnostic use in paroxysmal supraventricular tachycardia. *Ann Intern Med.* 1979;91:161–166.

Question

A 44-year-old man with history of Wolff-Parkinson-White ablation presents with recurrent palpitations. Tachycardia is induced using isoproterenol with periods of spontaneous aberrancy.

What is the mechanism of the difference in the postpacing interval after ventricular overdrive pacing?

A) Phase III block in AV node

B) Supernormal conduction in left bundle branch

C) Proximity to reentrant circuit

D) Rate dependent delay at site of pacing

Figure 2.E.1

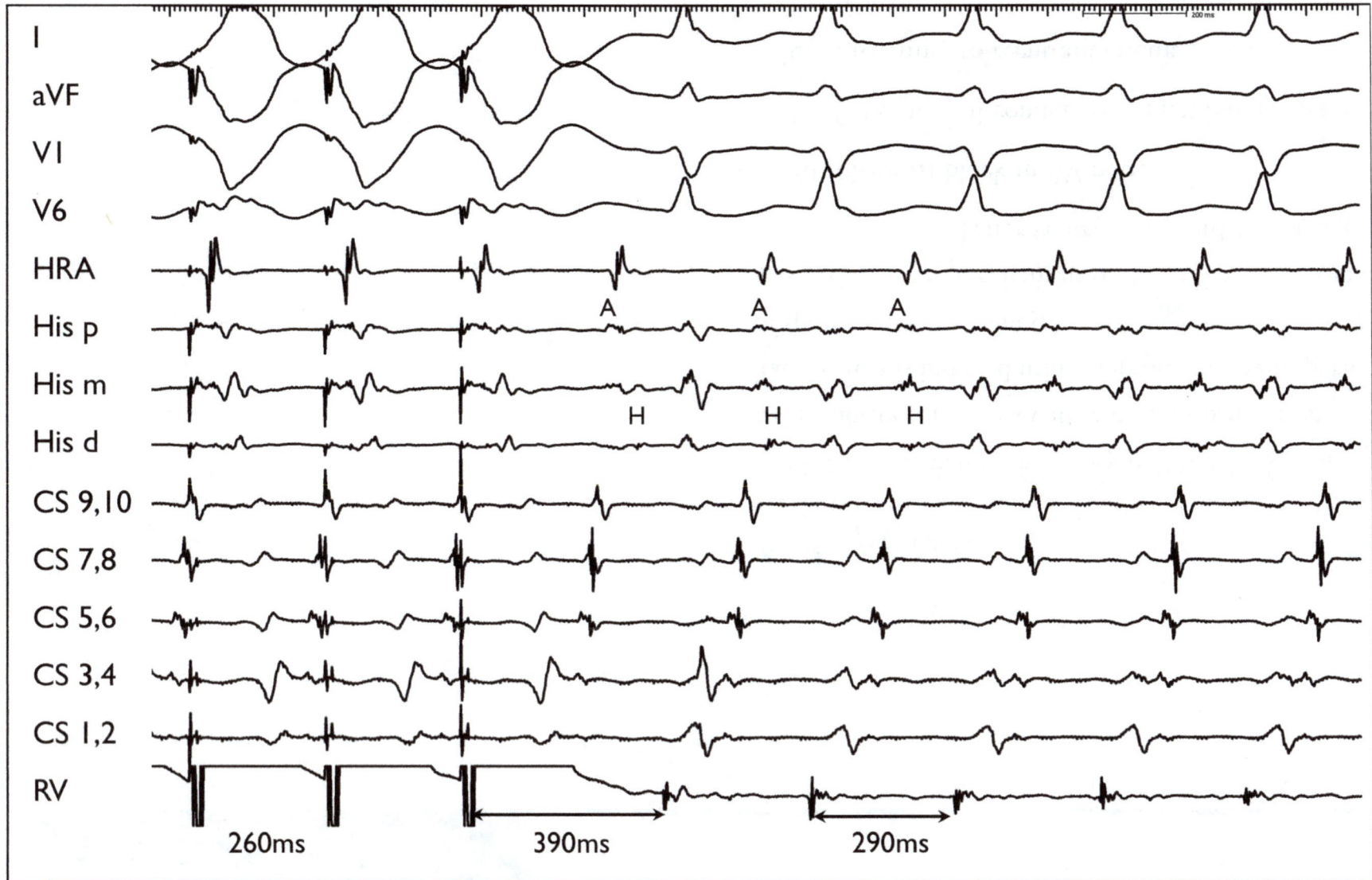

Figure 2.E.2

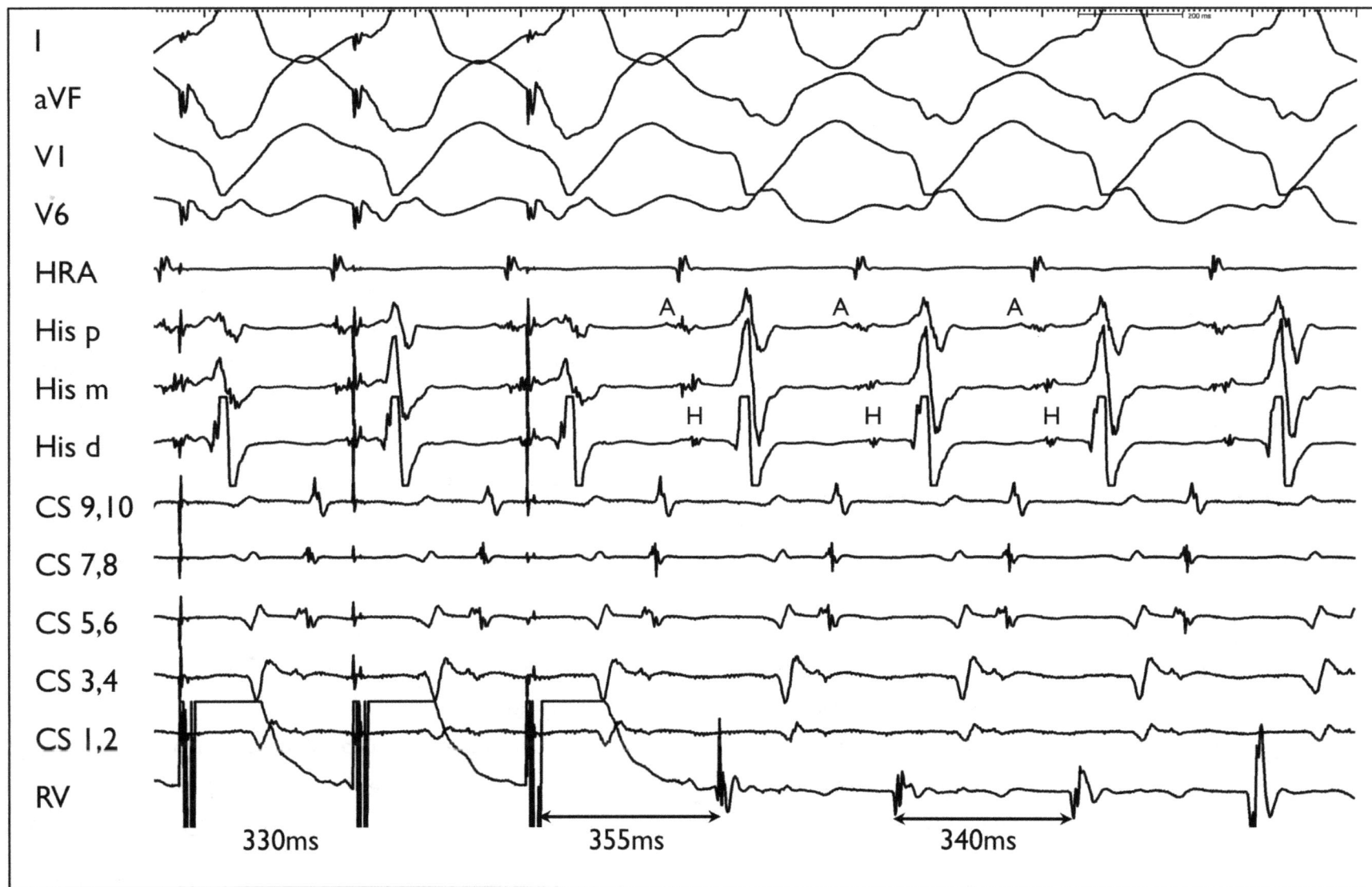

Answer

The correct answer is **C**. The distance of the pacing site from the circuit is responsible for the PPI difference.

Orthodromic reentry utilizing a concealed left lateral bypass tract is seen, with distal to proximal CS activation. The tachycardia cycle length is 50 ms longer in the presence of left bundle aberrancy, which proves participation of the bypass tract. Overdrive pacing from the same site in the RV apex results in a postpacing interval 100 ms longer than the tachycardia during narrow complex, which is only 15 ms in the presence of aberrancy. Although the pacing train is faster to entrain the narrow complex tachycardia, no significant differences are seen in the subsequent AH intervals, which obviates the need to correct for AV nodal decremental conduction. Although the VA time is longer during wide complex tachycardia, the postpacing interval is not affected, as the same paced VA time is present.

In the presence of left bundle branch block, the right bundle becomes a necessary part of the longer tachycardia circuit. Therefore, the RV apex becomes "closer" to the circuit, which results in a shorter PPI. With loss of aberrancy, the circuit only requires the left bundle for antegrade conduction, although passive conduction down the right bundle is also present.

References

1. Josephson ME. *Clinical Cardiac Electrophysiology: Techniques and Interpretations*, 4th ed. Philadelphia: Lippincott Williams & Wilkins; 2008.
2. Gonzalez-Torrecilla E, Arenal A, Atienza F, Osca J, Garcia-Fernandez J, Puchol A, et al. First postpacing interval after tachycardia entrainment with correction for atrioventricular node delay: a simple maneuver for differential diagnosis of atrioventricular nodal reentrant tachycardias versus orthodromic reciprocating tachycardias. *Heart Rhythm.* 2006;3(6):674–679.

Figure 2.E.3

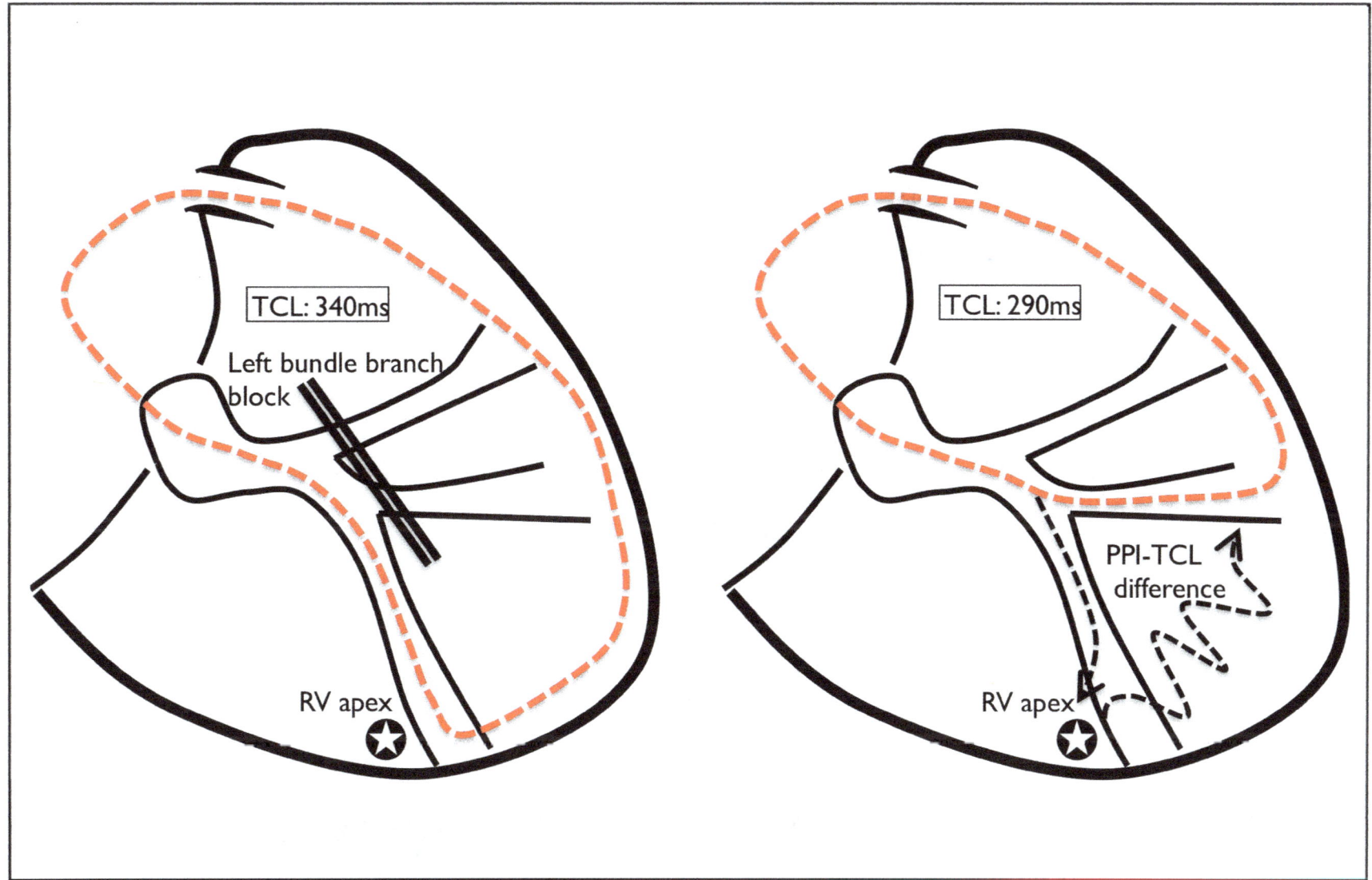

TCL: 340ms

Left bundle branch block

RV apex

TCL: 290ms

PPI-TCL difference

RV apex

Question

A 36-year-old man presented with documented narrow complex tachycardia. Which of the following arrhythmias is demonstrated by the tracing?

A) Atrial tachycardia

B) Atypical AVNRT with bystander

C) AVRT with bystander

D) AVRT with pathway involved in the circuit

Figure 2.F.1

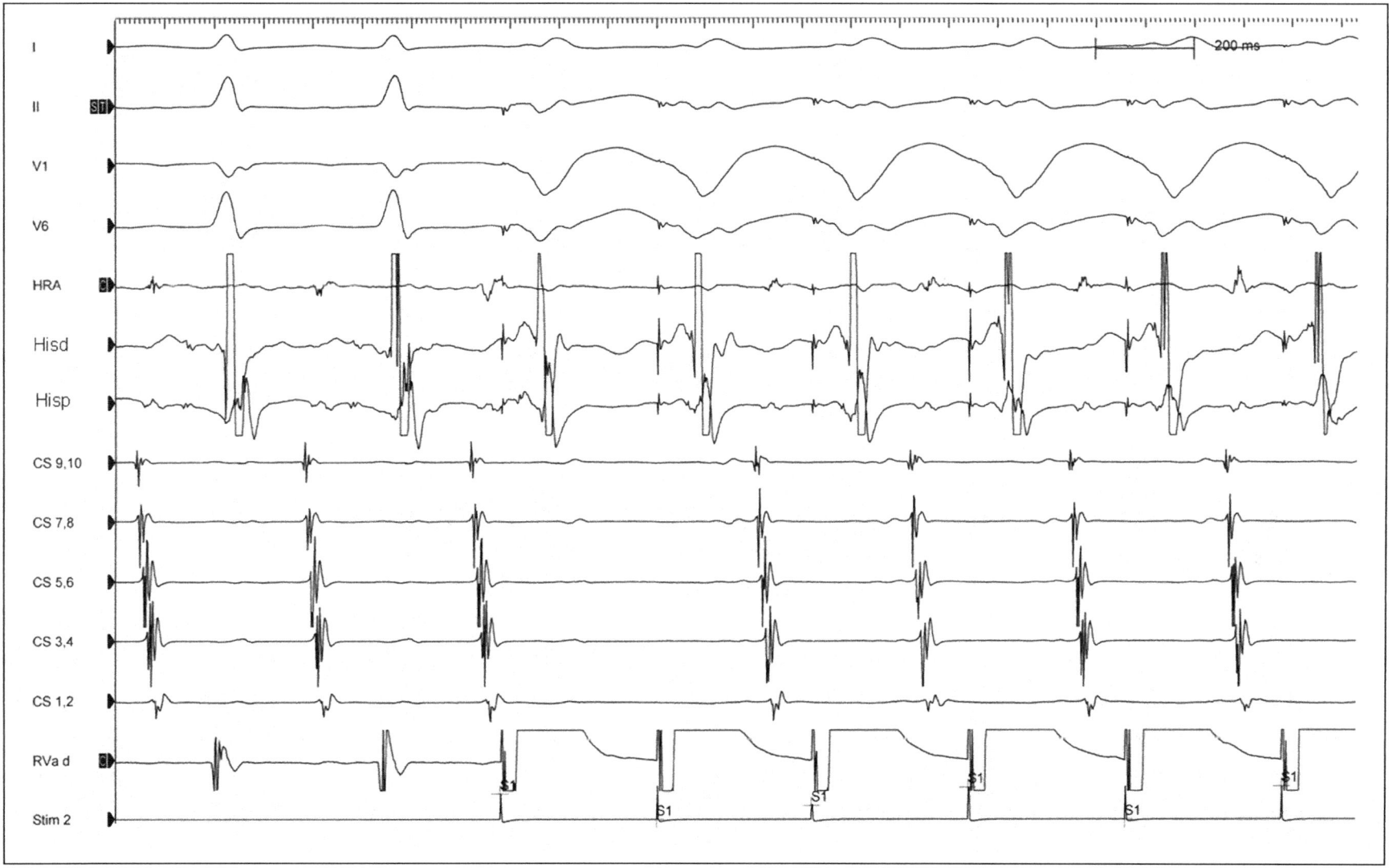

Answer

The correct answer is **D**. The tracing shows a narrow complex tachycardia (TCL 335 ms). The ventricle is paced at 320 ms to entrain the tachycardia. The His activation in the third beat is on time. The first paced beat is 30 ms prior to His activation, and since it does not alter the timing of His activation, the His bundle may be considered refractory. The QRS morphology of the first paced beat is different from the next captured beats, suggesting fusion on the first beat. The first paced V is not followed by atrial activity, and then the subsequent captured beats conduct retrogradely with 1:1 conduction. The tachycardia terminates with the first V paced beat, which is His synchronous, and termination occurs without conduction to the atrium. Atrial tachycardia cannot terminate without conduction to the atrium. His synchronous PVC may advance the next atrial activation in cases of AVNRT with a bystander pathway, but termination without conduction to the atrium is not consistent with the pathway being a bystander.

Termination of tachycardia by His synchronous PVC without conduction to the atrium indicates the presence of a bypass tract and in most cases the bypass tract is an integral part of the circuit except in rare cases of atypical AVNRT with a bystander retrogradely conducting nodofascicular or nodoventricular pathway inserting into the slow pathway. Under those circumstances, a PVC may terminate the tachycardia by resulting in concealed conduction into the slow pathway via the concealed nodofasicular or nodoventricular pathway.

References

1. Knight BP, Ebinger M, Oral H, et al. Diagnostic value of tachycardia features and pacing maneuvers during paroxysmal supraventricular tachycardia. *J Am Coll Cardiol.* 2000;36:574–582.

2. Veenhuyzen GD, Quinn FR, Wilton SB, Clegg R, Mitchell LB. Diagnostic pacing maneuvers for supraventricular tachycardia: part 1. *Pacing Clin Electrophysiol.* 2011;34:767–782.

3. Rosman JZ, John RM, Stevenson WG, et al. Resetting criteria during ventricular overdrive pacing successfully differentiate orthodromic reentrant tachycardia from atrioventricular nodal reentrant tachycardia despite interobserver disagreement concerning QRS fusion. *Heart Rhythm.* 2011;8:2–7.

4. Ho RT, Levi SA. An atypical long RP tachycardia: what is the mechanism? *Heart Rhythm.* 2013;10:1089–1090.

Figure 2.F.2

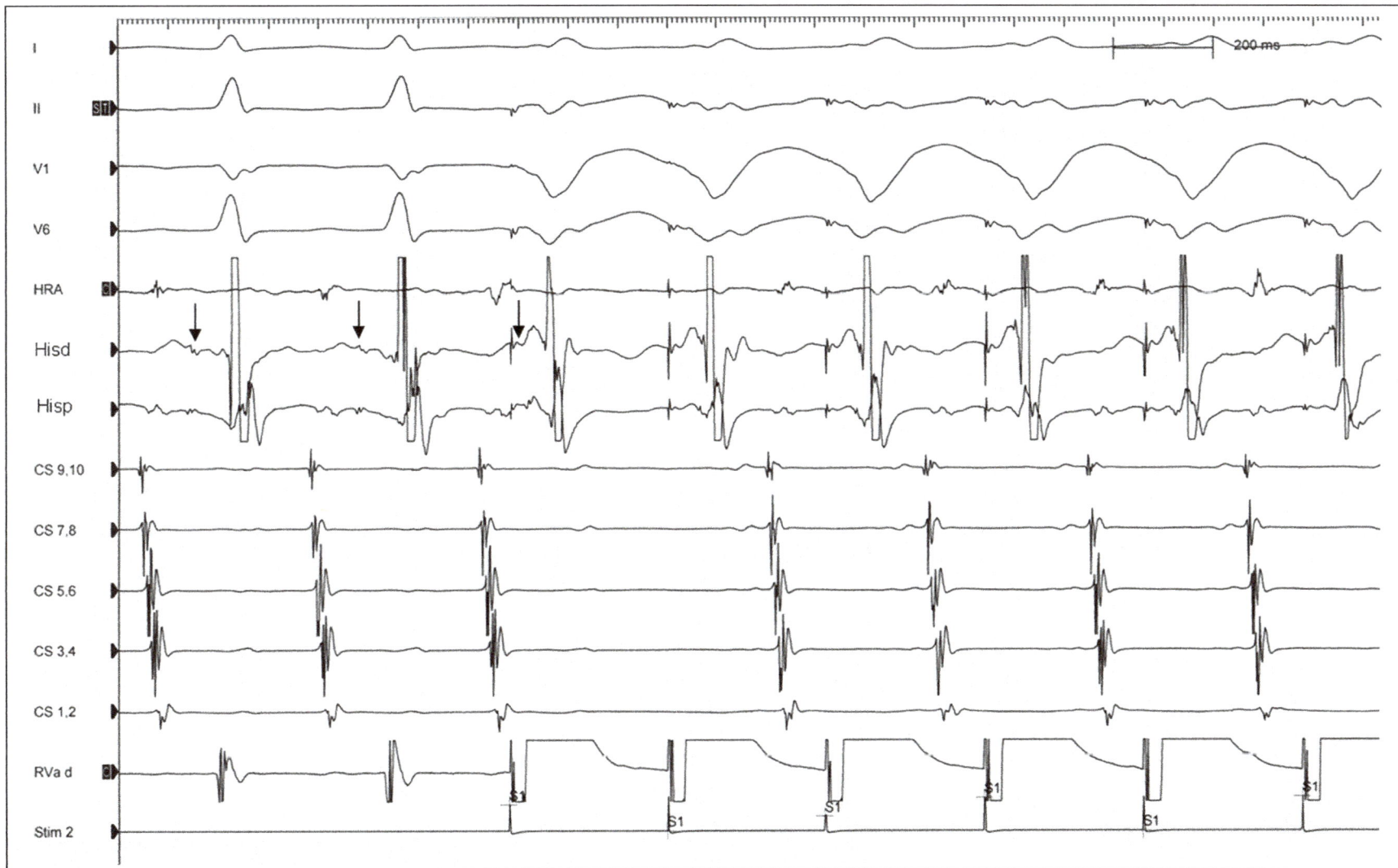

Question

An electrophysiology study is done for evaluation of recurrent narrow complex tachycardia. The following pacing maneuver shows:

A) Atypical AVNRT

B) Focal atrial tachycardia

C) Typical AVNRT

D) AVRT with right-sided pathway

E) AVRT with left-sided pathway

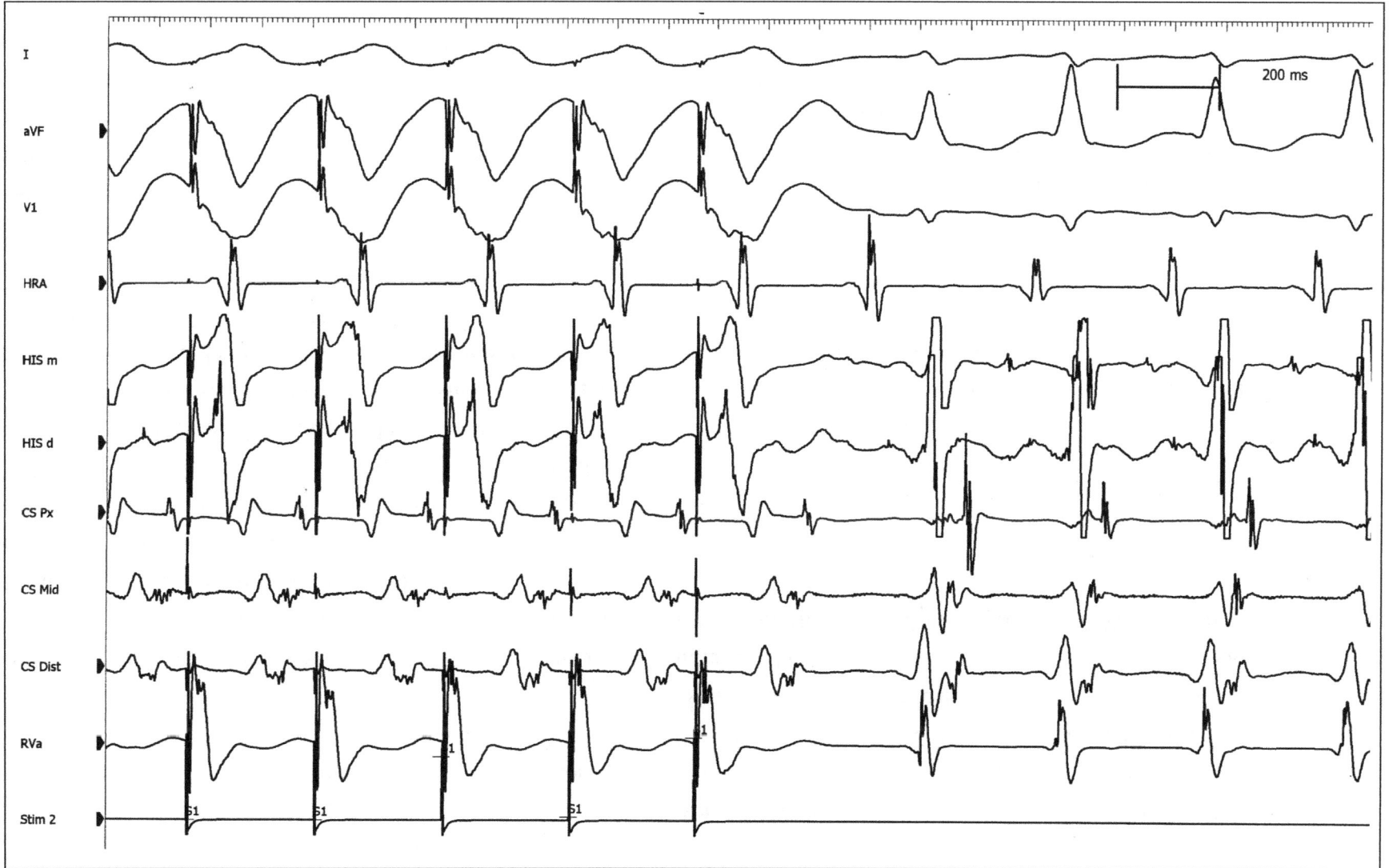

Figure 2.G.1

Answer

The correct answer is **E.**

The tracing shows a narrow complex tachycardia with long VA and HA intervals. VA interval > 60 ms rules out typical AVNRT.

Ventricular pacing is carried out to entrain the tachycardia. The atrial activation is accelerated to the tachycardia cycle length (TCL), and the tachycardia resumes after termination of pacing. At termination of pacing, the last paced QRS is followed by two atrial activations on the HRA tracing followed by a His and V, giving the appearance of VAAHV response (suggestive of atrial tachycardia). Careful evaluation of the tachycardia shows that the earliest atrial activation is in distal coronary sinus. High right atrium activation is late due to intra-atrial conduction delay (slanted arrow follows activation). The same pattern persists during V pacing. The first right atrial activation following the last V paced beat is delayed activation from the previous cycle, and the right atrium is most likely not part of the circuit and activated late as a bystander. Hence, this represents VAHV response. The PPI–TCL is 150 ms.

It is important to ensure there has been no significant change in the antegrade and retrograde conduction timing. In this case,

AH increases by ~40 ms postpacing. The corrected PPI–TCL is 110 ms, indicative of AVRT. The earliest atrial activation in the CS distal suggests AVRT mediated by left-sided pathway. The explanation for this unusual finding is that the patient has severe intra-atrial conduction delay, and thus, this is an example of an unusual mechanism causing a "pseudo-VAAV" pattern.

References

1. Knight B, Zivin A, Souza J, Flemming M, Pelosi F, Goyal R, et al. A technique for the rapid diagnosis of atrial tachycardia in the electrophysiology laboratory. *J Am Coll Cardiol.* 1999;33:775–781.

2. Michaud GF, Tada H, Chough S, Baker R, Wasmer K, Sticherling C, et al. Differentiation of atypical atrioventricular node re-entrant from orthodromic reciprocating tachycardia using a septal accessory pathway by the response to ventricular pacing. *J Am Coll Cardiol.* 2001;38:1163–1167.

3. Gonzalez-Torrecilla E, Arenal A, Atienza F, Osca J, Garcia-Fernandez J, Puchol A, et al. First postpacing interval after tachycardia entrainment with correction for atrioventricular node delay: a simple maneuver for differential diagnosis of atrioventricular nodal reentrant tachycardias versus orthodromic reciprocating tachycardias. *Heart Rhythm.* 2006;3:674–679.

Figure 2.G.2

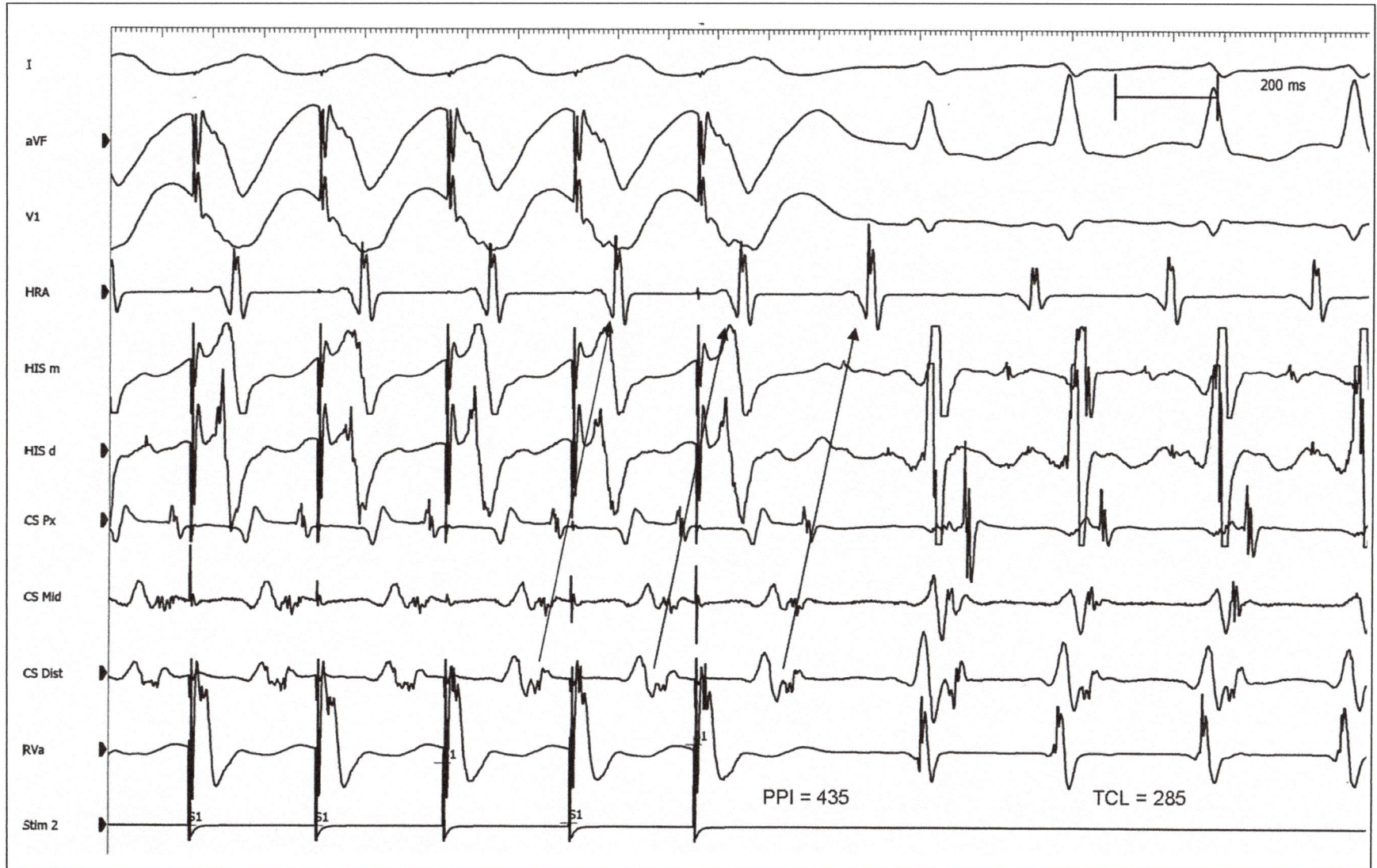

Case 2.H

Question

A 21-year-old man presents with recurrent palpitations and spontaneous wide complex tachycardia. What does this maneuver prove?

A) Ventricular tachycardia

B) Bundle branch reentry

C) Atriofascicular antidromic reentry

D) Bystander atriofascicular Mahaim pathway

Figure 2.H.1

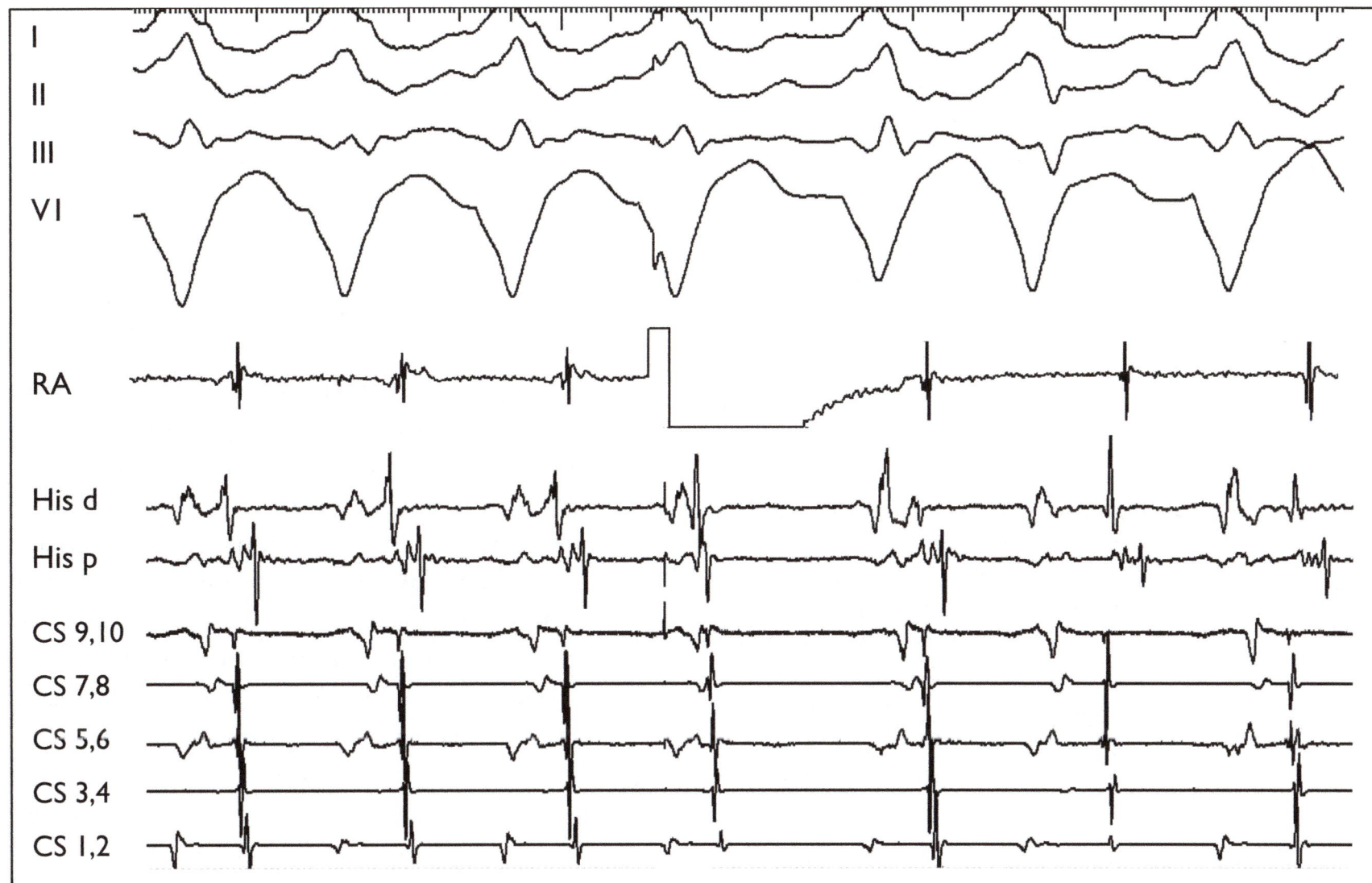

Answer

The correct answer is **C**. Antidromic tachycardia using an atriofascicular bypass tract is demonstrated.

A wide complex tachycardia with left bundle branch block morphology is seen. No apparent His is seen, which excludes bundle branch reentry. The earliest atrial electrogram is seen on the distal His catheter suggesting retrograde AV nodal conduction. A premature atrial beat delays the next tachycardia beat, which proves the presence and participation of a decremental atriofascicular pathway.

Myocardial VT should not be influenced by an atrial premature beat, and a bystander Mahaim should not delay the ongoing tachycardia. Such an extreme decrement is atypical of Mahaim atriofascicular antidromic tachycardia.

References

1. Tchou P, Lehmann MH, Jazayeri M, Akhtar M. Atriofascicular connection or a nodoventricular Mahaim fiber? Electrophysiologic elucidation of the pathway and associated reentrant circuit. *Circulation*. 1988;77(4):837.

2. Sternick EB, Lokhandwala Y, Timmermans C, Rodriguez LM, Gerken LM, Scarpelli R, et al. The atrioventricular interval during pre-excited tachycardia: a simple way to distinguish between decrementally or rapidly conducting accessory pathways. *Heart Rhythm*. 2009;6(9):1351–1358.

Figure 2.H.2

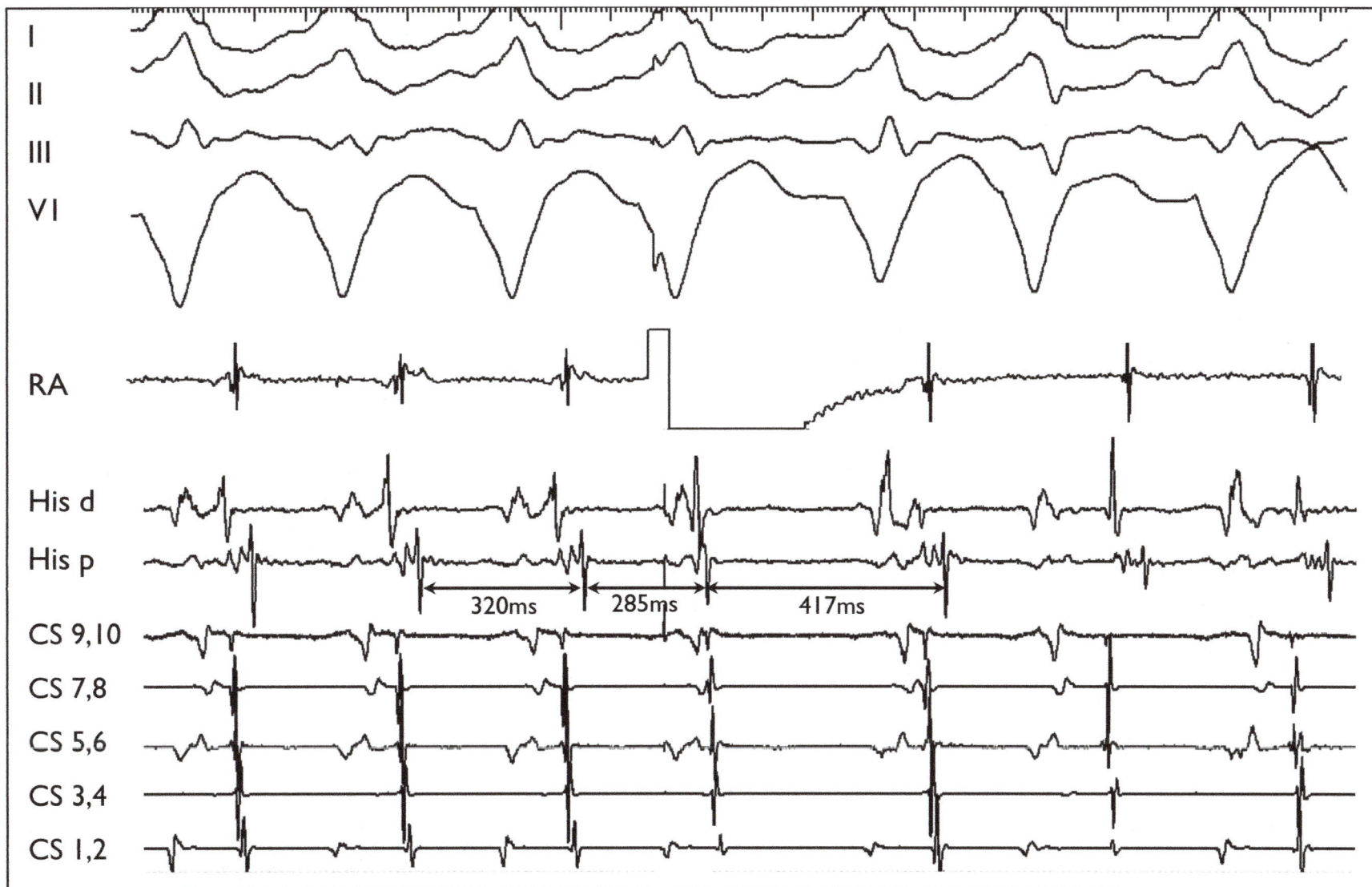

Question

A 20-year-old man with documented SVT underwent catheter ablation.

What is the most likely explanation for the observed response?

A) Typical and atypical AV nodal reentrant tachycardia are present

B) Atrial tachycardia and atrioventricular reentrant tachycardia are present

C) Atrial tachycardia and AV nodal reentrant tachycardia are present

D) Atrioventricular reentrant tachycardia and AV nodal reentrant tachycardia are present

E) Atrioventricular reentrant tachycardia is present utilizing two distinct retrograde accessory pathways

Figure 2.I.1

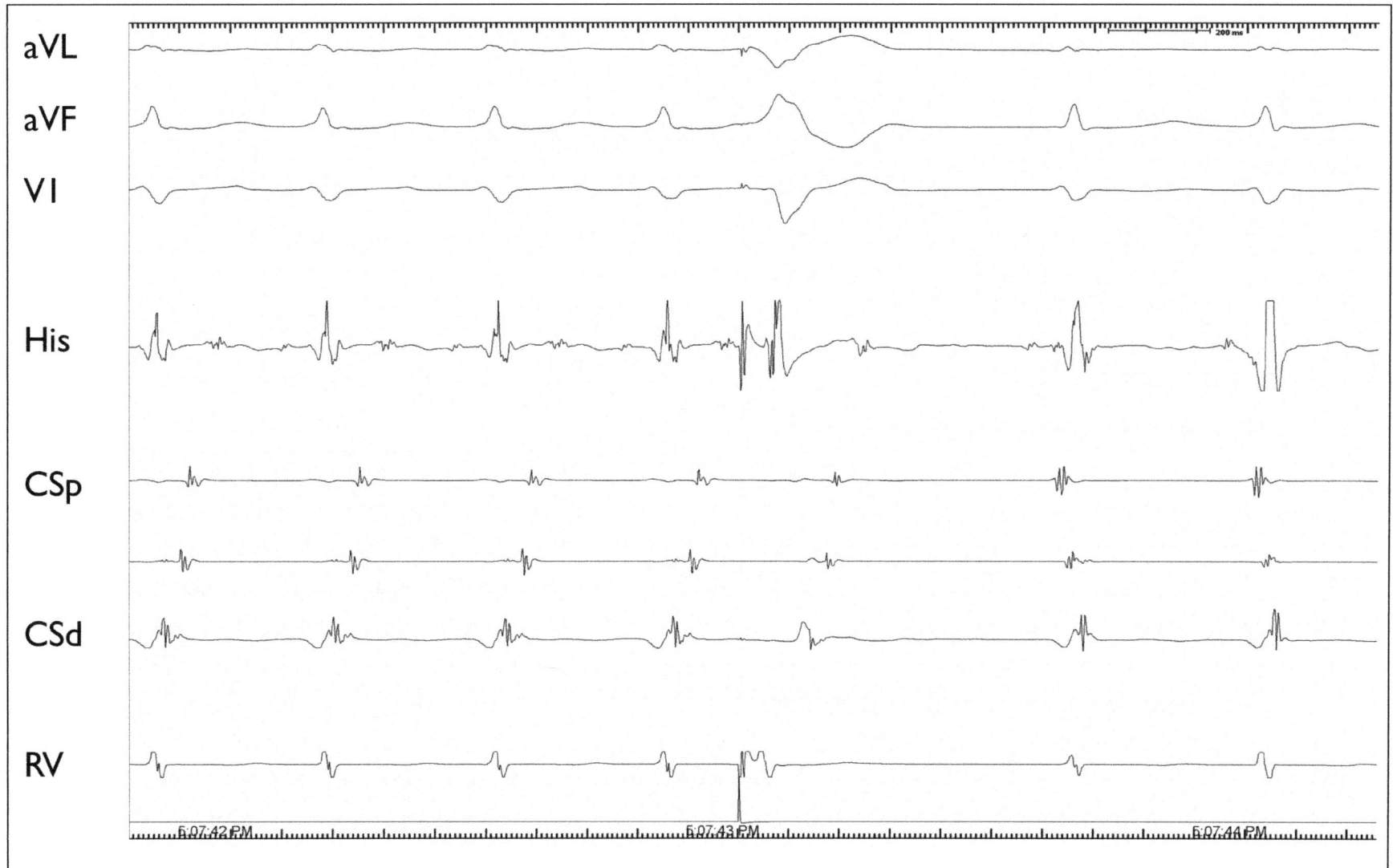

Answer

The correct answer is **D**. Two distinct SVTs are present on this tracing. The atrial activation sequence is eccentric during the initial tachycardia, earliest on the distal coronary sinus, ruling out AVNRT. An early PVC is delivered from the RV catheter, advancing the atrium with an identical activation sequence as the tachycardia. While it is possible that SVT1 (Figure 2.I.2) is a left atrial tachycardia and the PVC advances the atrium over a bystander left lateral accessory pathway coincidentally inserting near the AT site of origin, far more likely is AVRT utilizing a left lateral accessory pathway as the retrograde limb. The resulting premature atrial beat causes an AH jump, with shift to anterograde conduction over the slow AV nodal pathway and initiation of SVT2 (Figure 2.I.3). SVT2 has a concentric atrial activation sequence, as well as a VA time of 10 ms, ruling out AVRT. Given initiation with a jump to the slow pathway and VA time < 70, AVNRT is most likely.

SVT1 reproducibly terminated with an A, ruling out atrial tachycardia and confirming the diagnosis of AVRT.

Ventricular overdrive pacing during SVT2 resulted in a VAHV response, ruling out atrial tachycardia and confirming the diagnosis of AVNRT.

Figure 2.1.2

SVT1

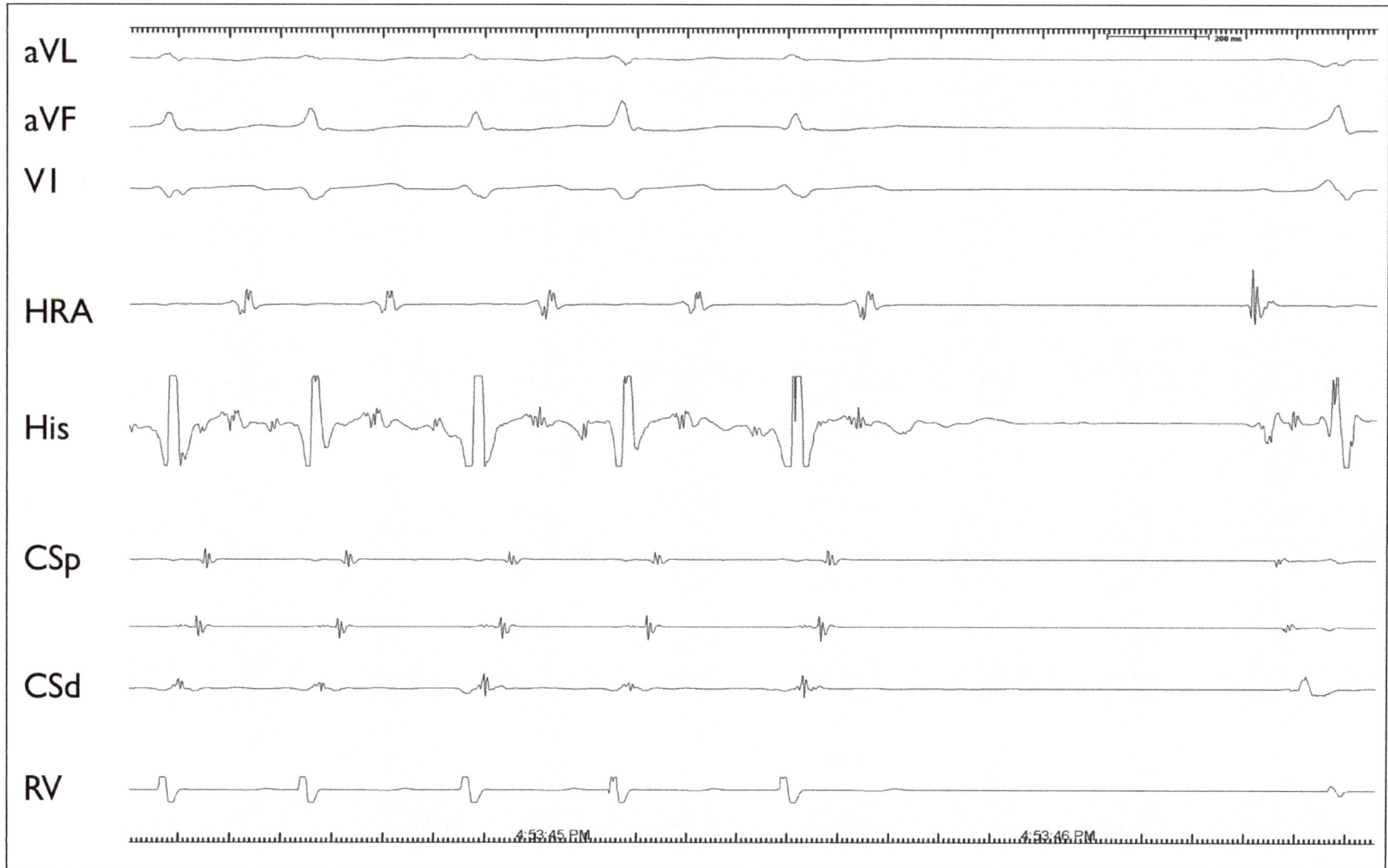

4:53:45 PM   4:53:46 PM

Figure 2.1.3

SVT2

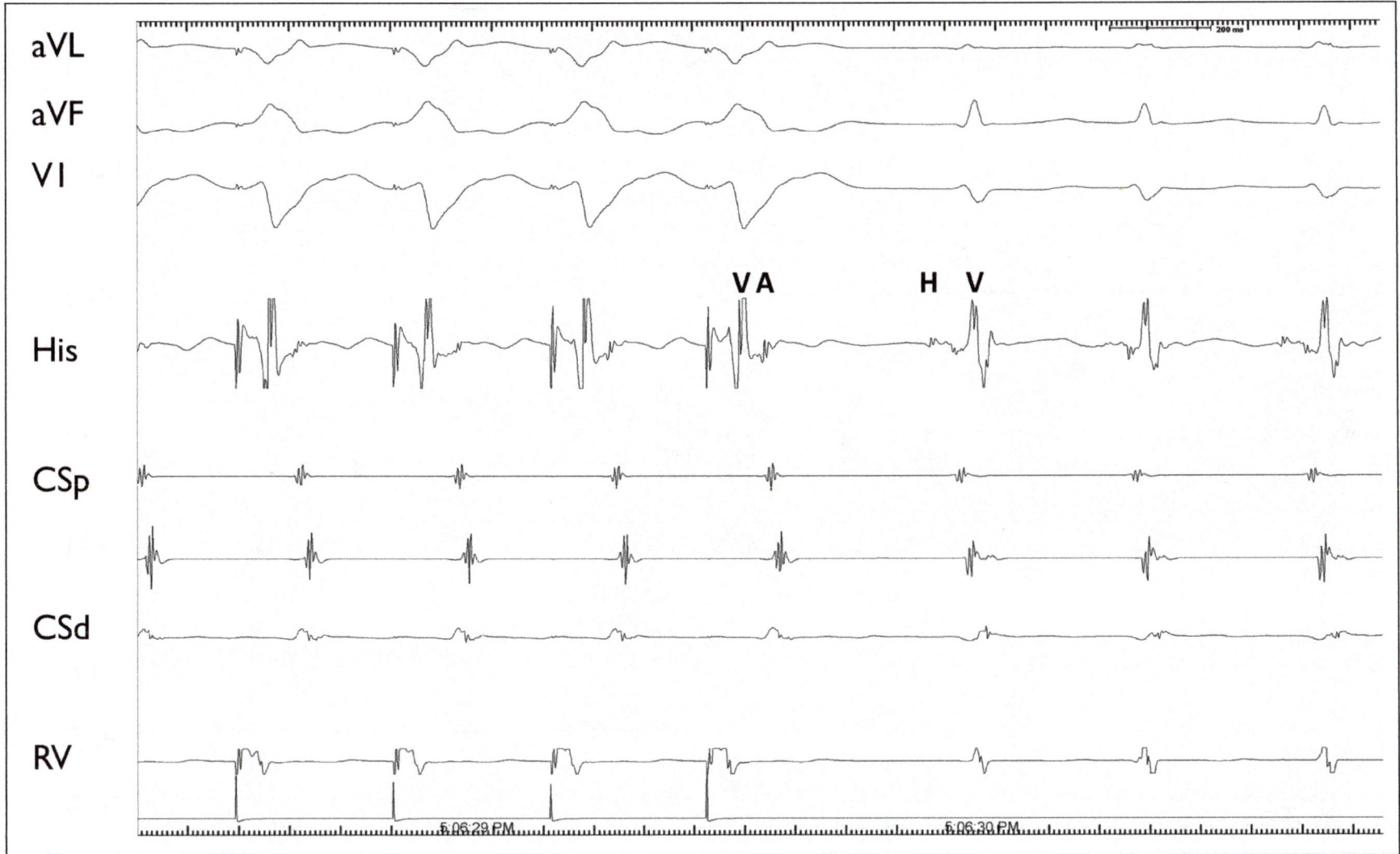

Reference

1. Knight BP, Ebinger M, Oral H, Kim MH, Sticherling C, Pelosi F, et al. Diagnostic value of tachycardia features and pacing maneuvers during paroxysmal supraventricular tachycardia. *J Am Coll Cardiol.* 2000;36:574–582.

Question

A 50-year-old man with hypertension has recurrent SVT after left total knee arthroplasty.

What is the most likely diagnosis?

A) ORT using a left free wall AP

B) ORT using a right free wall AP

C) Atrial tachycardia with a bystander AP near the site of AT

D) AVNRT with a bystander nodofascicular AP

Figure 2.J.1

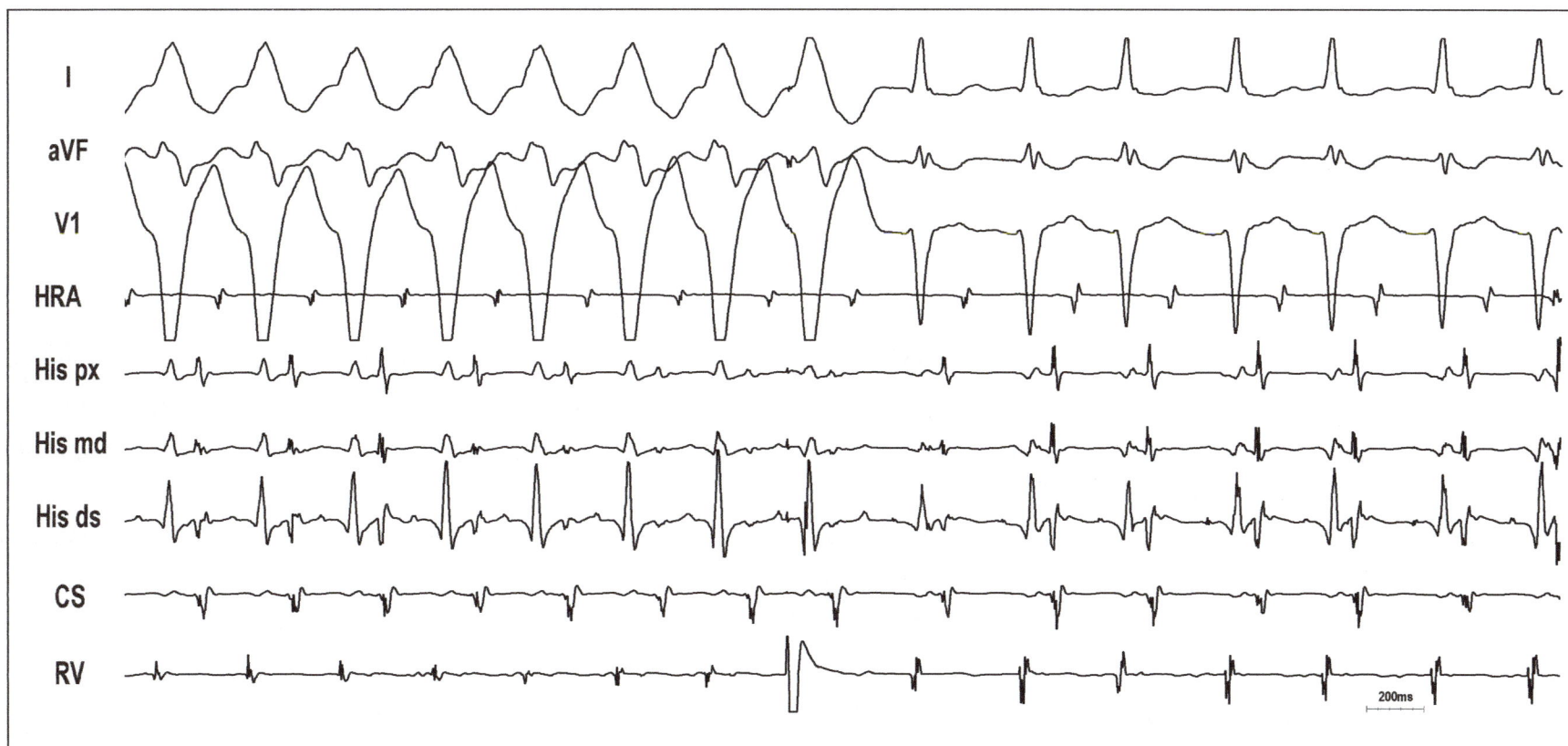

Answer

The correct answer is **A**. A LBBB tachycardia transitions to a slower, narrow complex tachycardia with cycle length alternans after a His-refractory VPD. The intrinsicoid during LBBB is rapid, His bundle potentials precede each QRS complex with normal HV intervals, and atrial activation is unchanged, suggesting a supra-ventricular mechanism with and without LBBB.

The His-refractory VPD not only preexcites the atrium (★) indicating the presence of an accessory pathway but also retro-gradely penetrates the LB, breaking the transseptal link perpetuating LBBB. The VA interval during LBBB is 27 ms longer than without LBBB, indicating not only that the His-Purkinje system is an integral part of tachycardia but also that the AP is left-sided (ipsilateral to BBB), a finding diagnostic of ORT using a left-sided AP and excluding AT, AVNRT, and ORT using a right-sided AP. Generally, the ORT cycle length shortens with loss of BBB ipsilateral to the AP (Coumel's sign) but can paradox-ically lengthen if the decrease in VA interval is counterbalanced by a greater increase in the AH interval due to decremental AV nodal conduction or switch to the SP, as seen here. Cycle length alternans results from alternating SP and FP conduction during ORT. The longer AH_{FP} intervals during narrow QRS complex compared to LBBB despite the slower rate is the result of conceal-ment from SP into the FP, rendering the latter relatively refractory during ongoing tachycardia.

Figure 2.J.2

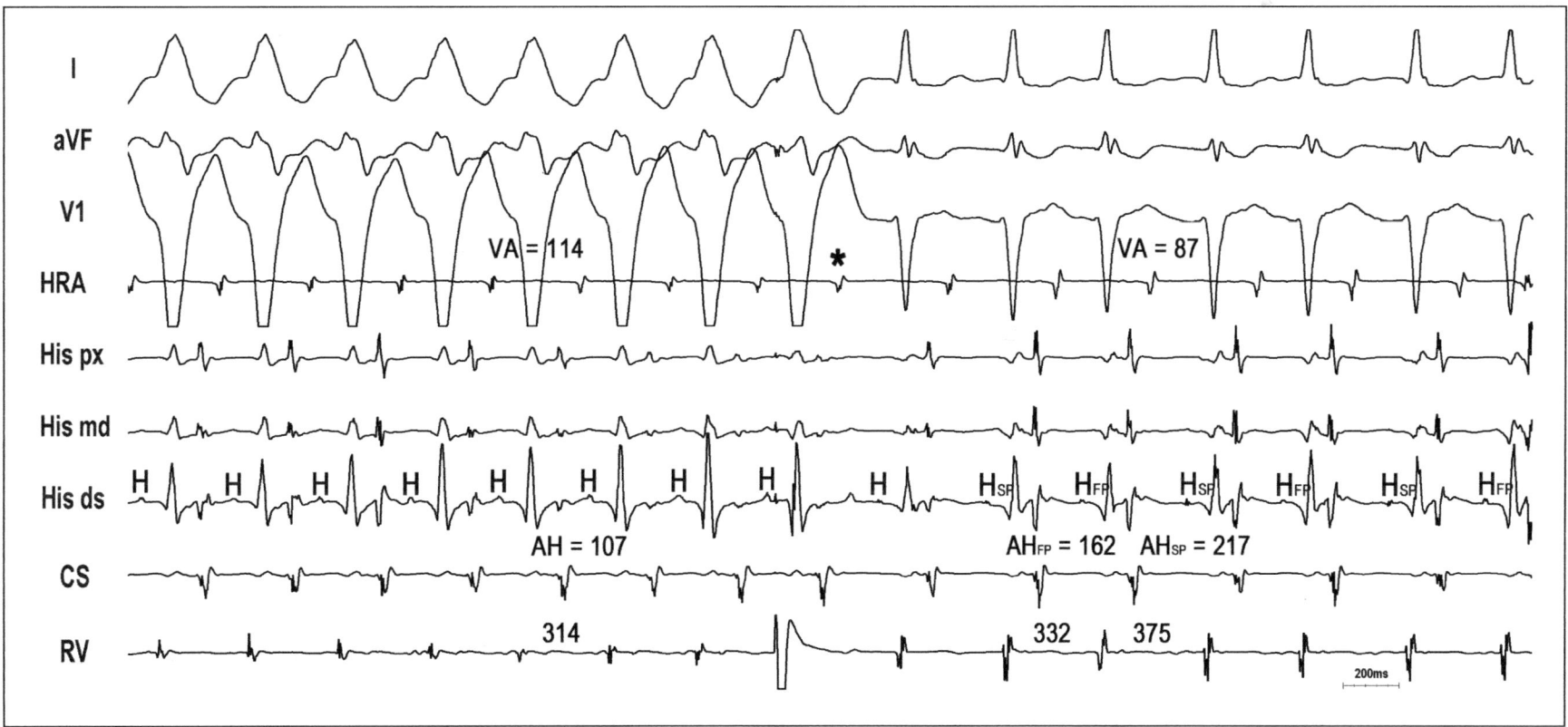

References

1. Benditt D, Benson W, Dunnigan A, Gornick C, Ring S, Almquist A, et al. Role of extrastimulus site and tachycardia cycle length in inducibility of atrial preexcitation by premature ventricular stimulation during reciprocating tachycardia. *Am J Cardiol*. 1987;60:811–819.

2. Spurrell R, Krikler D, Sowton E. Retrograde invasion of the bundle branches producing aberration of the QRS complex during supraventricular tachycardia studied by programmed electrical stimulation. *Circulation*. 1974;50:487–495.

3. Coumel P, Attuel P. Reciprocating tachycardia in overt and latent preexcitation. *Eur J Cardiol*. 1974;1:423.

Question

Based on the tracings, the most likely diagnosis is:

A) Typical AVNRT

B) AVRT

C) Atrial tachycardia

D) Atypical AVNRT

Figure 2.K.1

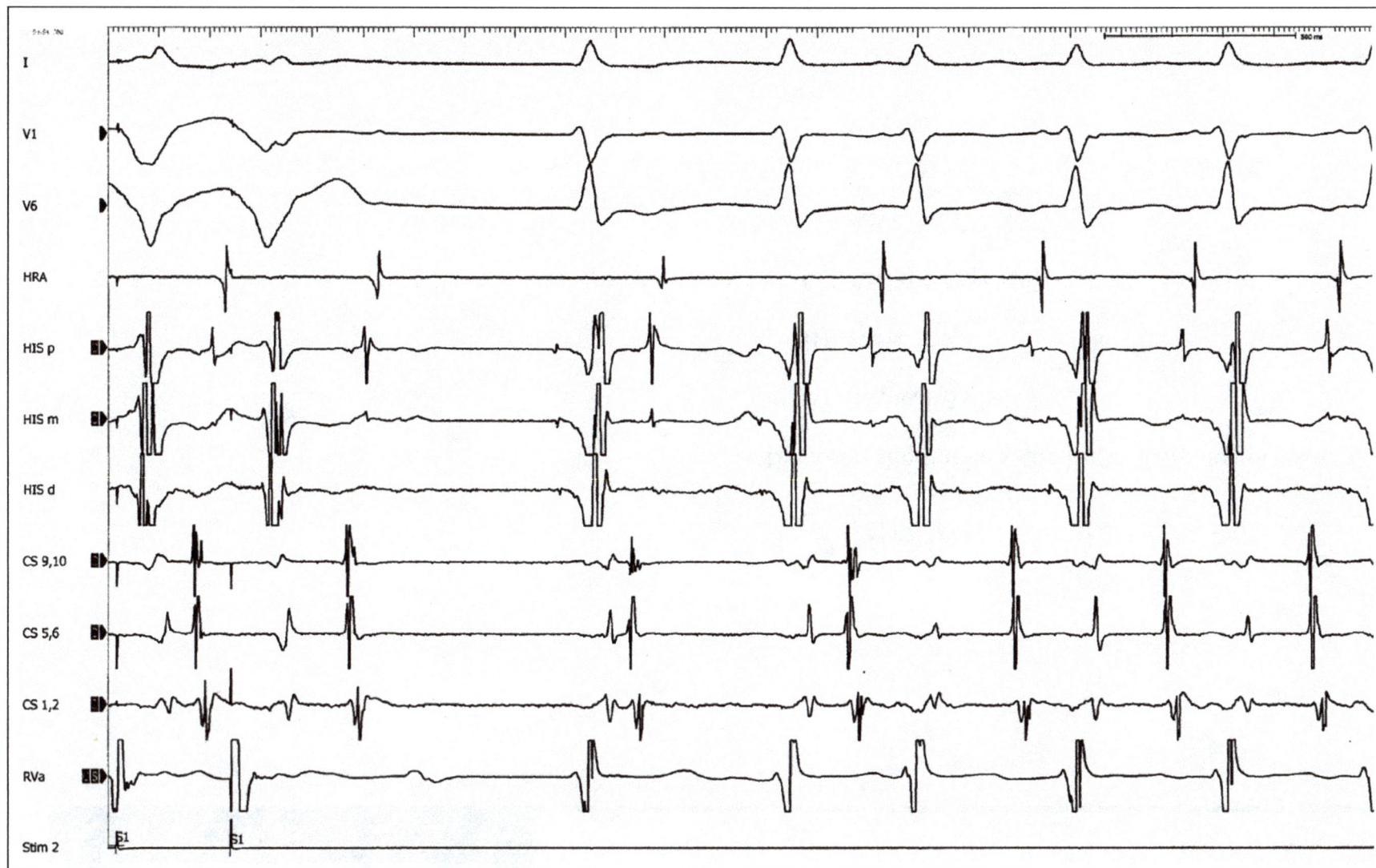

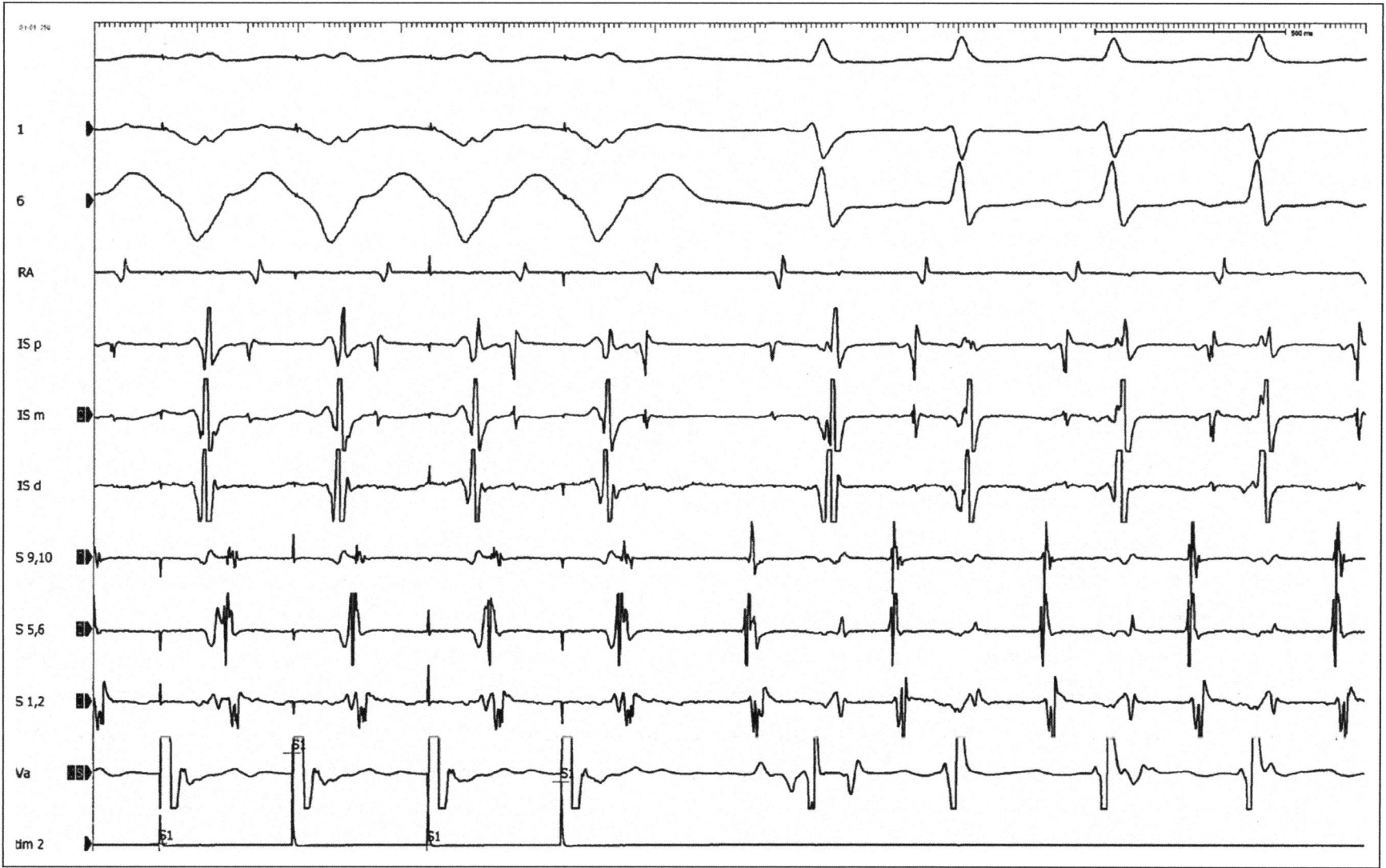

Figure 2.K.2

Answer

The correct answer is **D**. The first tracing shows ventricular pacing with 1:1 VA conduction with earliest atrial activity at the His and proximal coronary sinus (CS). The retrograde atrial activation then conducts with a long AH interval (~510 ms).

During the subsequent cycles the AH shortens and the VA prolongs. At first glance, this appears to be an atrial tachycardia with VA dissociation, but a closer analysis reveals that the relative changes in H–H drive the changes in A–As. If this were an atrial tachycardia, the As should drive the Vs. The change in VA may reflect the presence of separate retrograde pathways or more likely reflect the change in conduction due to shortening of the antegrade conduction time. The long septal VA time rules out typical AVNRT.

In the second tracing, the tachycardia is entrained from the ventricle (350 ms). At the termination of pacing, the tachycardia resumes with a VAAHV response. It is important to determine the last entrained atrial activity. Due to the long VA interval during pacing, the ventricular depolarization is linked to the atrial activity after the atrial depolarization that immediately follows the V. The pseudo VAAHV response makes the diagnosis of focal atrial tachycardia unlikely. AVRT is unlikely based on the first tracing where VA is variable at the beginning of the tachycardia. The PPI–TCL > 115 and SA–VA > 85 ms makes AVRT unlikely. His sync PVC delivered with 27 ms of inscribed His signal does not perturb the tachycardia.

Figure 2.K.3

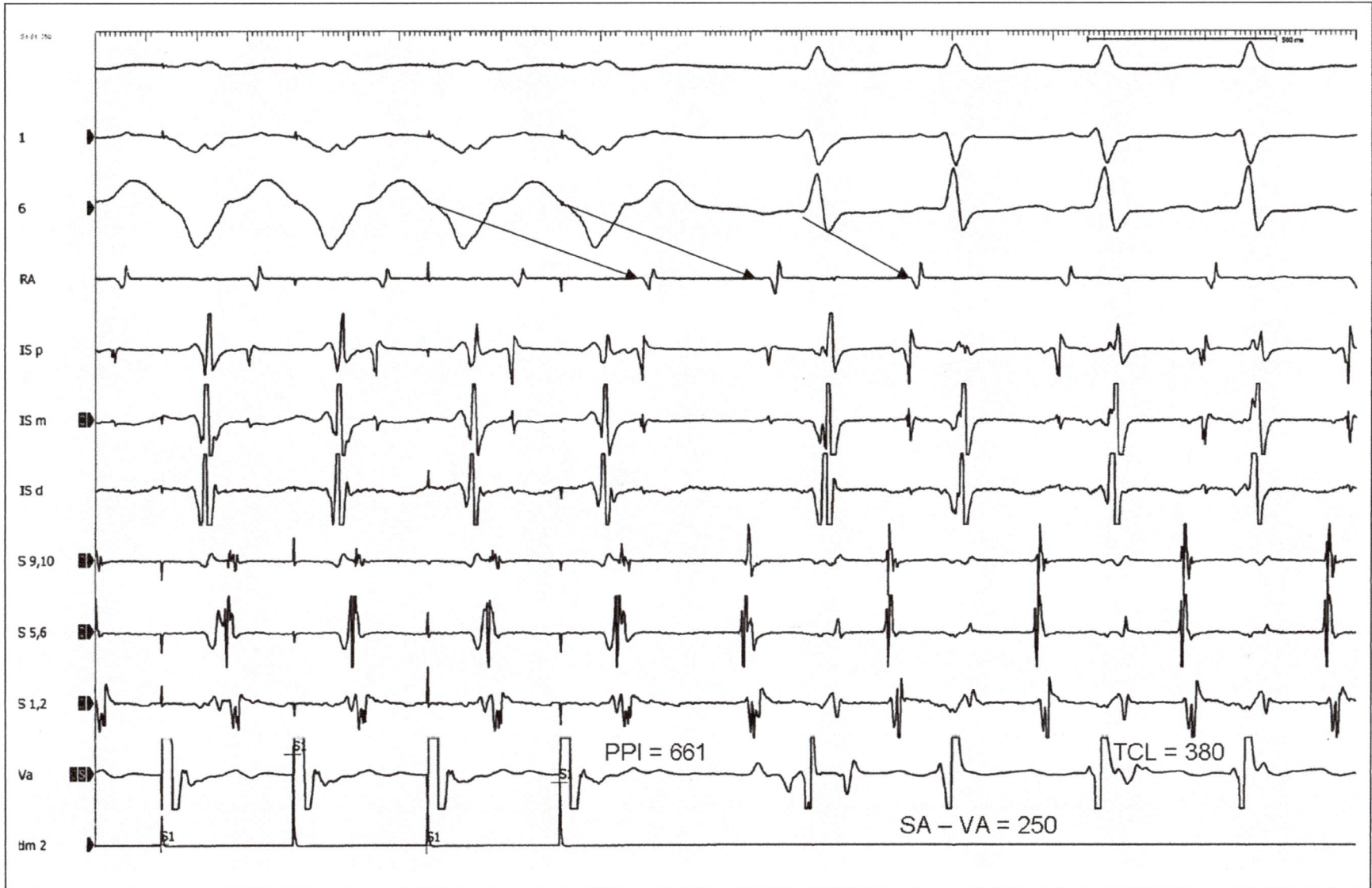

Figure 2.K.4

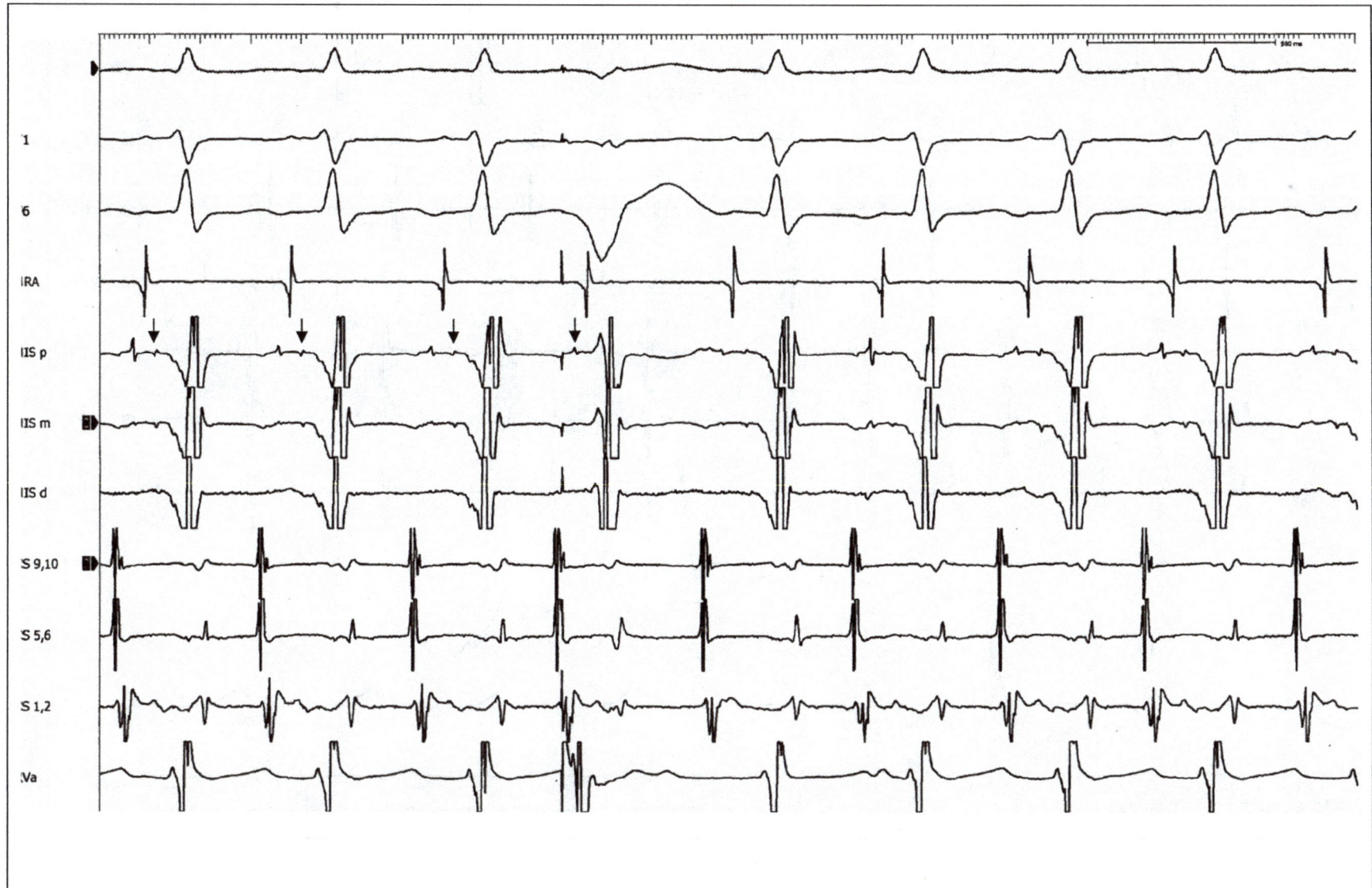

References

1. Bennett MT, Leong-Sit P, Gula LJ, et al. Entrainment for distinguishing atypical atrioventricular node reentrant tachycardia from atrioventricular reentrant tachycardia over septal accessory pathways with long-RP [corrected] tachycardia. *Circ Arrhythm Electrophysiol.* 2011;4:506–509.

2. Vijayaraman P, Lee BP, Kalahasty G, Wood MA, Ellenbogen KA. Reanalysis of the "pseudo A-A-V" response to ventricular entrainment of supraventricular tachycardia: importance of his-bundle timing. *J Cardiovasc Electrophysiol.* 2006;17:25–28.

3. Knight BP, Ebinger M, Oral H, et al. Diagnostic value of tachycardia features and pacing maneuvers during paroxysmal supraventricular tachycardia. *J Am Coll Cardiol.* 2000;36:574–582.

*Q*uestion

This tracing was made during an electrophysiology study from a 40-year-old woman with recurrent palpitations. The tracing demonstrates which of the following?

A) Atrial tachycardia

B) Atrial tachycardia with a bystander accessory pathway

C) AVRT

D) Atypical AVNRT with resetting

Figure 2.L.1

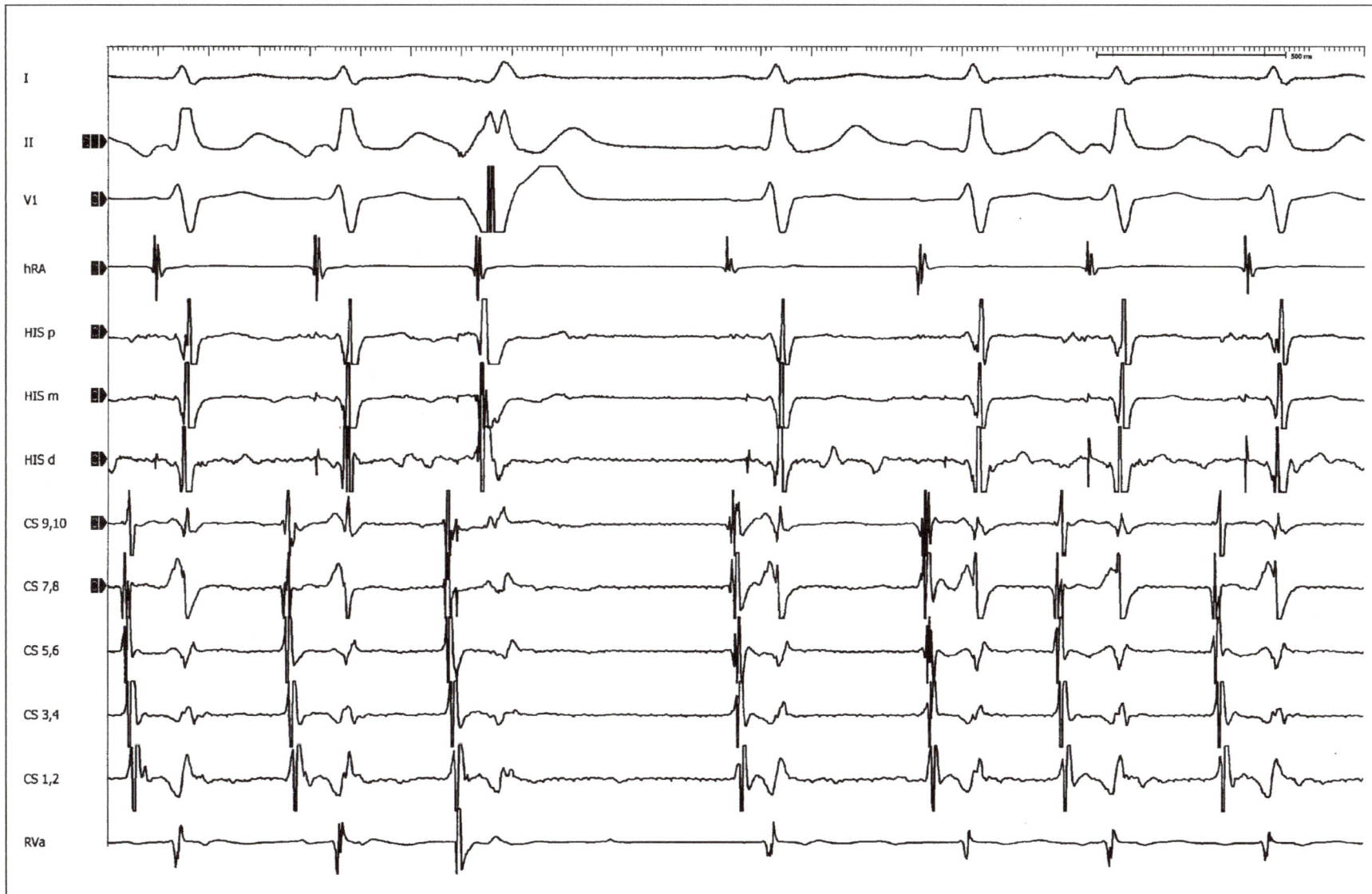

*A*nswer

The correct answer is **C**. The first two beats show a long RP tachy-cardia. The long HA and VA interval rules out typical AVNRT.

A PVC is delivered synchronous with His activation. It appears that the tachycardia continues after a pause; however, the atrial activation on the beat after the pause is different, with HRA being the earliest as opposed to earliest activation in the CS during the tachycardia. The sinus beat is followed by a PAC (note the difference in the P wave morphology and activation), which triggers the tachycardia. Termination of the tachycardia after the PVC occurs without conduction to the atrium.

Termination of an atrial tachycardia is not possible unless there is early atrial activation, even in the presence of a bystander pathway. Atypical AVNRT should not be affected by a His-synchronous PVC, except in the presence of a bystander concealed accessory pathway (AP), either atrioventricular (by advancing or delaying the A) or nodoventricular (without conduc-tion to the A). While it is conceivable that a His-refractory VPD can *advance* the atrium during atypical AVNRT with a bystander atrioventricular AP with a likely change in the atrial activation pattern (depending on the atrial insertion site of the AP), it is unlikely that a His-refractory VPD can *delay* the atrium during atypical AVNRT and a bystander AV AP, since atrial activa-tion over the AV nodal circuit would then preempt slow AP conduction.

Termination of a long-RP tachycardia by His-synchronous PVC without conduction to the atrium indicates the presence of a bypass tract—and, in most cases, the bypass tract is an integral part of the circuit, except in rare cases of atypical AVNRT with a bystander retrogradely conducting nodofascicular or nodoven-tricular pathway inserting into the slow pathway. In such cases, the PVC may terminate the tachycardia by resulting in concealed conduction in the slow pathway. Practically speaking for examina-tions, this phenomenon is proof of the presence and participation of an accessory pathway in the tachycardia.

References

1. Ho RT, Frisch DR, Pavri BB, Levi SA, Greenspon AJ. Electrophysiological features differentiating the atypical atrioventricular node-dependent long RP supraventricular tachycardias. *Circ Arrhythm Electrophysiol.* 2013;6:597–605.

2. Ho RT, Levi SA. An atypical long RP tachycardia: what is the mechanism? *Heart Rhythm.* 2013;10:1089–1090.

Question

A 46–year–old man undergoes electrophysiologic evaluation because of recurrent palpitations despite nadolol therapy. What is the most likely explanation for the high-frequency potential (arrow) observed during tachycardia?

A) High-frequency component of the atrial electrogram

B) High-frequency component of the ventricular electrogram

C) Second His bundle potential

D) Accessory pathway potential

Figure 2.M.1

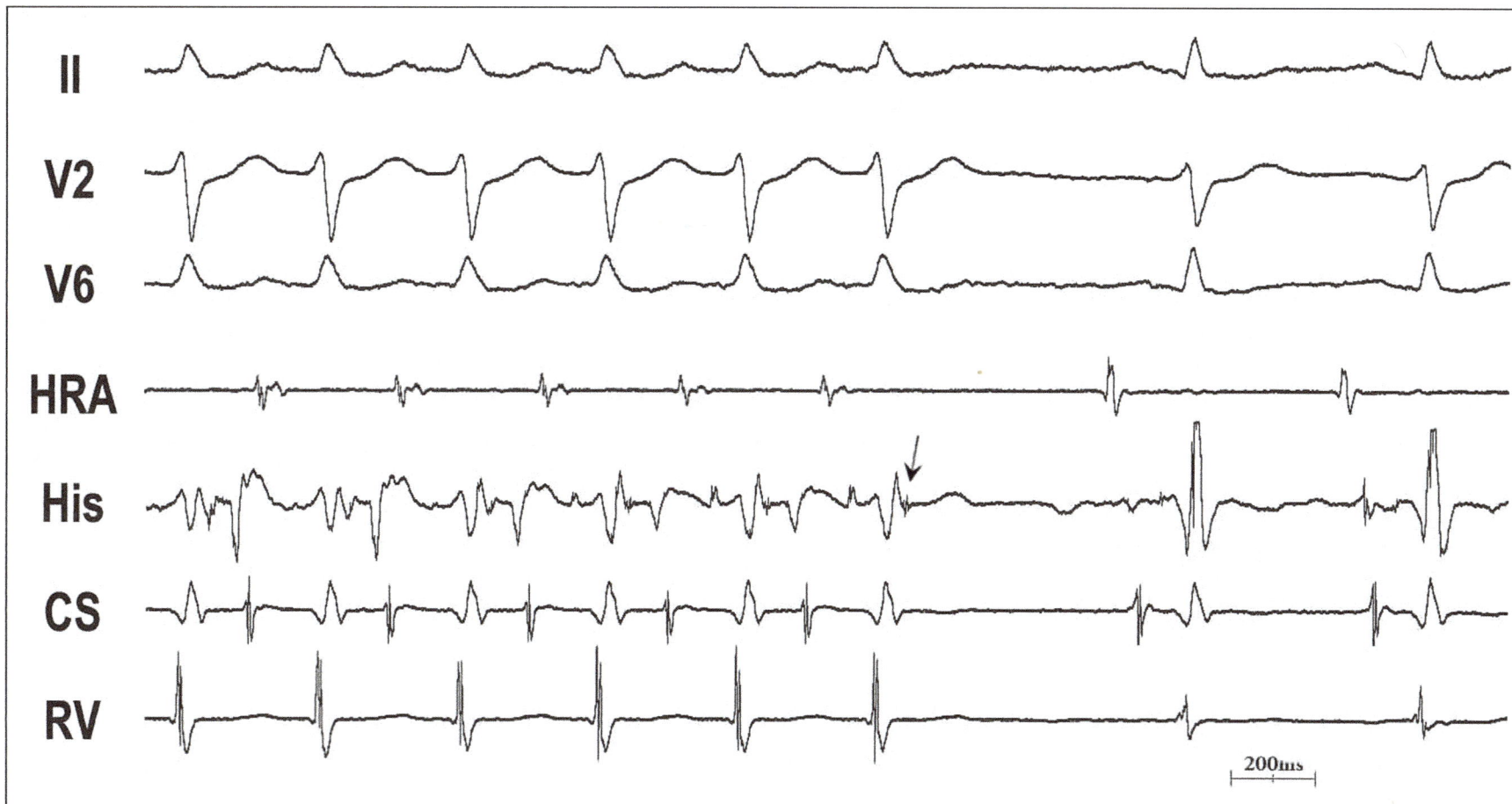

Figure 2.M.2

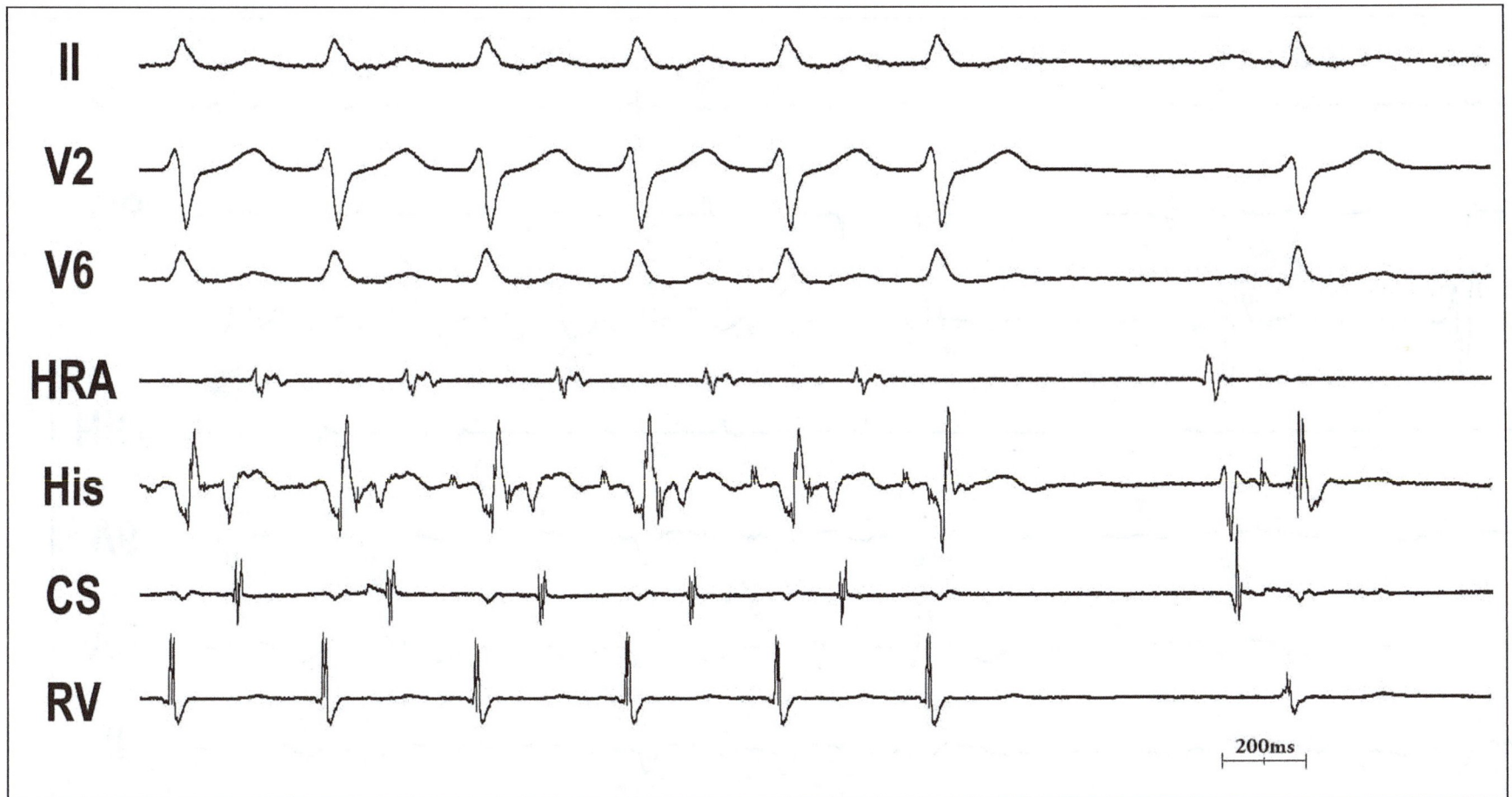

Figure 2.M.3

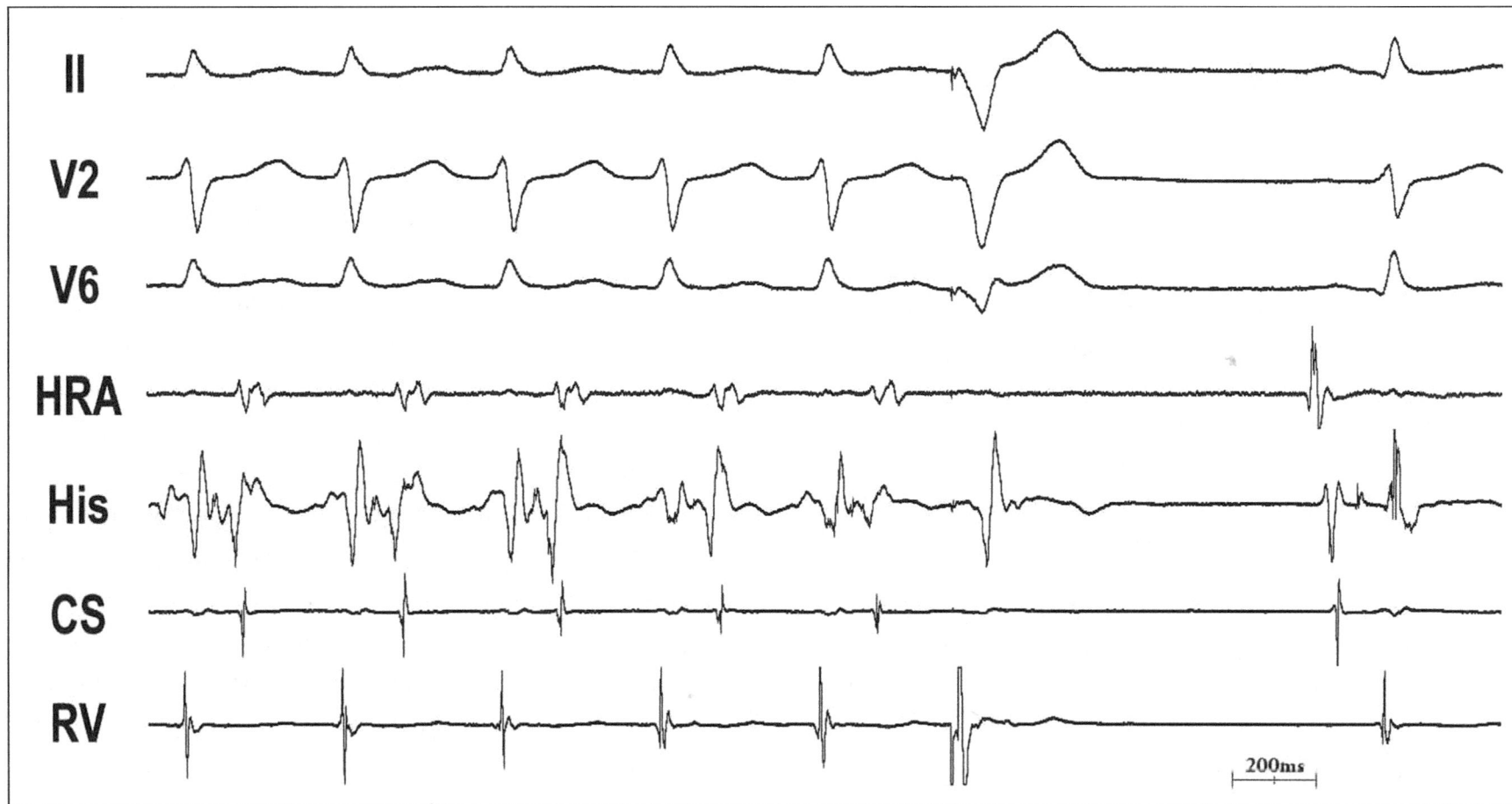

Answer

The correct answer is **D**. Figure 2.M.1 and Figure 2.M.2 show two episodes of a narrow complex tachycardia terminating with a QRS complex. The His bundle catheter records a high-frequency potential between the ventricular and atrial electrogram that persists during the first termination. Its persistence despite loss of atrial activation indicates that this potential is not a part of the atrial electrogram. During the second termination, it is absent. Its absence despite presence of ventricular activation indicates that it is not a part of the ventricular electrogram. While dual AV-node physiology with simultaneous FP and SP conduction can generate two His bundle potentials for a given P wave, H_1–H_2 intervals must exceed His-Purkinje refractoriness and generally exceed 300 ms. The short interval (129 ms) between the His bundle and second potential makes it physiologically impossible to be a second His bundle electrogram. The potential of interest is an accessory pathway potential recorded during ORT using a parahisian AP.

ORT was terminated by a His-refractory VPD with VA block (bottom) and spontaneously with retrograde block at the atrial (top) and ventricular (middle) insertion sites of the AP.

References

1. Kuch KH, Friday KJ, Kunze KP, Schluter M, Lazzara R, Jackman WM. Sites of conduction block in accessory atrioventricular pathways. Basis for concealed accessory pathways. *Circulation*. 1990;82:407–417.

2. Jackman W, Friday K, Scherlag B, Dehning M, Schechter E, Reynolds D, et al. Direct endocardial recording from an accessory atrioventricular pathway: localization of the site of block, effect of antiarrhythmic drugs, and attempt at nonsurgical ablation. *Circulation*. 1983;68:906–916.

3. Lin F-C, Yeh S-J, Wu D. Determinants of simultaneous fast and slow pathway conduction in patients with dual atrioventricular nodal pathways. *Am Heart J*. 1985;109:963–970.

Figure 2.M.4

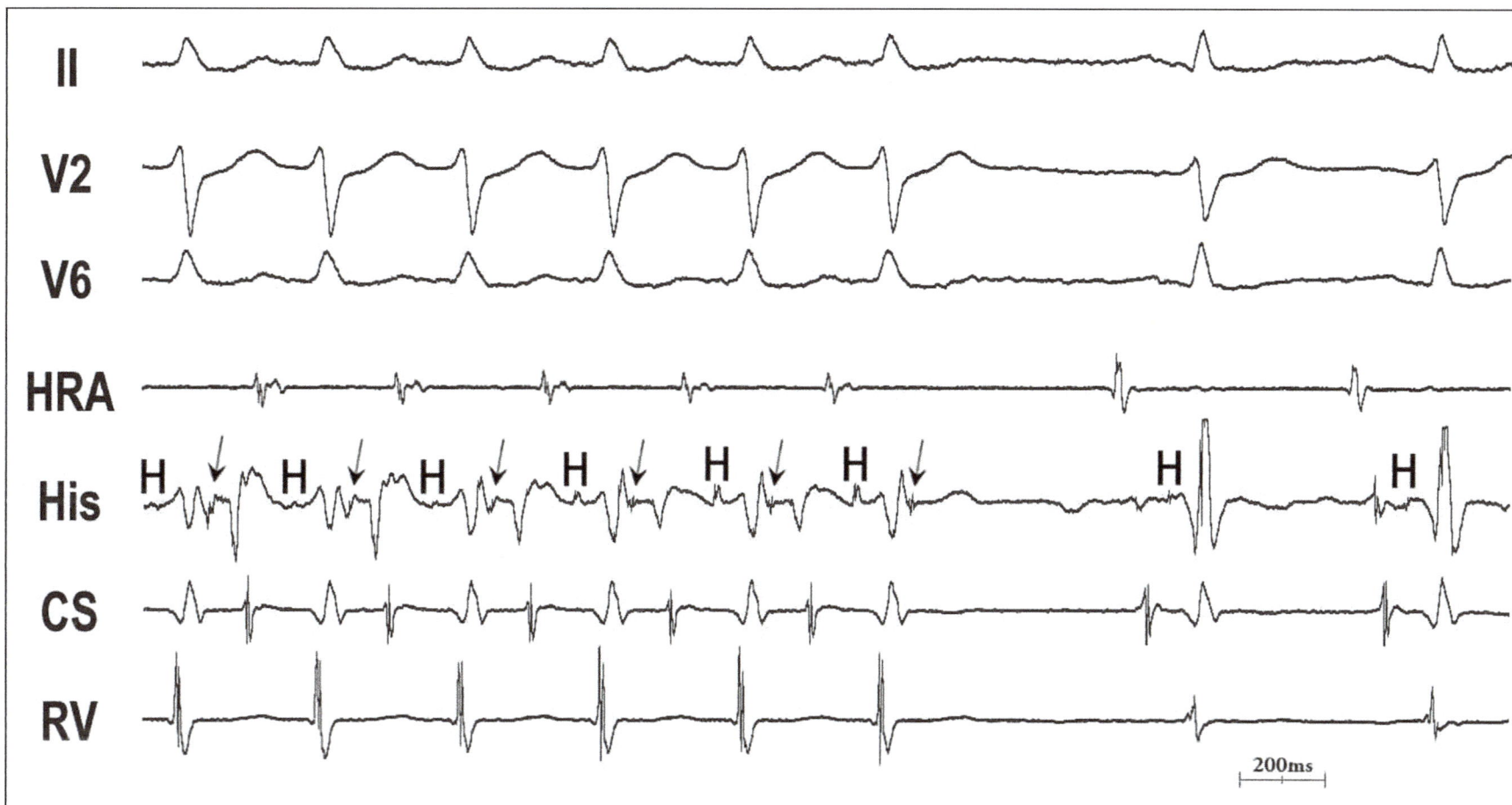

Figure 2.M.5

Figure 2.M.6

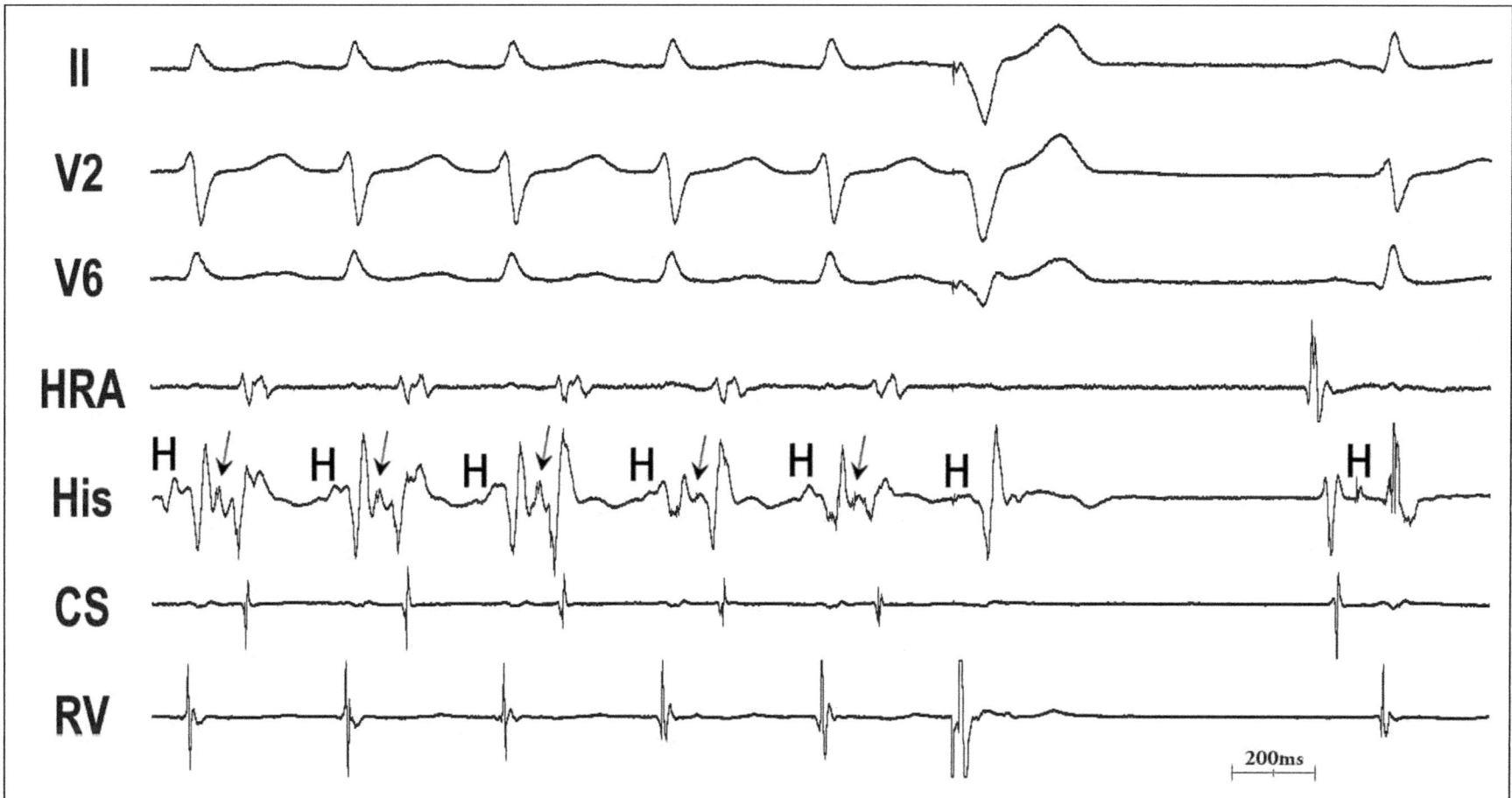

*Q*uestion

Ablation is likely to be successful at

A) High right atrium (HRA)

B) Posterior mitral annulus

C) Right superior pulmonary vein (RSPV)

D) Left superior pulmonary vein (LSPV)

Figure 2.N.1

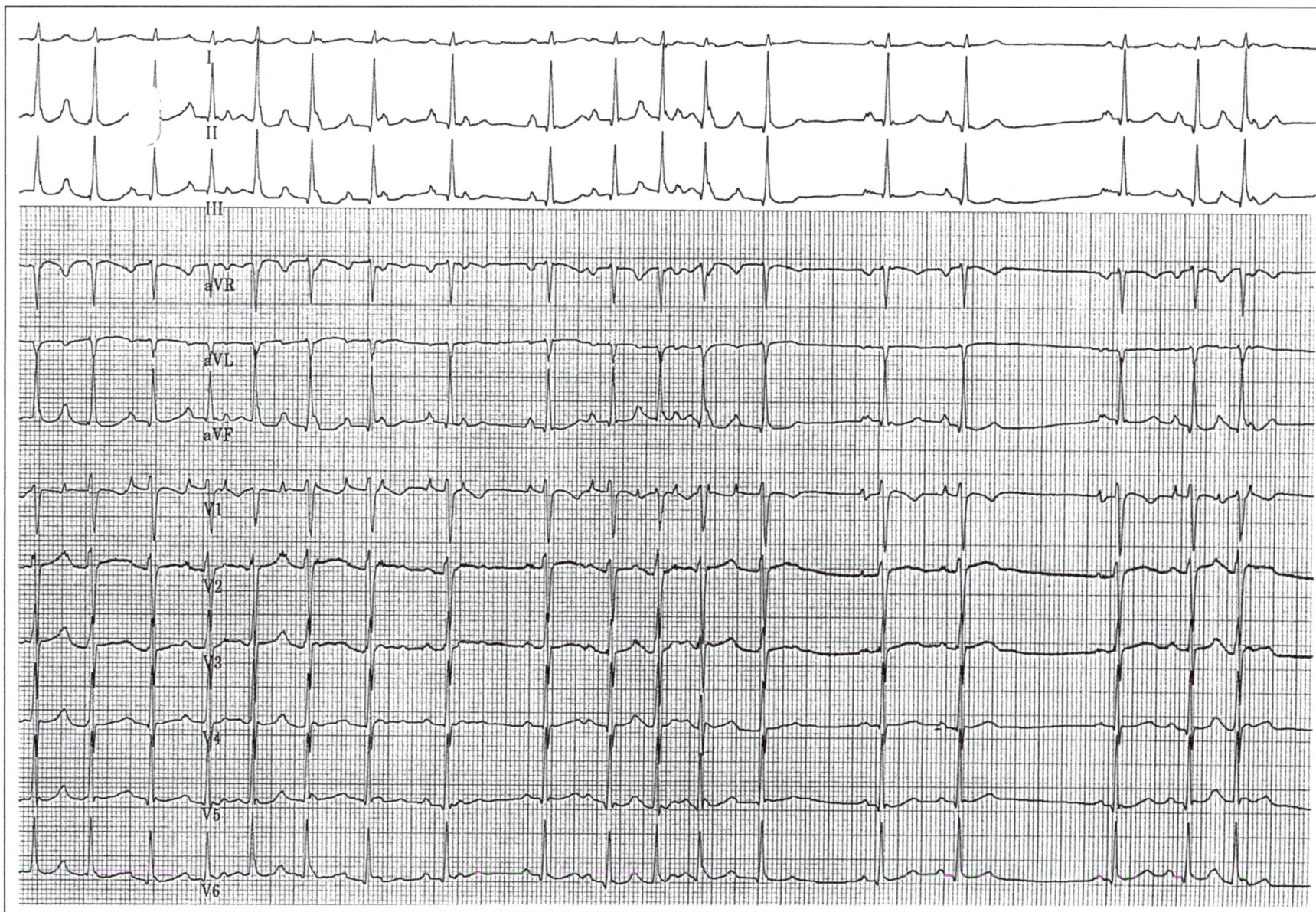

Answer

The correct answer is **C**. The patient has an atrial tachycardia with variable conduction to the ventricle. The P waves preceding the 14th and 16th QRS complexes (or 15th and 17th P waves, since two AT complexes are nonconducted) are sinus beats with biphasic P waves and inferiorly directed in V_1.

The P-wave morphology in V_1 during the atrial tachycardia is very narrow and peaked. The P waves are positive across the precordial leads and positive in I. The P-wave morphology in V_1 is distinctive feature of RSPV tachycardia. The P-wave duration of atrial tachycardia from the left PV is wider and may be negative in I because of left-to-right vector of atrial activation.

The first beat is a sinus beat (note the P-wave morphology on the first beat), then there is spontaneous initiation of tachycardia.

The ablation catheter electrogram shows two distinct potentials. The wider initial complex, which is the far-field atrial activity, is followed by a sharp potential, which represents the near-field pulmonary vein potential (marked by arrowheads). The pulmonary vein potential follows the P wave by ~40 ms.

At the onset of tachycardia, there is reversal of the complexes, with the pulmonary vein potential preceding the atrial activity and is ahead of the P wave by ~70 ms. This confirms that the RSPV is the source of the atrial tachycardia and the catheter is located near the source of the arrhythmia. Ablation at this site resulted in acceleration of the tachycardia for a few beats and then termination within 2 seconds.

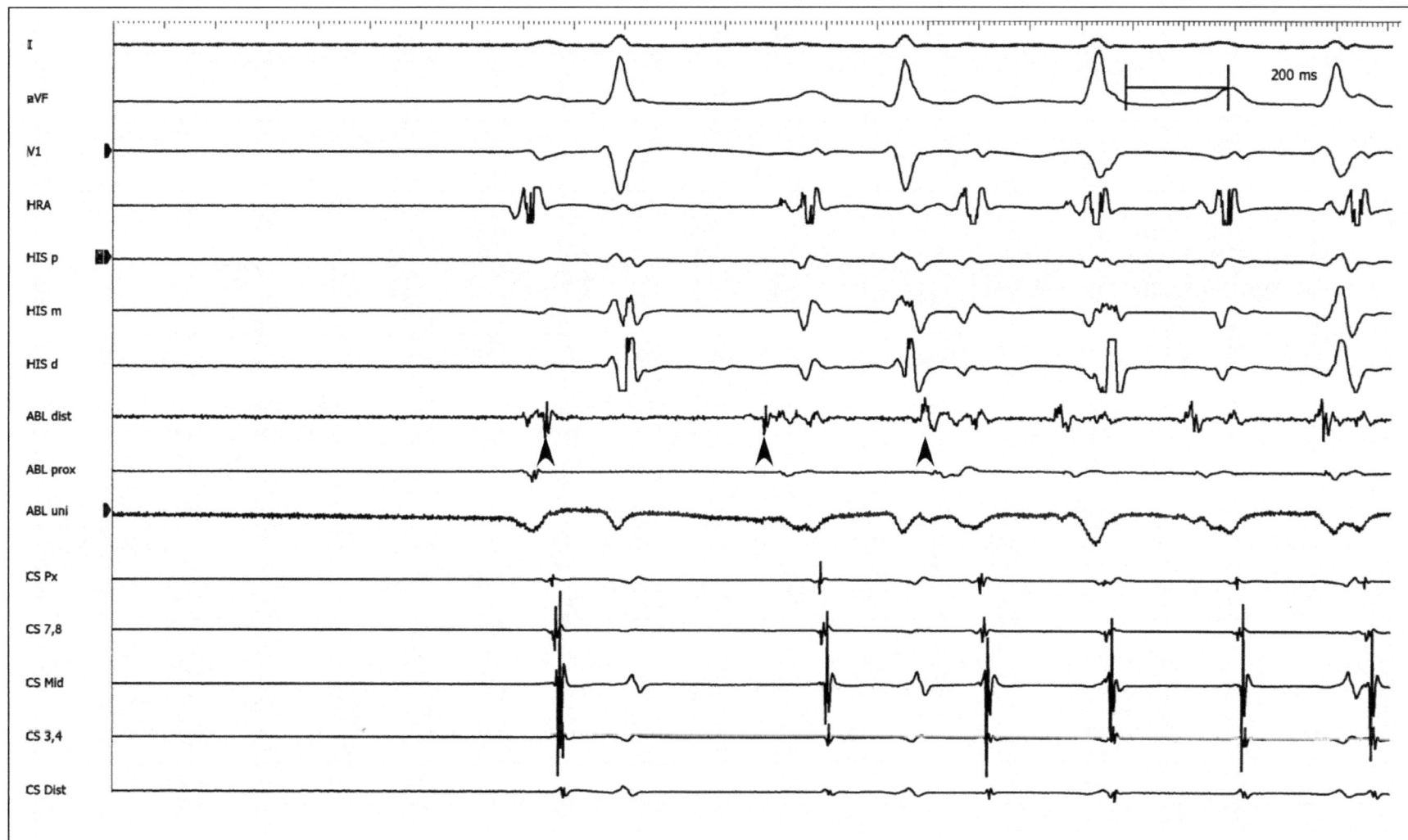

Figure 2.N.2

Figure 2.N.3

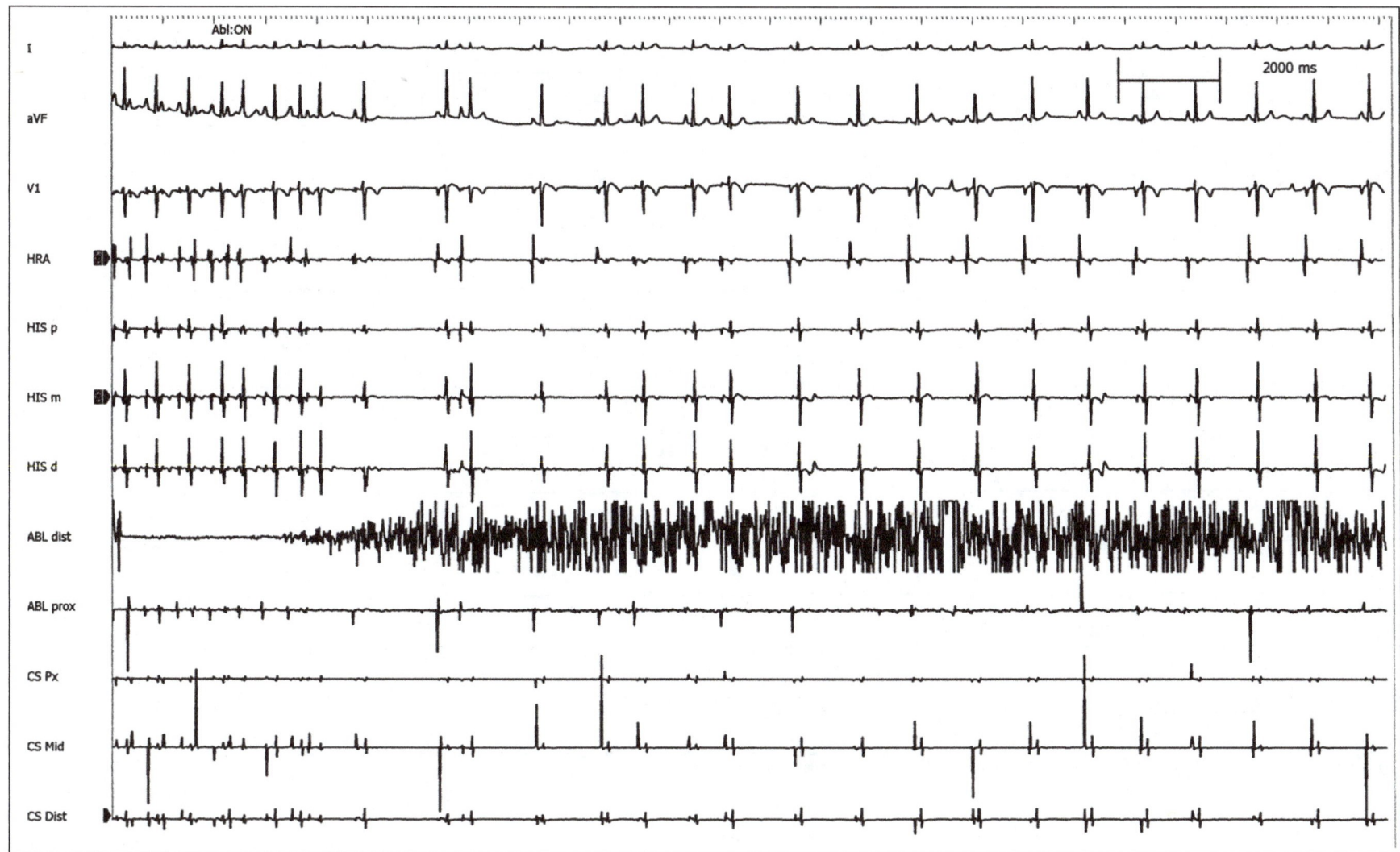

References

1. Kistler PM, Roberts-Thomson KC, Haqqani HM, et al. P-wave morphology in focal atrial tachycardia: development of an algorithm to predict the anatomic site of origin. *J Am Coll Cardiol.* 2006;48:1010–1017.

2. Roberts-Thomson KC, Kistler PM, Kalman JM. Focal atrial tachycardia I: clinical features, diagnosis, mechanisms, and anatomic location. *Pacing Clin Electrophysiol.* 2006;29:643–652.

Case 2.0

Question

A 24-year-old man presents with recurrent palpitations despite metoprolol therapy.

Based on the figure, what is the single most likely diagnosis?

A) Atrial tachycardia arising from the noncoronary cusp of the aortic valve

B) Atrioventricular nodal reentrant tachycardia

C) Orthodromic reentrant tachycardia using a septal accessory pathway

D) Atrial tachycardia originating from the fossa ovalis

Figure 2.O.1

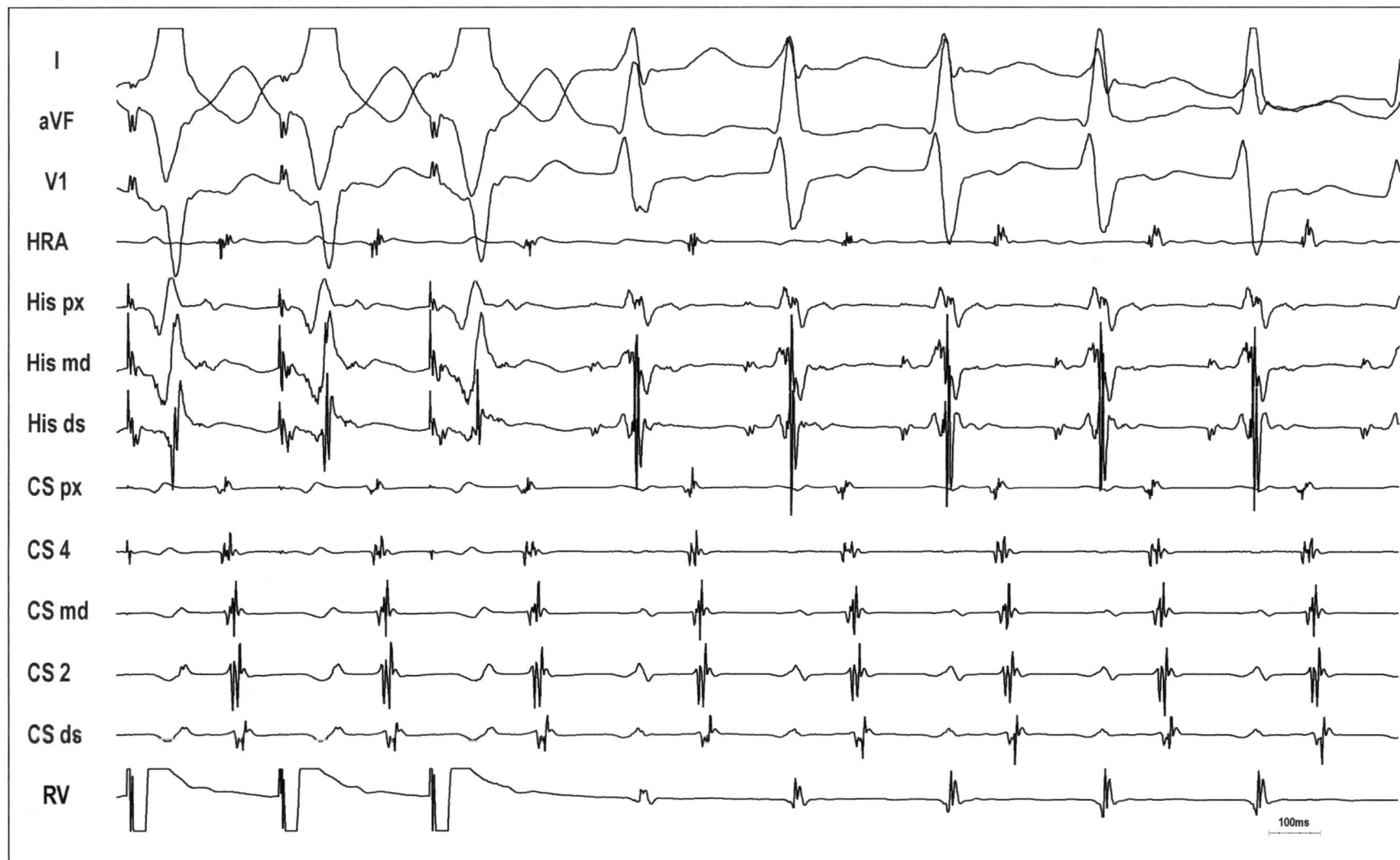

Answer

The correct answer is **C**. The figure shows entrainment of tachycardia from the ventricle with acceleration of the atrium to the pacing cycle length. Atrial activation is midline (earliest at the His bundle region). Upon pacing cessation, the response of tachycardia is "AVA," excluding atrial tachycardia. The short PPI–TCL (75 ms) and ΔVA ($V_{entrain} - V_{SVT}$) of 30 ms during entrainment also help differentiate ORT from AVNRT, but were not specifically provided because diagnosis can be established by the simple observation alone that pacing entrains tachycardia with orthodromic capture of the His bundle with the morphology of entrained His bundle electrograms identical to that of tachycardia. (The collision point between each [n] orthodromic and [n+1] antidromic wavefronts is below, rather than above, the His bundle and is essentially equivalent to continuous resetting of tachycardia by His-refractory VPDs.) Such a finding cannot occur with pure AVNRT and identifies the presence of an AP. Identifying His bundle potentials during pacing can be very helpful in establishing the mechanism of a supraventricular tachycardia.

References

1. Michaud GF, Tada H, Chough S, et al. Differentiation of atypical atrioventricular node re-entrant from orthodromic reciprocating tachycardia using a septal accessory pathway by the response to ventricular pacing. *J Am Coll Cardiol.* 2001;38:1163–1167.

2. Knight B, Zivin A, Souza J, et al. A technique for the rapid diagnosis of atrial tachycardia in the electrophysiology laboratory. *J Am Coll Cardiol.* 1999;33:775–781.

3. Ho RT, Mark GE, Rhim ES, Pavri BB, Greenspon AJ. Differentiating atrio-ventricular nodal reentrant tachycardia from atrio-ventricular reentrant tachycardia by ΔHA intervals during entrainment from the ventricle. *Heart Rhythm.* 2008;5:83–88.

Figure 2.0.2

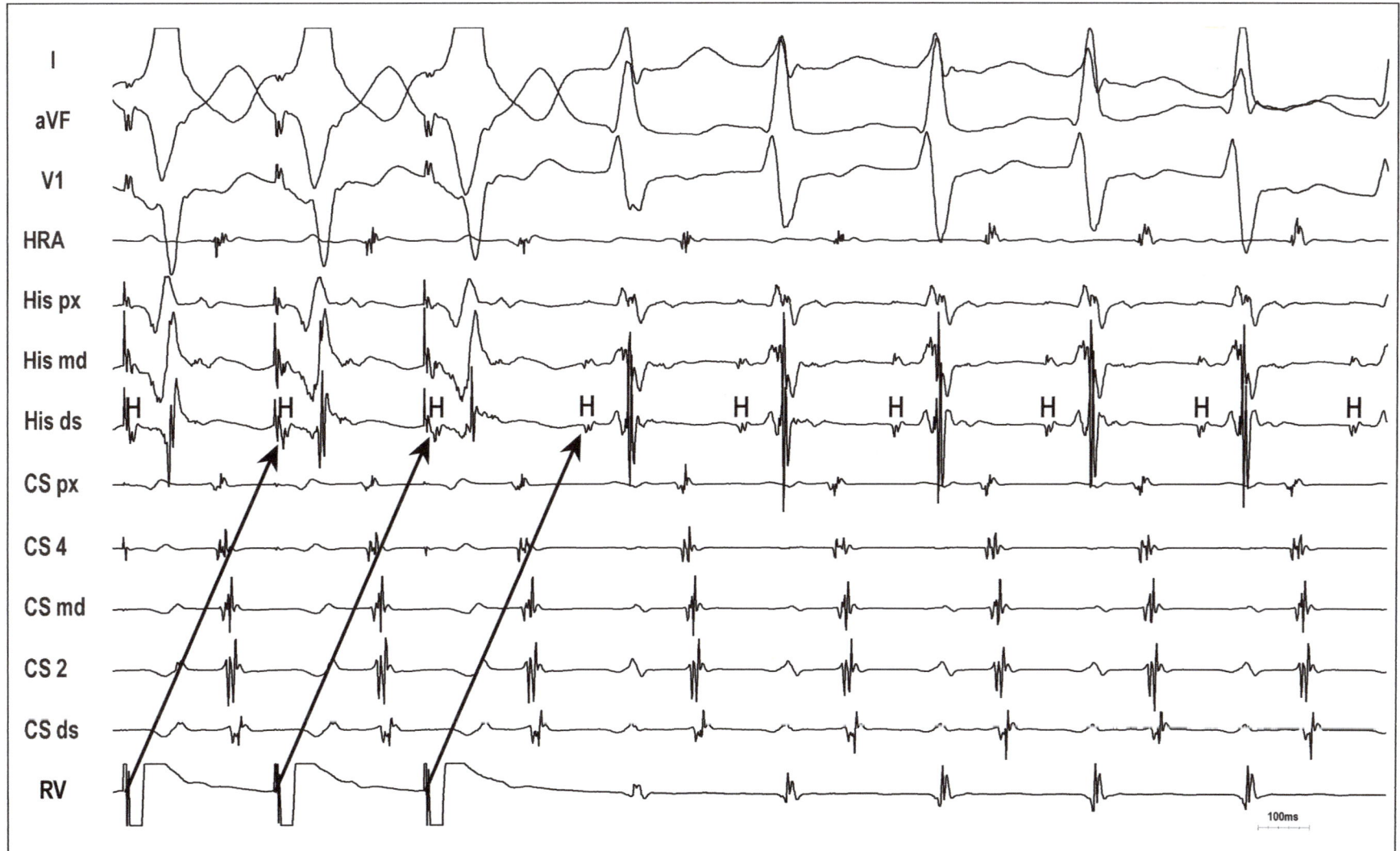

Question

A 64-year-old man with a history of alcohol abuse undergoes electrophysiologic study because of recurrent palpitations and lightheadedness.

What is the most likely mechanism of his induced arrhythmia?

A) Orthodromic reentrant tachycardia using a slowly conducting atrioventricular accessory pathway (PJRT)

B) Atypical AVNRT

C) Atypical AVNRT with a bystander nodofascicular AP inserting into the SP of the AV node

D) Atypical AVNRT with a bystander nodofascicular AP inserting into the FP of the AV node

Figure 2.P.1

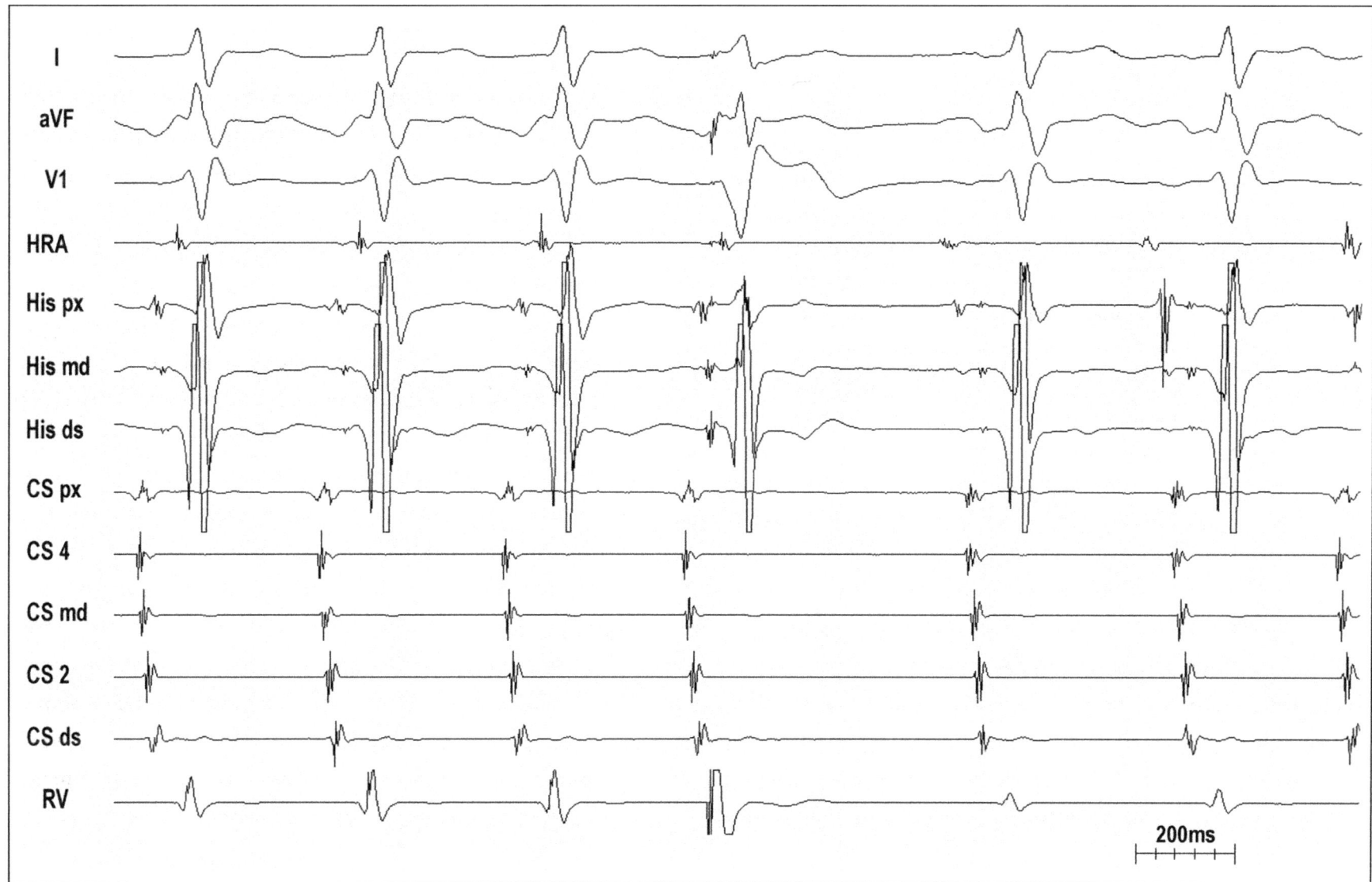

200ms

Answer

The correct answer is **C**. The figure shows a long RP tachycardia with midline atrial activation earliest near the ostium of the coronary sinus, the differential diagnosis of which includes: 1) ORT using a slowly conducting posteroseptal atrioventricular AP (permanent junctional reciprocating tachycardia [PJRT]) or nodofascicular AP (nodofascicular reciprocating tachycardia [NFRT]); 2) atypical AVNRT with or without a concealed nodofascicular AP; and 3) AT. A His-refractory VPD terminates tachycardia with VA block, indicating the presence of an AP and excluding pure AVNRT and AT without proving AP participation in tachycardia. The AH interval is very short (25 ms) and paradoxically shorter than that during sinus rhythm. This indicates that the AH interval is actually a pseudo-interval, resulting from simultaneous (not sequential) activation of the atrium and His bundle as occurs with atypical AVNRT but not PJRT. A His-refractory VPD can terminate atypical AVNRT with VA block in the presence of a nodofascicular AP inserting into the retrograde limb (SP) of tachycardia. The VPD penetrates the excitable gap of tachycardia after the tachycardia wavefront passes the lower turnaround point of the circuit. Its antidromic wavefront collides with tachycardia while its orthodromic

wavefront fails to conduct over the remaining distal portion of the SP. A nodofascicular AP inserting into the antegrade FP would terminate atypical AVNRT with AV block. While NFRT is another possibility, it is not listed as an option. Reproducible termination of a supraventricular tachycardia by His-refractory VPDs is an extremely valuable finding proving the presence (but not necessarily participation) of an AP during tachycardia.

References

1. Ho RT, Frisch DF, Pavri BB, Levi SA, Greenspon AJ. Electrophysiologic features differentiating the atypical atrioventricular node-dependent long RP supraventricular tachycardia. *Circ Arrhythm Electrophysiol.* 2013;6:597–605.
2. Coumel P. Junctional reciprocating tachycardias. The permanent and paroxysmal forms of A-V nodal reciprocating tachycardias. *J Electrocardiol.* 1975;8:79–90.
3. Man KC, Niebauer M, Daoud E, Strickberger SA, Kou W, Williamson BD, Morady F. Comparison of atrial-His intervals during tachycardia and atrial pacing in patients with long RP tachycardia. *J Cardiovasc Electrophysiol.* 1995;6:700–710.

Figure 2.P.2

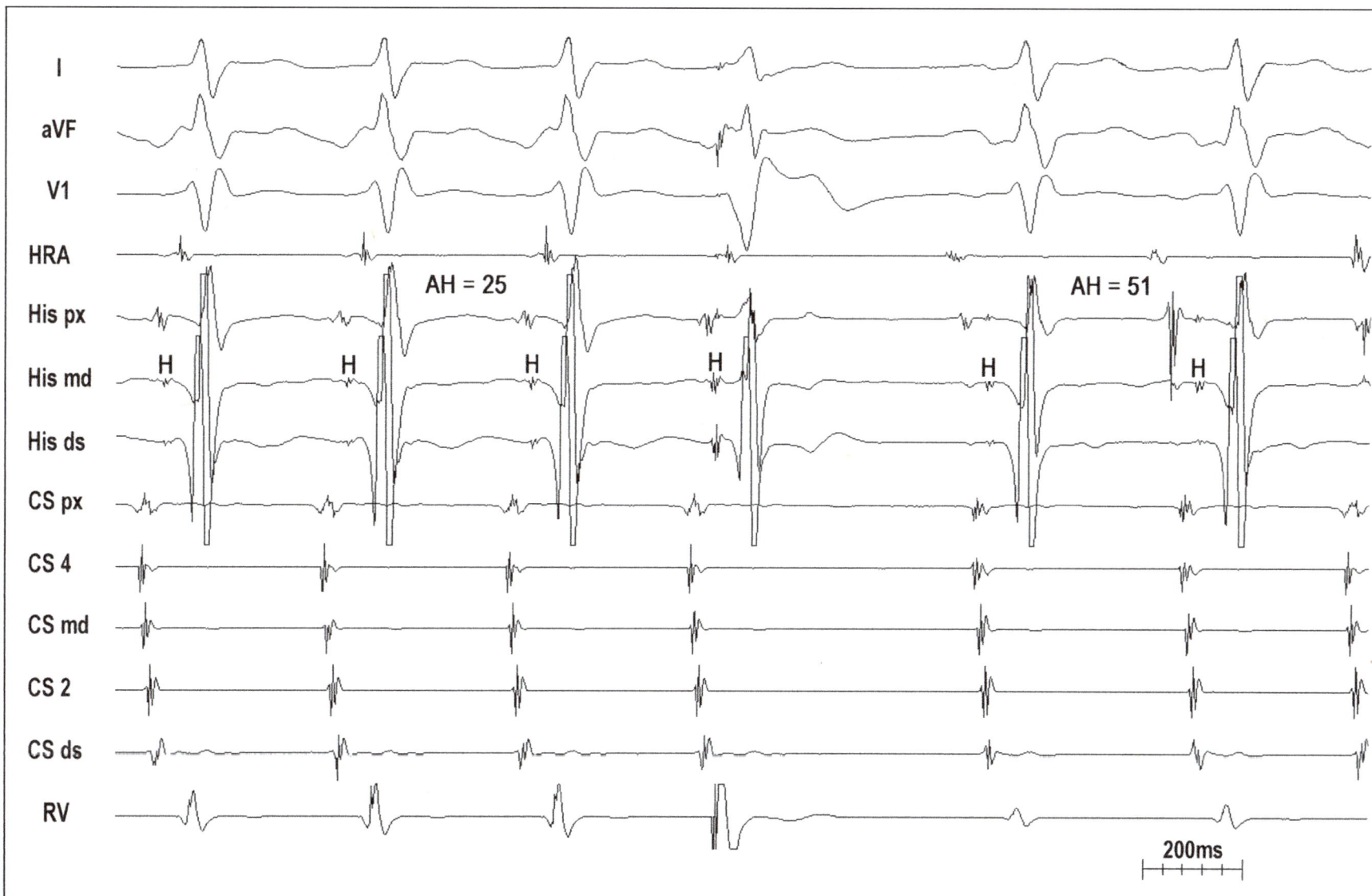

Question

A 35-year-old woman with GERD undergoes electrophysiologic study for an incessant tachycardia unresponsive to atenolol therapy.

Which of the following locations would most likely result in successful ablation of her tachycardia?

A) Noncoronary cusp of the aortic valve

B) Left-sided input of the AV node

C) Posteroseptum of the right atrium

D) Left superior pulmonary vein

Figure 2.Q.1

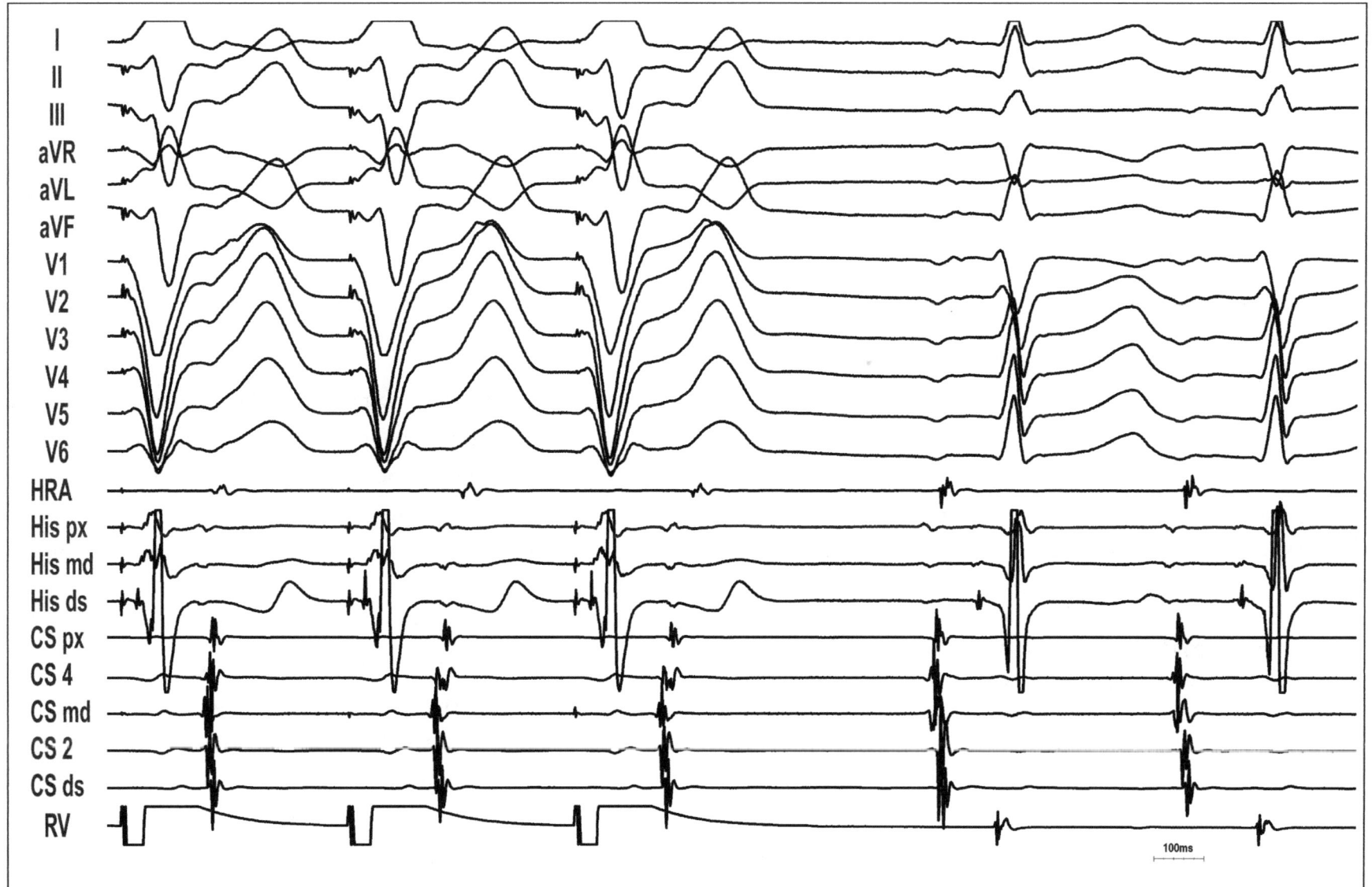

Answer

The correct answer is **A**. The figure shows entrainment of a narrow complex tachycardia from the ventricle with acceleration of the atrium to the pacing rate. The response of tachycardia upon pacing cessation is a true "AAV" response favoring an atrial tachycardia. The unusual P-wave morphology (biphasic (−/+) in the inferior leads and V_1) and early activation at the His bundle region (simultaneous with P-wave onset) is due to origin from the noncoronary cusp of the aortic valve. Atrioventricular nodal reentrant tachycardia produces an "AVA" response to entrainment and different P-wave morphology (negative inferiorly, positive in V_1). A left superior pulmonary vein tachycardia produces positive P-waves in V_1 and inferiorly and generally demonstrates distal to proximal CS activation.

References

1. Ouyang F, Ma J, Ho SY, et al. Focal atrial tachycardia originating from the non-coronary aortic sinus: Electrophysiologic characteristics and catheter ablation. *J Am Coll Cardiol*. 2006;48:122–131.

2. Knight B, Zivin A, Souza J, Flemming M, Pelosi F, Goyal R, Man C, Strickberger A, Morady F. A technique for the rapid diagnosis of atrial tachycardia in the electrophysiology laboratory. *J Am Coll Cardiol*. 1999;33:775–781.

3. Kistler PM, Kalman JM. Locating focal atrial tachycardias from P-wave morphology. *Heart Rhythm*. 2005;2:561–564.

Figure 2.Q.2

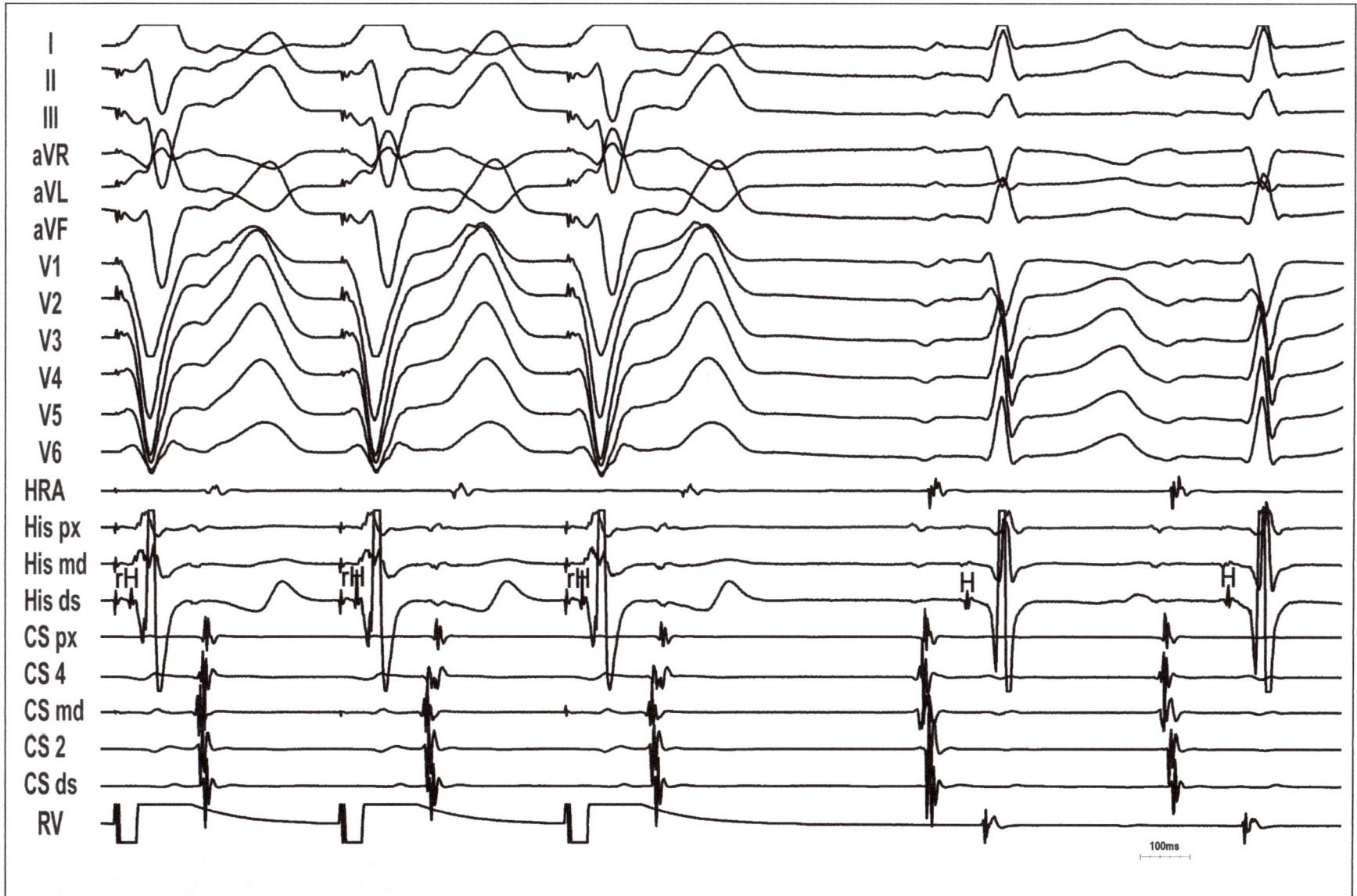

Question

A 22-year-old woman with a bicuspid aortic valve undergoes electrophysiologic evaluation for recurrent palpitations with lightheadedness. Rapid ventricular pacing initiates the following tachycardia.

What is the single most likely diagnosis?

A) Atrial tachycardia

B) Orthodromic reentrant tachycardia

C) Atrioventricular nodal reentrant tachycardia

D) Fascicular ventricular tachycardia

Figure 2.R.1

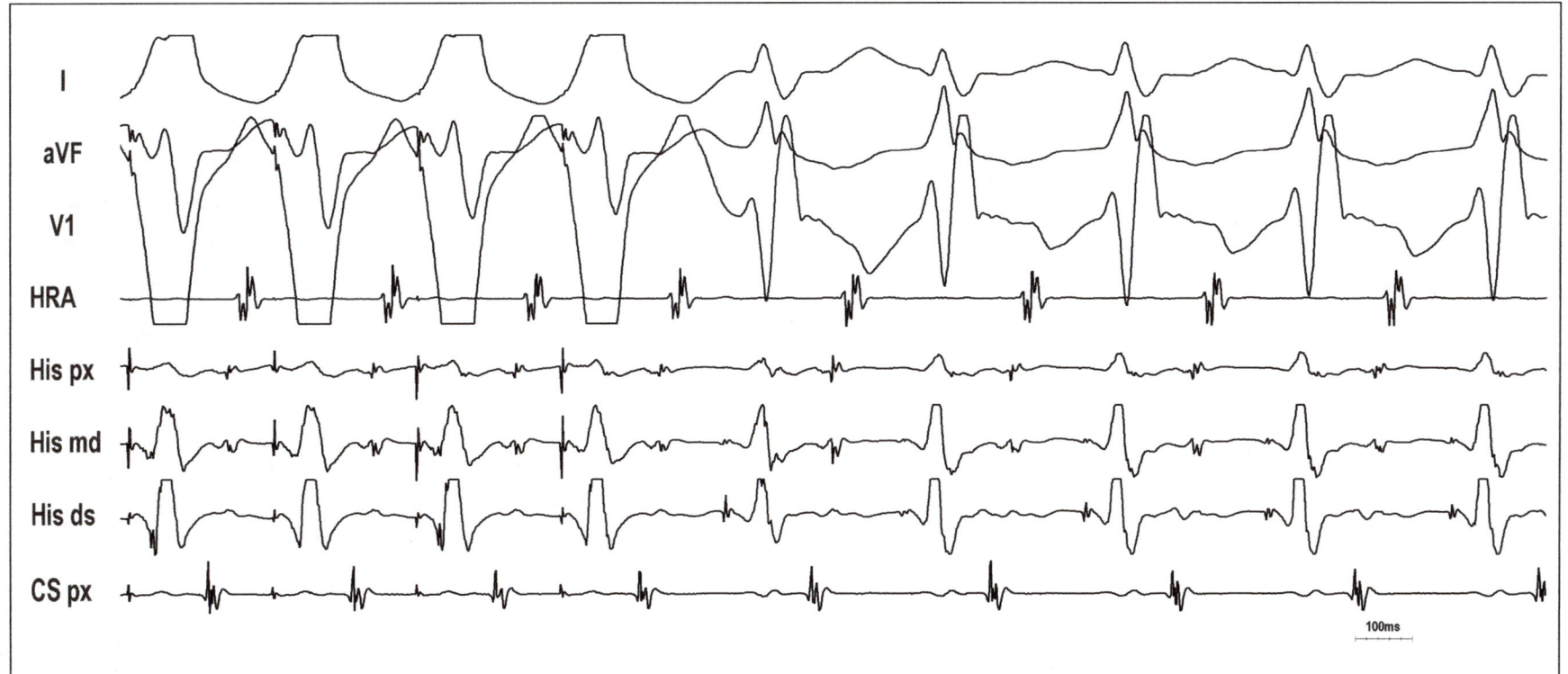

100ms

Answer

The correct answer is **B**. The figure shows initiation of a tachycardia with incomplete RBBB morphology. His bundle potentials precede each QRS with proximal-to-distal His bundle activation and normal HV intervals, indicating a supraventricular tachycardia. Rapid ventricular pacing with 1:1 retrograde conduction to the atrium initiates tachycardia with an identical atrial activation pattern after an "AVA" response, excluding atrial tachycardia. Rapid pacing, however, results in 2:1 retrograde activation of the His bundle, indicating that the retrograde atrial activation pattern is not linked to His bundle activation, which excludes conduction over the AV node. Retrograde conduction, therefore, occurs over an accessory pathway, indicating a diagnosis of ORT.

An alternative possibility to retrograde capture of the His bundle is that the His bundle is activated orthodromically in a 2:1 fashion (the "AH" interval during pacing is similar to the first AH interval of tachycardia) but such an explanation further establishes ORT.

While the PPI–TCL could be helpful if the RV pacing channel is displayed, the short ΔVA ($V_{pacing} - V_{SVT}$) of 13 ms further corroborates the diagnosis of ORT. Identifying His bundle potentials during pacing can be very helpful in establishing the mechanism of a supraventricular tachycardia.

References

1. Knight B, Zivin A, Souza J, Flemming M, Pelosi F, Goyal R, et al. A technique for the rapid diagnosis of atrial tachycardia in the electrophysiology laboratory. *J Am Coll Cardiol.* 1999;33:775–781.
2. Michaud GF, Tada H, Chough S, et al. Differentiation of atypical atrioventricular node re-entrant from orthodromic reciprocating tachycardia using a septal accessory pathway by the response to ventricular pacing. *J Am Coll Cardiol.* 2001;38:1163–1167.
3. Ho RT, Mark GE, Rhim ES, Pavri BB, Greenspon AJ. Differentiating atrio-ventricular nodal reentrant tachycardia from atrio-ventricular reentrant tachycardia by ΔHA intervals during entrainment from the ventricle. *Heart Rhythm.* 2008;5:83–88.

Figure 2.R.2

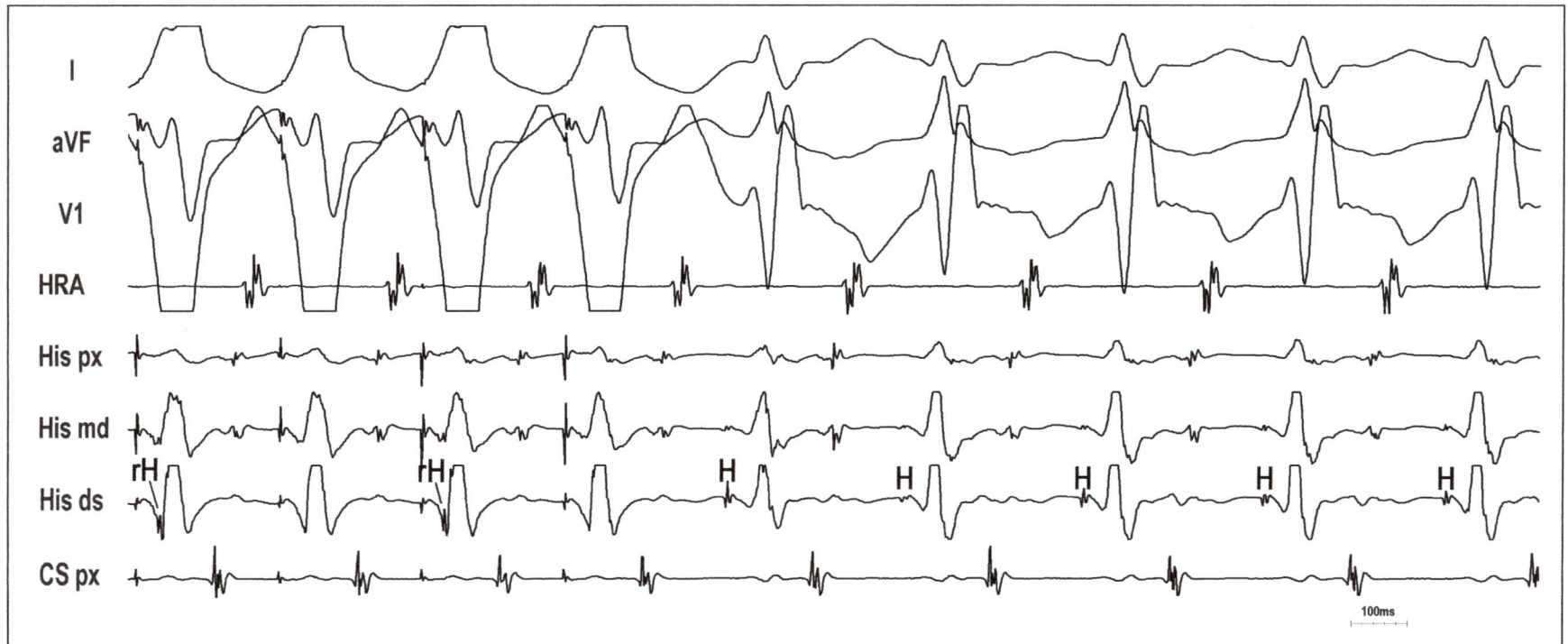

Question

A 39-year-old man presents with a severe dilated cardiomyopathy and congestive heart failure (ejection fraction = 20%). On telemetry, he has nearly incessant episodes of a wide complex tachycardia, which was recorded during electrophysiologic study.

What is the most likely diagnosis?

A) Scar-related ventricular tachycardia

B) Bundle branch reentrant tachycardia

C) Dual antegrade response tachycardia

D) Antidromic tachycardia using a left-sided atrioventricular AP

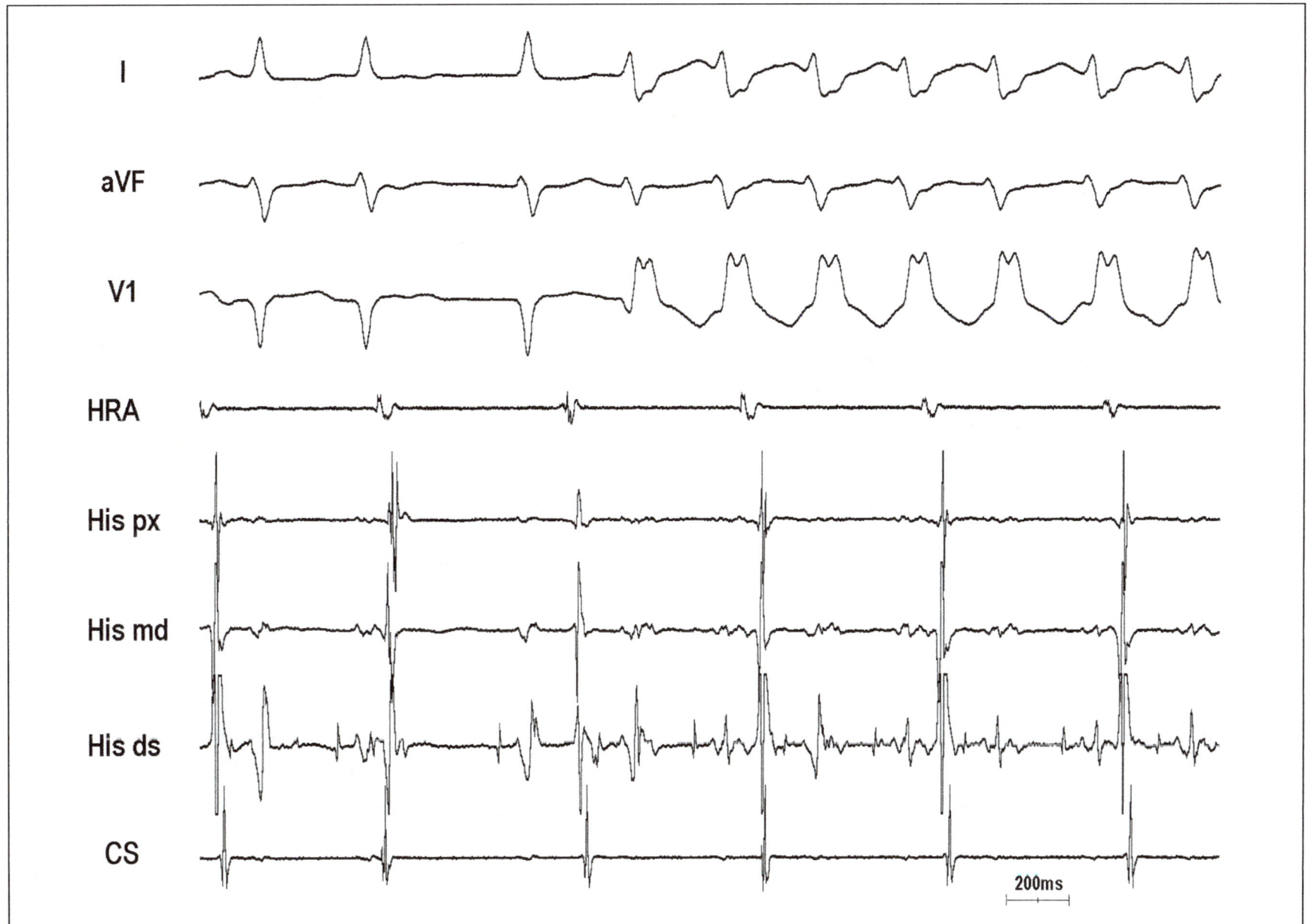

Answer

The correct answer is **C**. A spontaneous RBBB morphology tachycardia initiates after a "long–short" sequence. While its morphology is unusual for aberration, His bundle potentials precede each QRS complex with prolonged HV intervals, excluding scar-related VT. Bundle branch reentrant tachycardia is the only VT where His bundle potentials precede each QRS with normal or prolonged HV intervals. Its typical form (counterclockwise bundle branch activation) shows LBBB morphology but atypical BBRT has RBBB morphology. Bundle branch reentrant tachycardia, however, is generally associated with BBB and HV prolongation during sinus rhythm (neither of which are present here) and cannot explain the 1:2 atrioventricular relationship (except the second sinus complex) occurring both before and during tachycardia. The absence of 1:1 AV relationship exclude antidromic tachycardia using an atrioventricular AP. The diagnosis is dual antegrade response tachycardia ("double fire") resulting from simultaneous conduction over the FP and SP of the AV node, resulting in a tachycardia-induced cardiomyopathy. Exposure of the BBB to a "long–short" sequence induces HV prolongation and BBB—the latter being perpetuated by transseptal linking. The second sinus complex generates only a single response due to SP conduction because of the previous short HA_{SP} interval. Prior concealment from the SP into the FP renders the FP functionally refractory upon arrival of the second sinus complex. Note that as the HA_{SP} interval shortens during the tracing, the AH_{FP} steadily increases.

References

1. Csapo G. Paroxysmal nonreentrant tachycardia due to simultaneous conduction in dual atrioventricular nodal pathways. *Am J Cardiol*. 1979;49:1033–1045.
2. Lin F-C, Yeh S-J, Wu D. Determinants of simultaneous fast and slow pathway conduction in patients with dual atrioventricular nodal pathways. *Am Heart J*. 1985;109:963–970.
3. Wang N. Dual atrioventricular nodal nonreentrant tachycardia: a systematic review. *Pacing Clin Electrophysiol*. 2011;34:1671–1681.

Figure 2.S.2

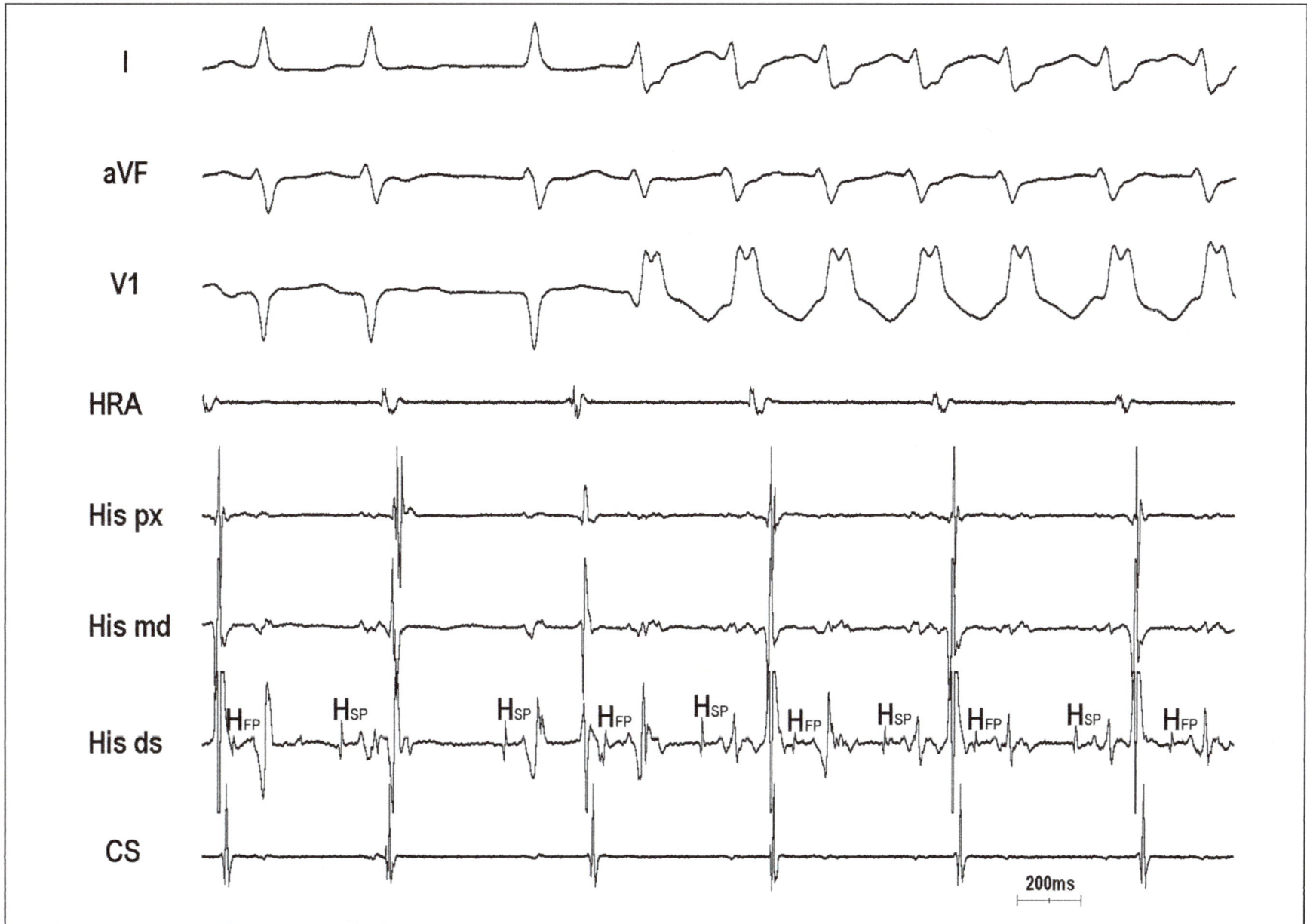

Question

A 39-year-old male with an unremarkable past medical history undergoes electrophysiologic study because of recurrent rapid palpitations.

Which of the following is shown in the figure?

A) A bundle branch reentrant beat initiating left AT

B) A bundle branch reentrant beat initiating AVNRT with left-sided inputs into the AV node

C) A bundle branch reentrant beat initiating ORT using a left free wall and left posteroseptal AP

D) Two accessory pathways (right and left)

Figure 2.T.1

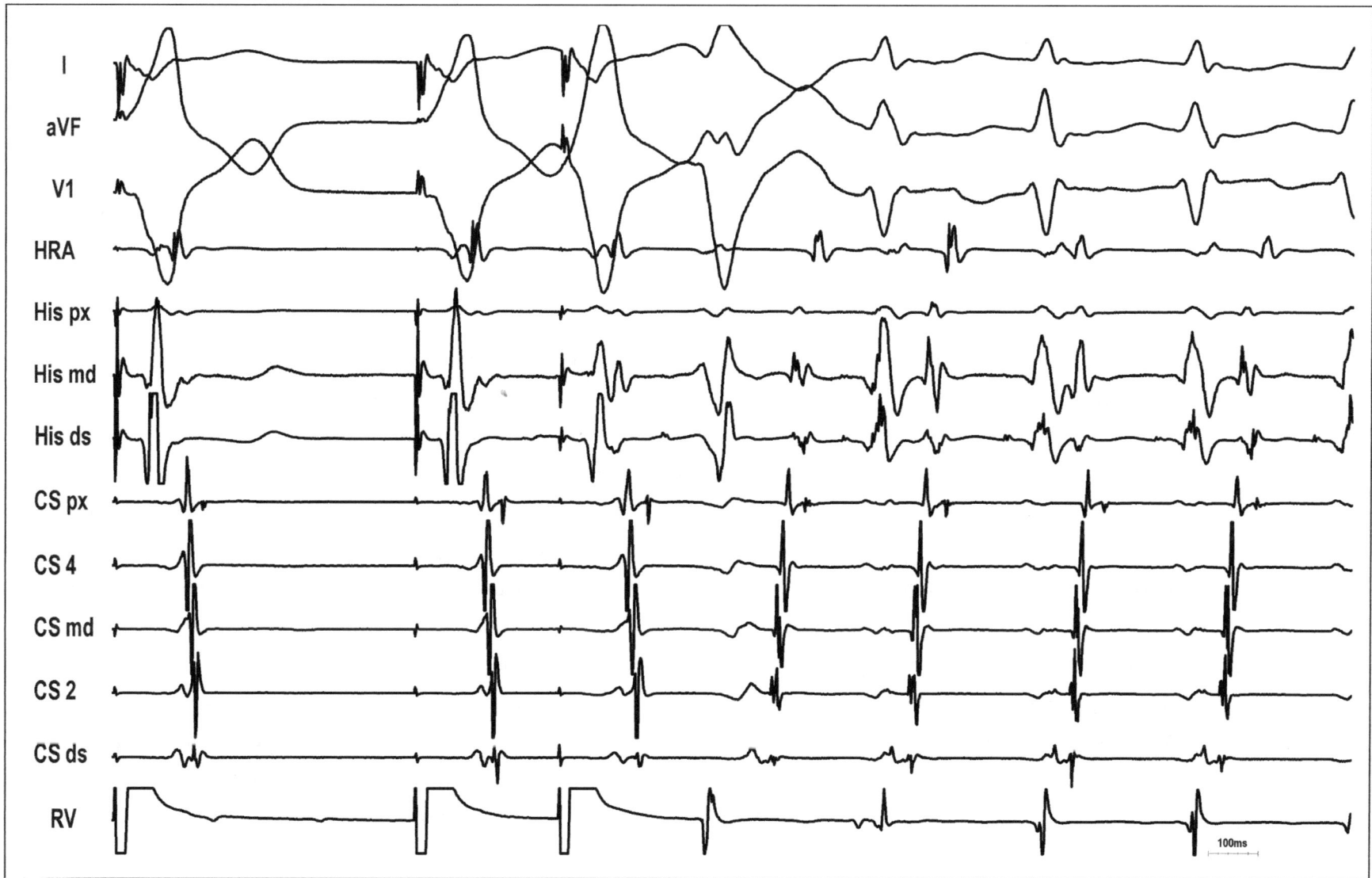

Answer

The correct answer is **D**. A single ventricular extrastimulus induces a VH jump and typical bundle branch reentrant beat, which conducts retrogradely to the atrium with an eccentric pattern (earliest at CS ds) followed by a narrow complex tachycardia with the same atrial activation sequence after an "AVA" response. Such findings, coupled with the observation during tachycardia that changes in the AH interval precede and predict the AA interval (AV-node dependence), exclude AT. While left-sided inputs to the AV node can produce an eccentric atrial activation pattern, its location along the lateral mitral annulus is unusual and could not have been generated by the BBR beat, which failed to conduct retrogradely to the His bundle; it is the preceding ventricular extrastimulus (S2) that retrogradely conducted to the His bundle and induced the VH jump. Initiation of ORT using a left-sided AP is facilitated by typical BBR beats because transseptal conduction to the AP and retrograde block in the left bundle provide the critical "VA" delay and unidirectional block, respectively required for reentry. Note that the VA interval following the BBR beat is longer than during tachycardia. The ventricular drive train and extrastimulus, however, conduct to the atrium with a different activation pattern that is right eccentric (earliest at the HRA, arrows) and precedes the VH jump, indicating the presence of a right-sided AP. During tachycardia, coronary sinus activation is continuous from distal to proximal (i.e., no other left atrial exit site), excluding a concomitant left posteroseptal AP, although momentary conduction over both the right- (4th arrow) and left-sided AP occurs during ORT.

Figure 2.T.2

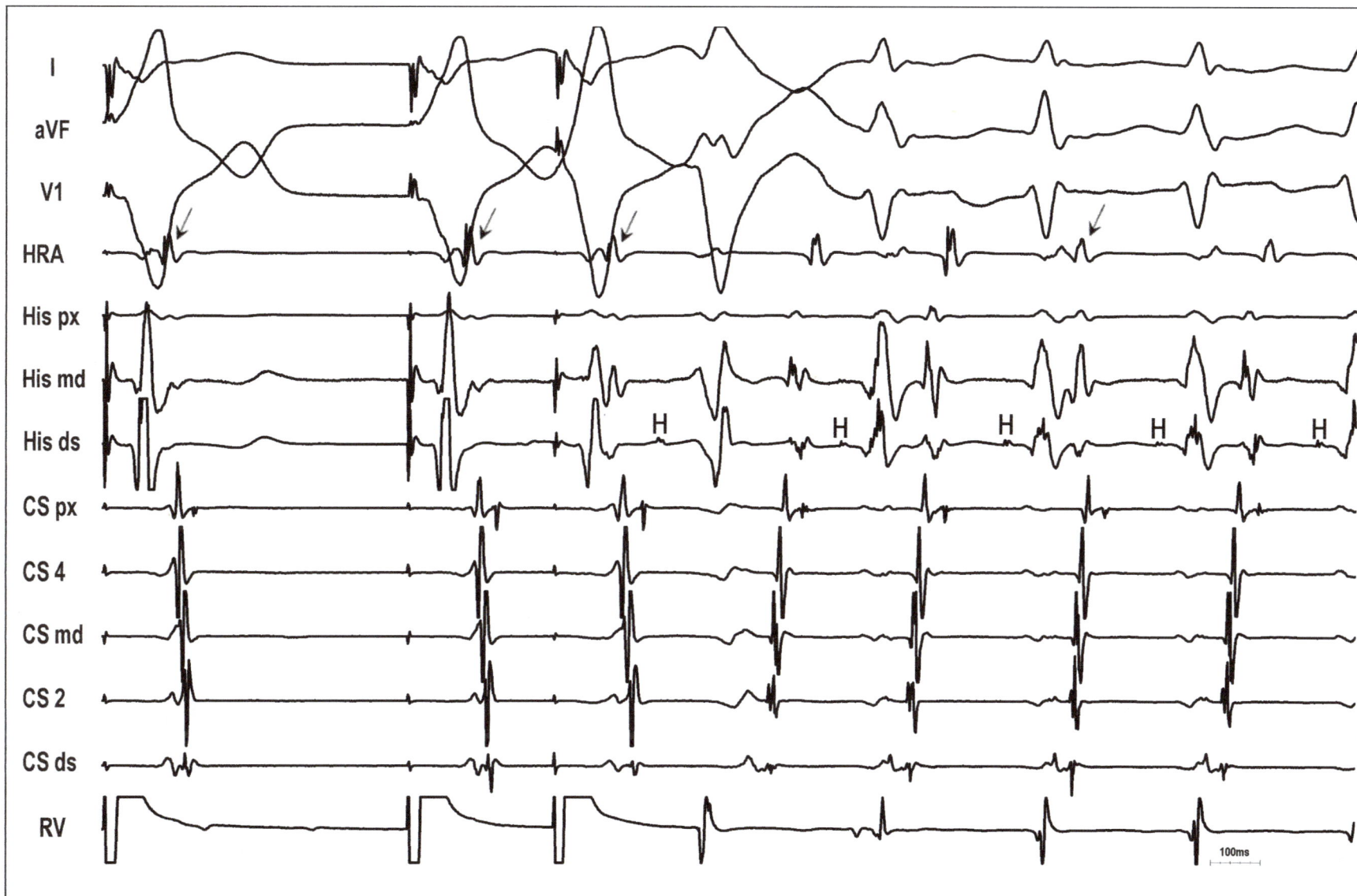

References

1. Colavita PG, Packer DL, Pressley JC, Ellenbogen KA, O'Callaghan WG, Gilbert MR, German LD. Frequency, diagnosis and clinical characteristics of patients with multiple accessory pathways. *Am J Cardiol.* 1987;59:601–606.

2. Josephson M, Scharf D, Kastor J, Kitchen J. Atrial endocardial activation in man. *Am J Cardiol.* 1977;39:972–981.

3. Kapa S, Henz BD, Dib C, et al. Utilization of retrograde right bundle branch block to differentiate atrioventricular nodal from accessory pathway conduction. *J Cardiovasc Electrophysiol.* 2009;20:751–758.

Question

A 67-year-old man with a dilated cardiomyopathy (ejection fraction = 15%) and prior ICD implantation received multiple shocks for SVT.

Which ablation site(s) would likely prevent recurrent inappropriate ICD therapy?

A) Slow pathway of the AV node

B) Fossa ovalis and right superior pulmonary vein

C) Posteroseptum of right atrium and lateral mitral annulus

D) Cavotricuspid isthmus and ostium of the coronary sinus

Figure 2.U.1

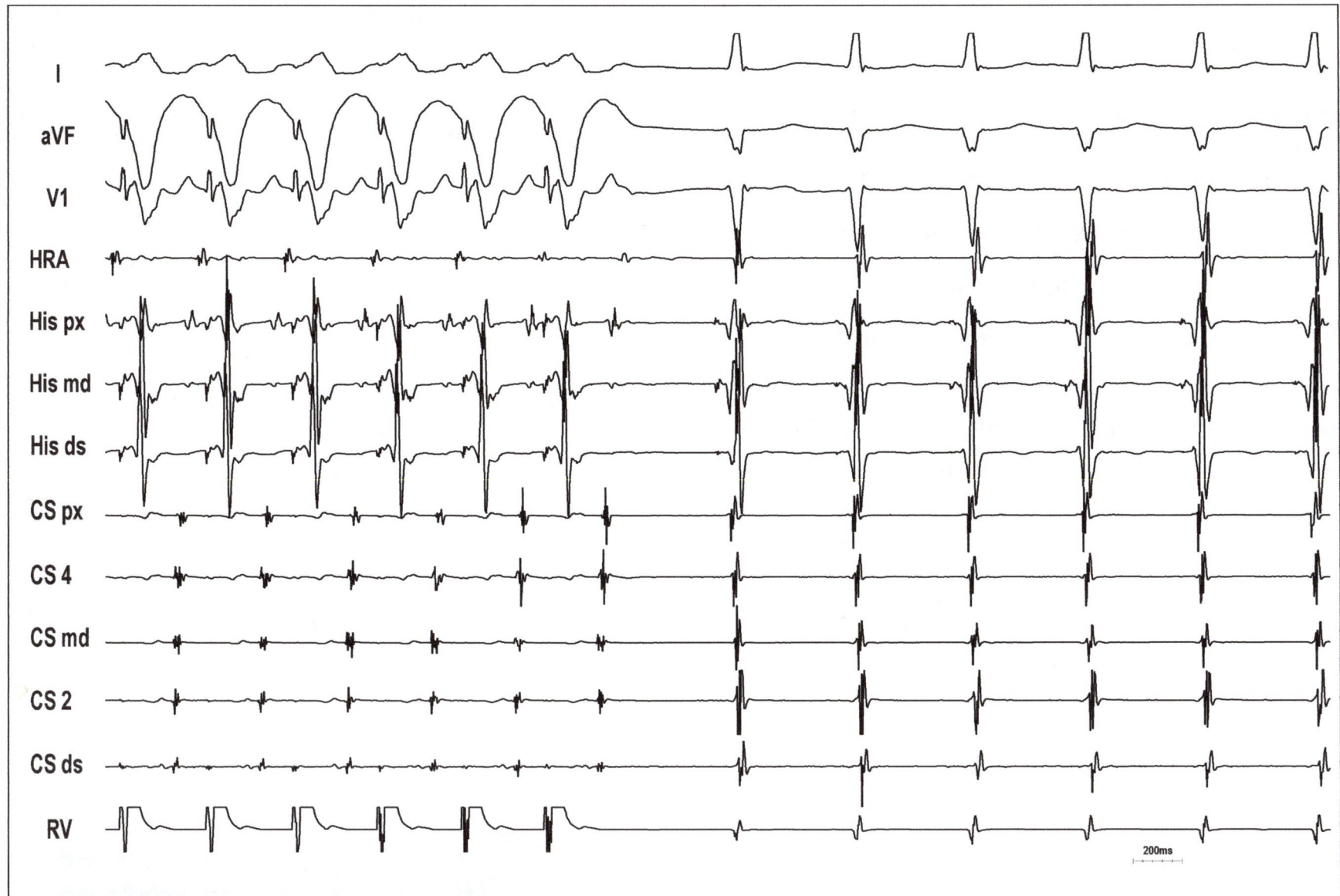

Figure 2.U.2

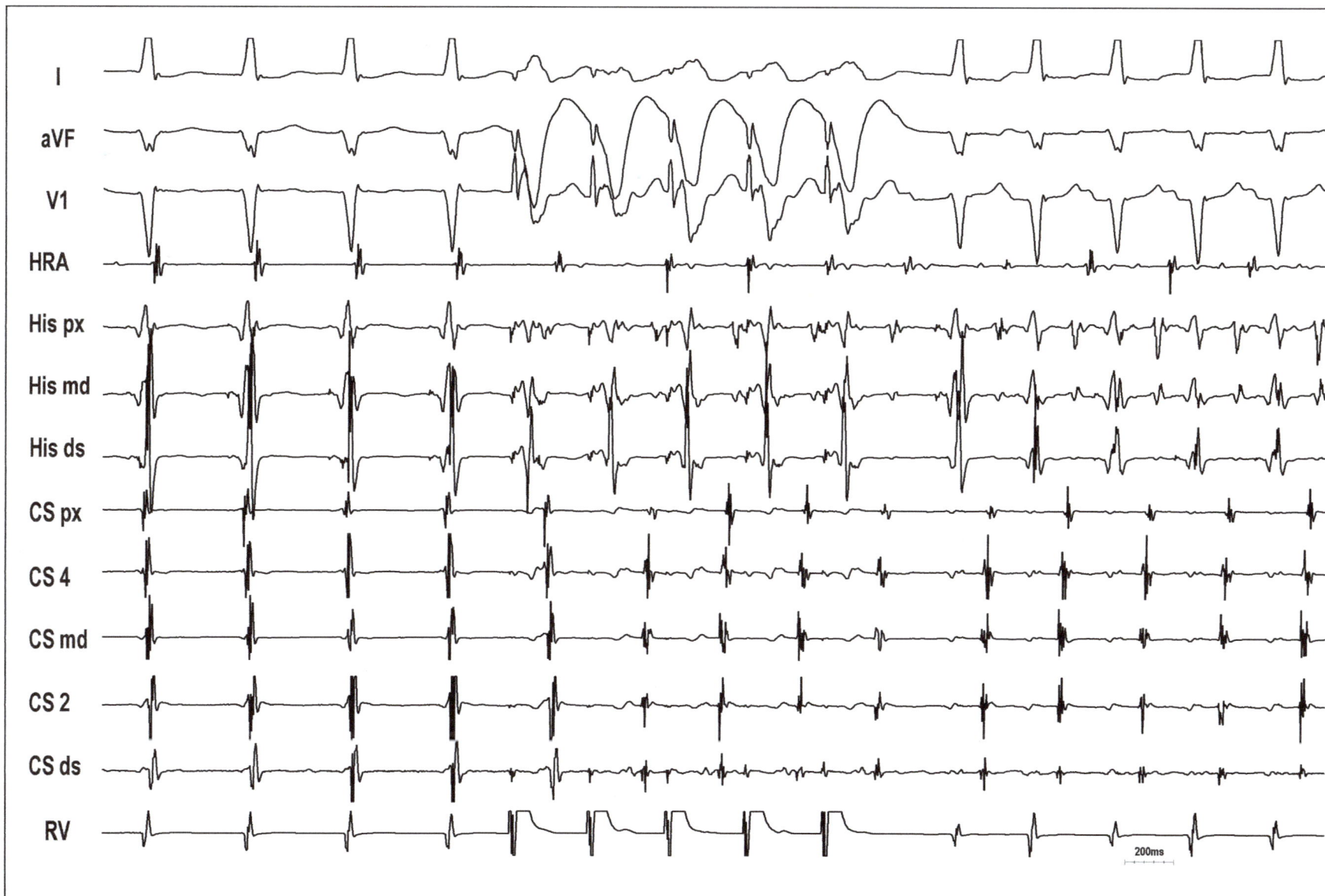

Answer

The correct answer is **C**. The top panel shows rapid ventricular pacing conducting to the atrium with eccentric atrial activation earliest along the lateral mitral annulus, consistent with a left free wall AP. Pacing, however, initiates a narrow complex tachycardia after a long AH interval that has a midline atrial activation pattern simultaneous with the ventricle, consistent with AVNRT and excluding ORT. The bottom panel shows rapid ventricular pacing into the tachycardia, the second paced complex of which terminates tachycardia with VA block, excluding the possibility of AT with a long PR interval that mimics AVNRT. After termination of tachycardia, pacing stimuli conduct retrogradely over the AP to then initiate ORT with the same atrial activation pattern after an "AVA" response. Of the anatomic sites listed, ablation of the SP of the AV node (posteroseptum of the right atrium) and AP (lateral mitral annulus) would prevent these two supraventricular tachycardias.

Figure 2.U.3

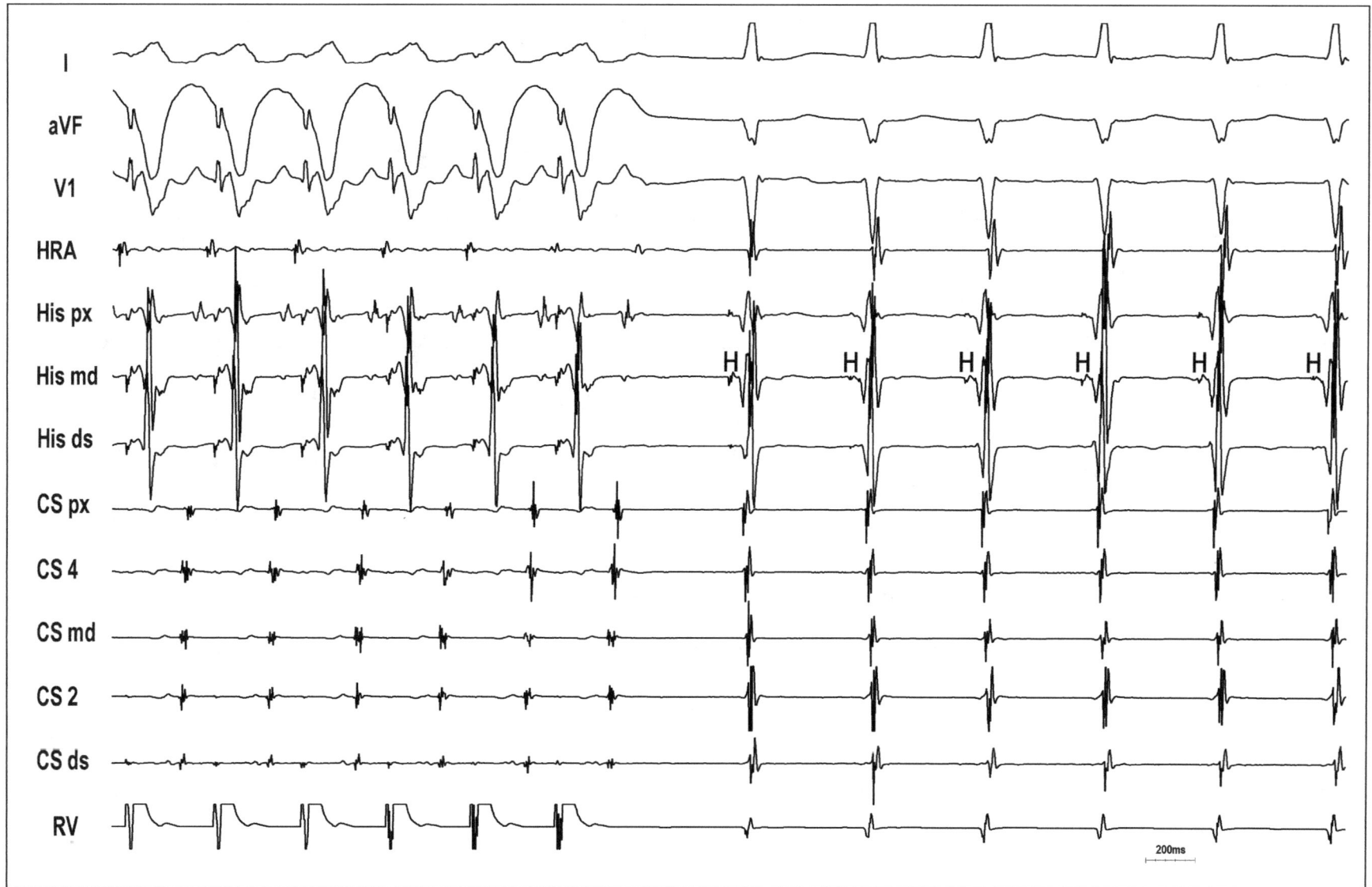

Figure 2.U.4

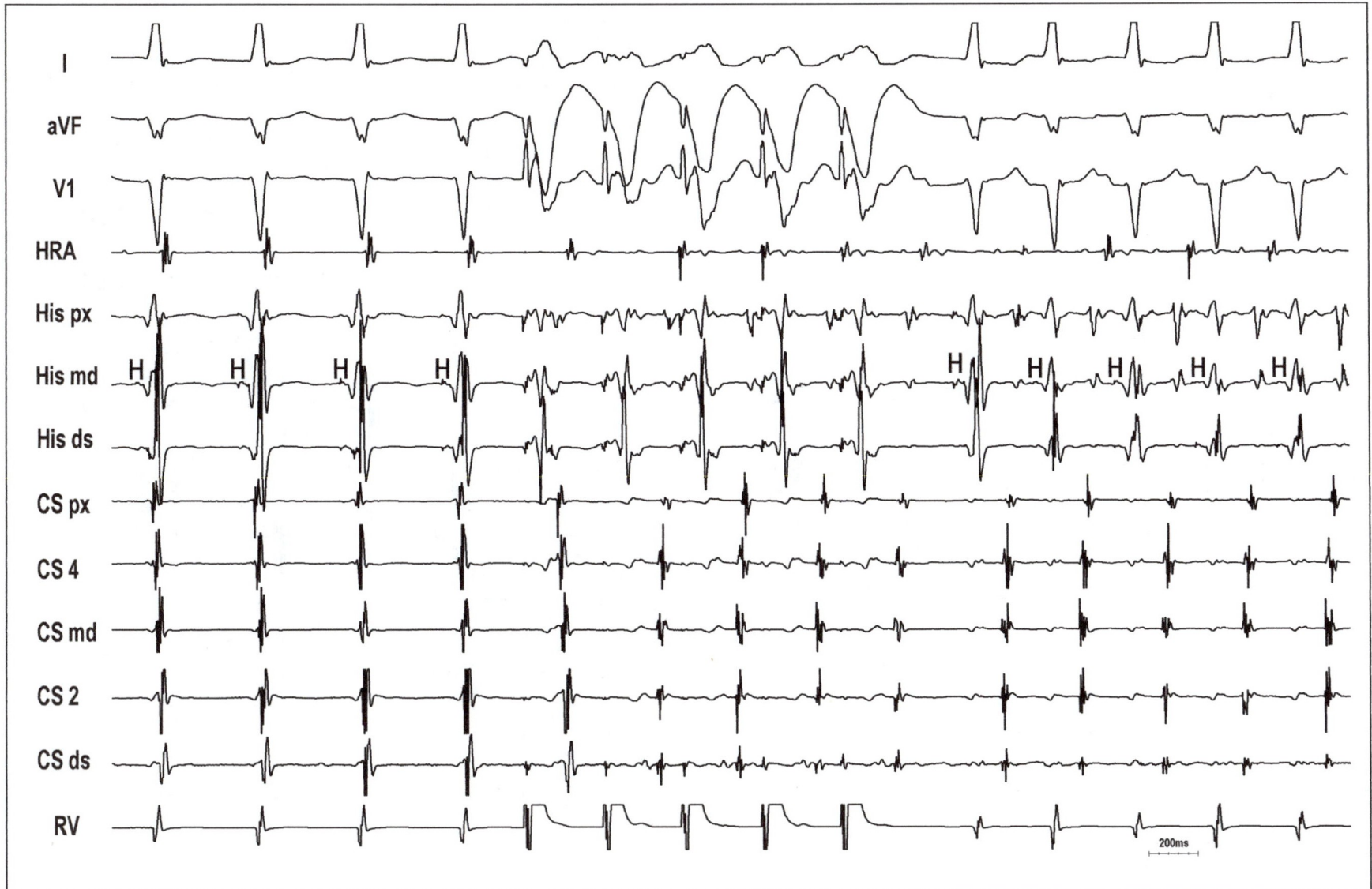

References

1. Knight BP, Ebinger M, Oral H, et al. Diagnostic value of tachycardia features and pacing maneuvers during paroxysmal supraventricular tachycardia. *J Am Coll Cardiol.* 2000;36:574–582.

2. Josephson M, Scharf D, Kastor J, Kitchen J. Atrial endocardial activation in man. *Am J Cardiol.* 1977;39:972–981.

3. Wellens H, Durrer D. Patterns of ventriculo-atrial conduction in the Wolff-Parkinson-White syndrome. *Circulation.* 1974;49:22–31.

Question

A 27-year-old man presented with recurrent palpitations and wide complex tachycardia. The tracing was obtained during EPS.

Which of the following is the most likely explanation for his wide complex tachycardia?

A) AVNRT with a bystander right-sided accessory pathway

B) AT over a right-sided accessory pathway

C) Antidromic tachycardia over an atriofascicular accessory pathway

D) Fascicular VT

Figure 2.V.1

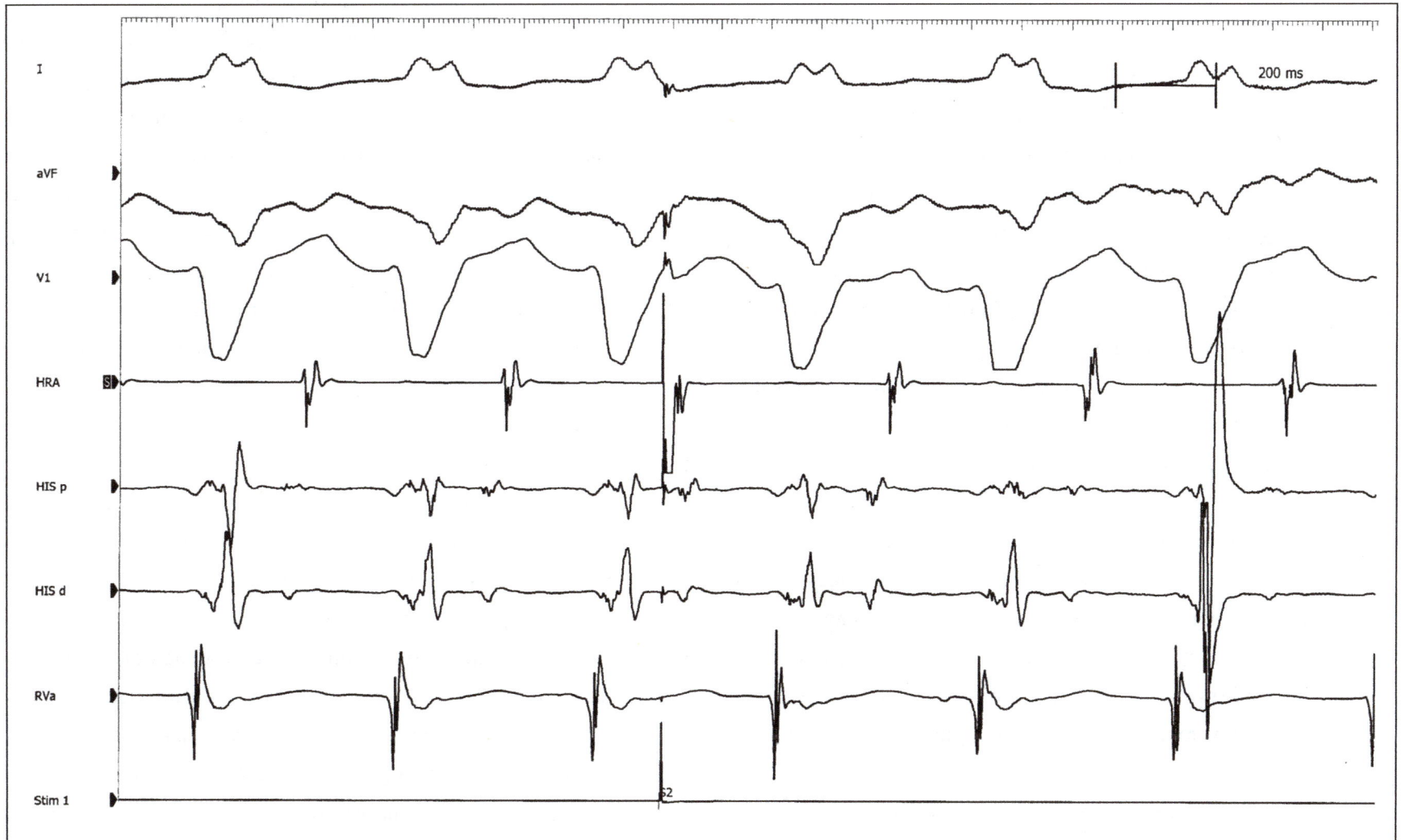

Answer

Correct answer is **C**. The tracing shows a wide complex tachycardia with a tachycardia cycle length of 415 ms. The differential diagnoses of a wide complex tachycardia with a short HV interval consist of ventricular tachycardia or a regular preexcited tachycardia. For a regular preexcited tachycardia, we must consider the following possibilities: 1) atrial flutter or atrial tachycardia over a bypass tract; 2) antidromic tachyardia; 3) AVNRT with a bystander bypass tract; 4) multiple accessory pathways with antegrade conduction over one pathway and retrograde conduction over a different pathway; or 5) antegrade conduction over an accessory pathway with retrograde conduction over a bystander nodofascicular or nodoventricular pathway.

In cases of wide complex tachycardia, the presence of AV dissociation favors ventricular tachycardia as well as certain forms of AVNRT and AVRT with either a nodoventricular or a nodofascicular retrograde pathway, which may also show VA dissociation. (AVNRT and AVRT with a retrograde nodoventricular/fascicular AP would have a narrow QRS complex unless aberration or bystander preexcitation was also present.) In this case the VA interval is fixed and there is 1:1 VA conduction. The HV interval is –35 ms. The HA interval is 170 ms. The long HA makes AVNRT unlikely because during AVNRT the H and

A are activated simultaneously and is usually short (for typical AVNRT).

Bundle branch VT and fascicular VT commonly show a LBBB pattern, as seen in this case. The HV interval is generally the same, slightly shorter or longer than in sinus rhythm, and in general is somewhat longer than 40–60 ms. In fascicular VT, the HV may be short or negative, as it is in this case.

Atriofascicular pathways insert in or near the distal RB or the distal RV myocardium. Therefore RV apical activation is earlier than the right ventricular activation on the His bundle, which is the case here, and **thus we have an atriofascicular and not an atrioventricular accessory pathway**.

The key maneuver here is introduction of a PAC from the right atrium without perturbing the His bundle atrial activation timing. Here, the PAC advances the tachycardia and the subsequent V, thus showing that an AV connection is present. The next V advances or resets the tachycardia—advances the A, proving resetting, showing this is a macroreentrant tachycardia; the diagnosis of an atriofascicular is the most likely here. VT should not be reset by a PAC from the right atrium. (Pathway was ablated on the lateral tricuspid annulus.)

Figure 2.V.2

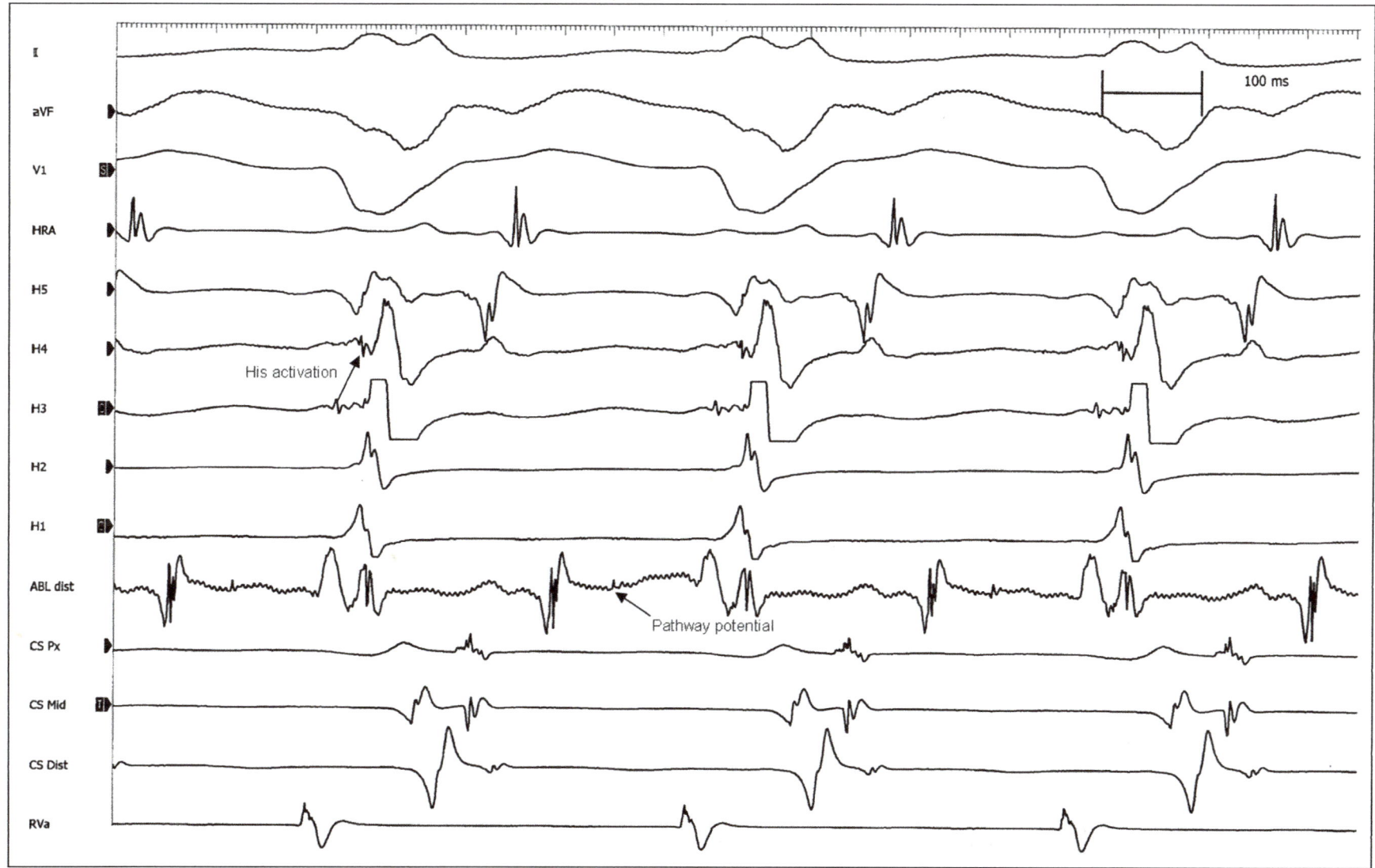

References

1. Haïssaguerre M, Cauchemez B, Marcus F, et al. Characteristics of the ventricular insertion sites of accessory pathways with anterograde decremental conduction properties. *Circulation*. 1995;91:1077–1085.

2. Tchou P, Lehmann MH, Jazayeri M, Akhtar M. Atriofascicular connection or a nodoventricular Mahaim fiber? Electrophysiologic elucidation of the pathway and associated reentrant circuit. *Circulation*. 1988;77:837–848.

3. Kottkamp H, Hindricks G, Shenasa H, et al. Variants of preexcitation—specialized atriofascicular pathways, nodofascicular pathways, and fasciculoventricular pathways: electrophysiologic findings and target sites for radiofrequency catheter ablation. *J Cardiovasc Electrophysiol*. 1996;7:916–930.

Question

Which of the following statements best describes the phenomenon demonstrated by these tracings?

A) Presence of a left–sided fasciculoventricular pathway

B) Presence of a left–sided atrioventricular accessory pathway

C) Presence of a decremental, left–sided atrioventricular accessory pathway

D) Presence of a left–sided accessory atrioventricular pathway and an ectopic left atrial pacemaker

Figure 2.W.1

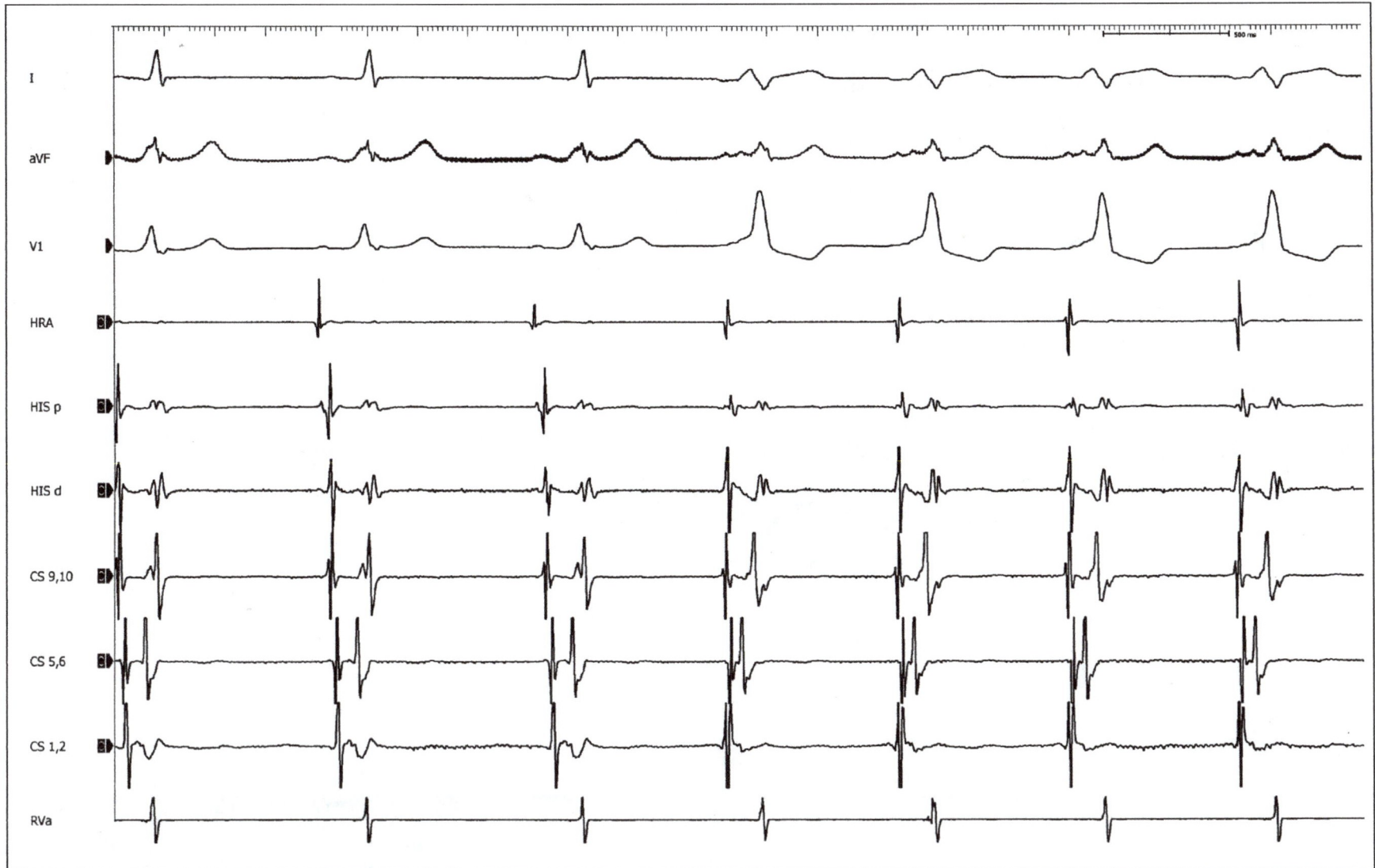

Figure 2.W.2

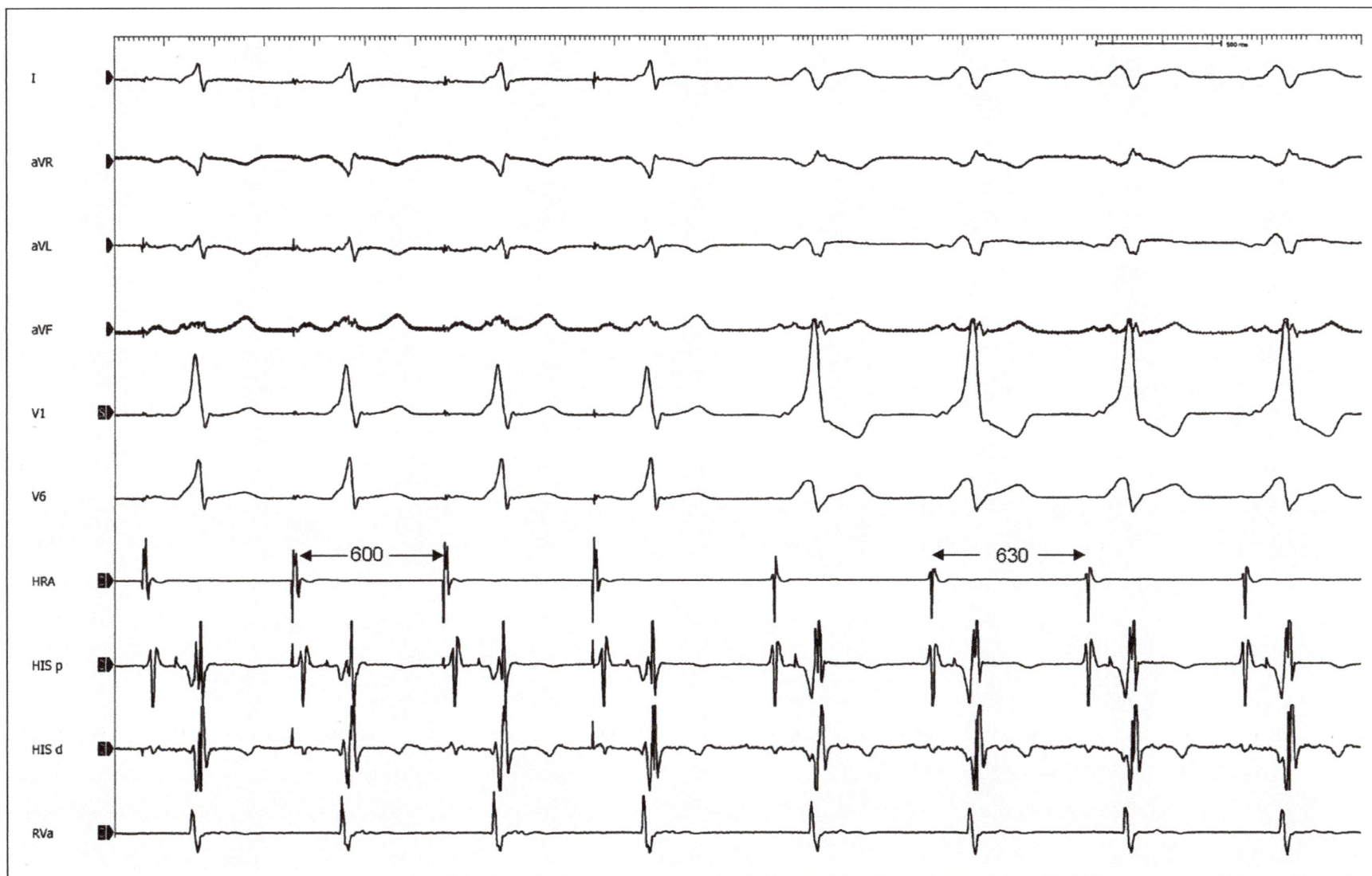

Answer

The correct answer is **D**. The top tracing shows three beats with minimal preexcitation and four beats with more marked preexcitation. The pattern of preexcitation has not changed, just the degree of preexcitation. The bottom tracing shows during the initial portion atrial pacing at a cycle length of 600 ms. After the termination of pacing, the spontaneous atrial rhythm resumes.

The QRS morphology during this spontaneous atrial rhythm shows a greater degree of preexcitation with a positive delta wave in V_1 and a prominent R wave, suggesting the presence of a left-sided pathway. The HV interval is negative during atrial rhythm.

During atrial pacing at a faster rate, the degree of preexcitation is lower, and the HV interval increases to 0 ms. Therefore, it appears that the pathway may be decremental in nature.

However, there is a more likely explanation shown by careful review of both the top and bottom tracings. In these tracings, carefully observe the atrial activation sequence. The atrial activation sequence is changed when atrial pacing is terminated. Specifically, during sinus rhythm the high right atrial electrogram is early, while during the rhythm to the right of both the top and bottom tracing, we can see the timing of the atrial electrograms change. Specifically, focusing on the top tracing, the mid coronary sinus electrogram is on time with the high right atrial electrogram (marked by circle) proving the presence of an ectopic focus in the left atrium (compare to sinus beat marked by ★). This ectopic focus is nearer to the accessory pathway and was in fact a left atrial rhythm, and thus demonstrates a greater degree of preexcitation.

Figure 2.W.3

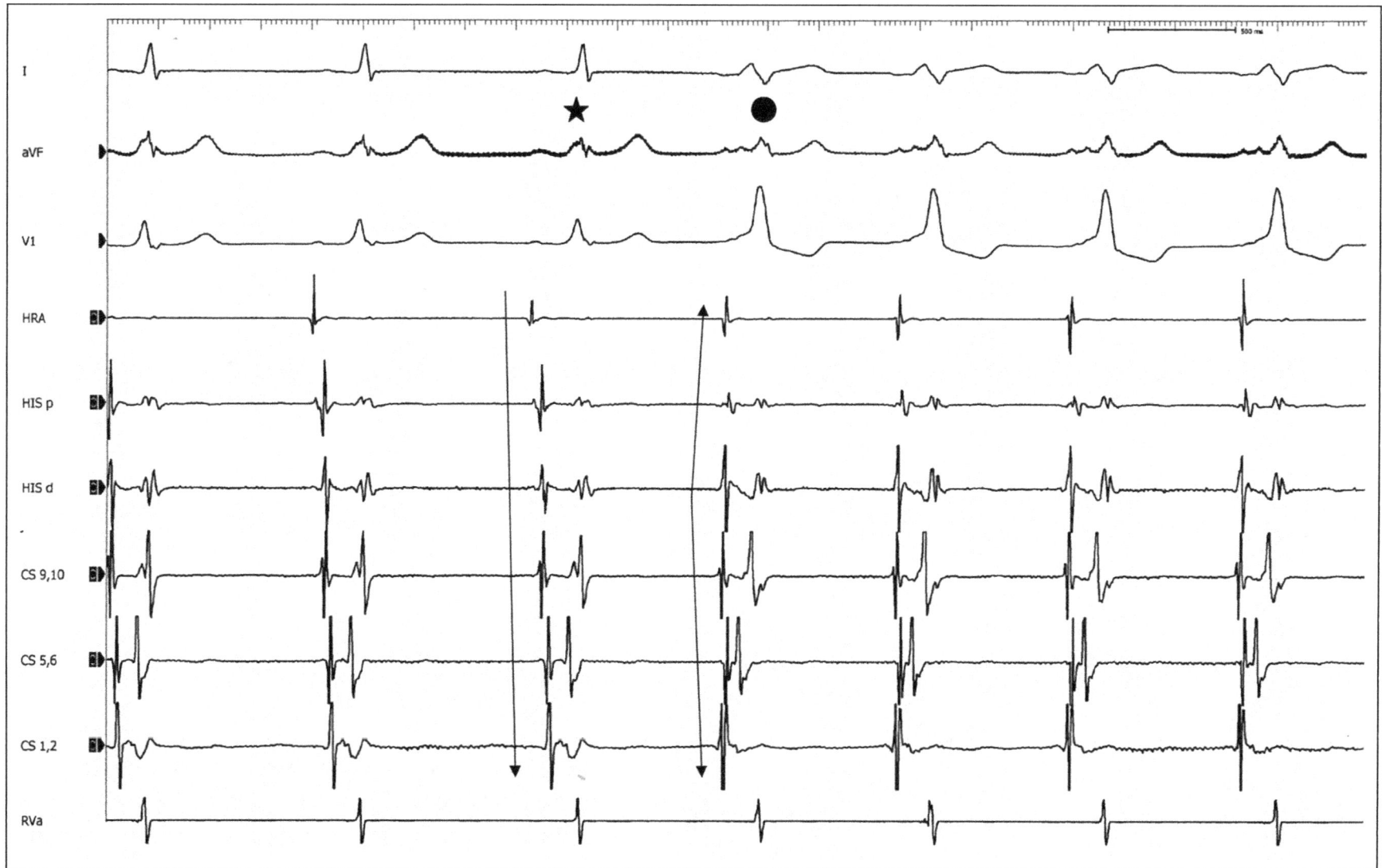

Reference

1. Arruda MS, McClelland JH, Wang X, et al. Development and valida-
    tion of an ECG algorithm for identifying accessory pathway ablation
    site in Wolff-Parkinson-White syndrome. *J Cardiovasc Electrophysiol.*
    1998;9:2–12.

Question 1

Tachycardia is induced in a 36-year-old man with prior ablation of the posterior fascicular ventricular tachycardia that resulted in iatrogenic left bundle branch block.

Which of the following is the most likely diagnosis based on the pacing maneuver?

A) Junctional tachycardia

B) AV node reentry

C) Orthodromic reentry using a concealed nodoventricular bypass tract

D) Bundle branch reentry

E) Cannot be determined

Figure 2.X.1

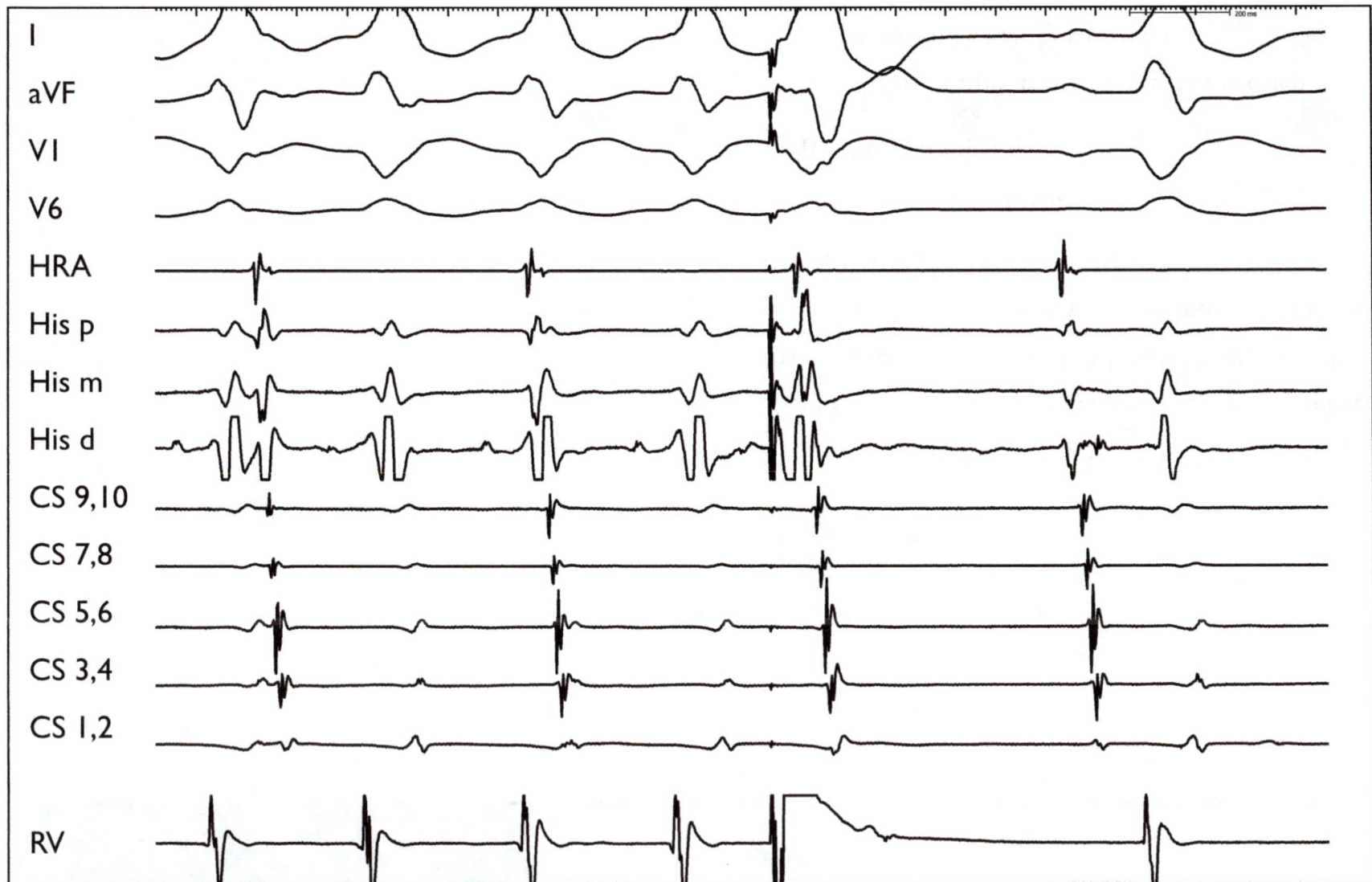

Figure 2.X.2

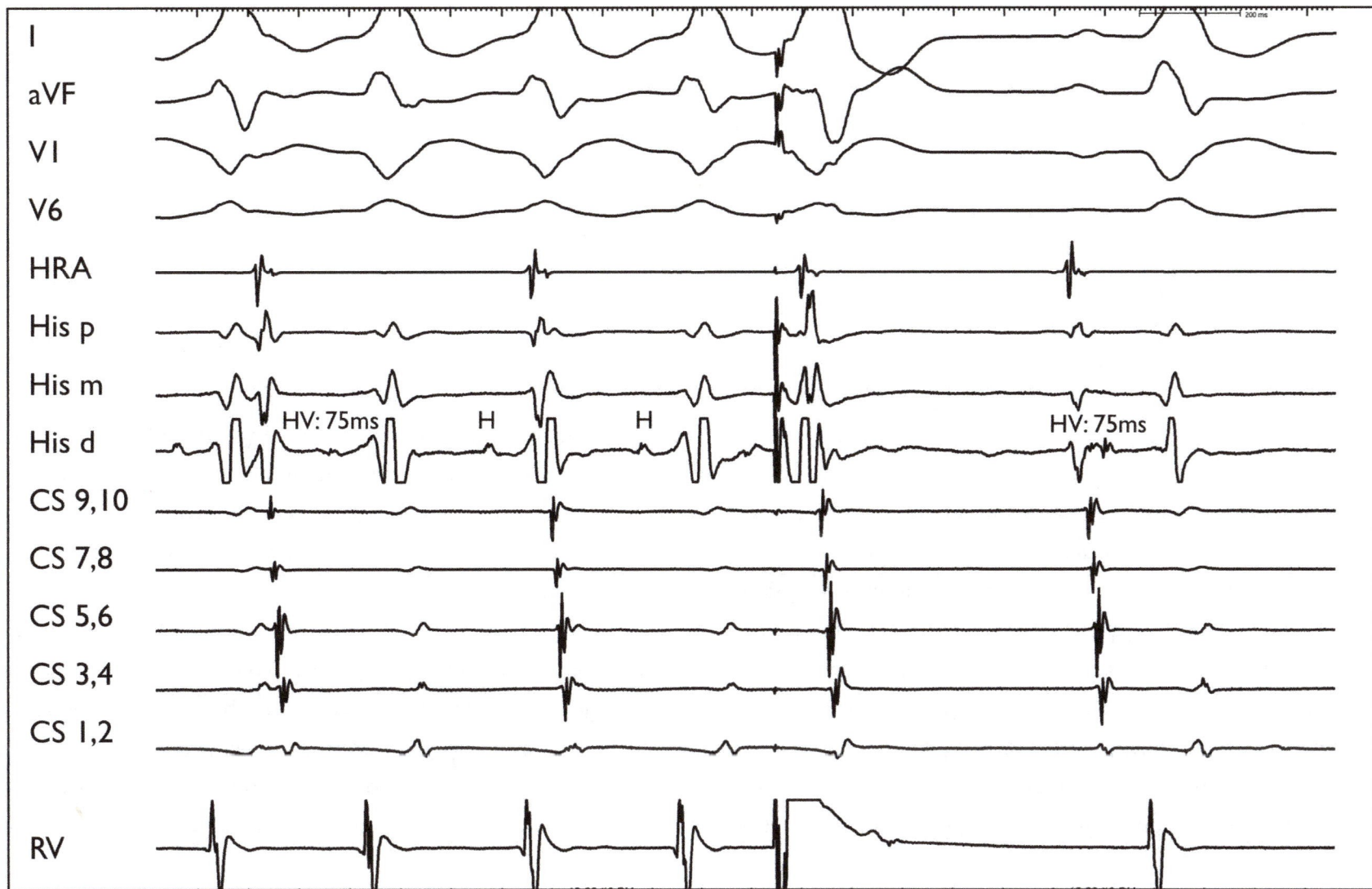

Figure 2.X.2

Answer 1

The correct answer is **E**. It cannot be determined and further testing is necessary to establish the diagnosis.

A left bundle branch tachycardia with AV dissociation is seen. All four options do not require the atrium for maintenance of tachycardia. A PVC delivered during His refractoriness results in termination of the PVC without conduction up to the His bundle or atrium. After termination, the baseline left bundle branch block pattern is seen during sinus rhythm with a prolonged HV interval of 75 ms.

A His-refractory PVC should not effect junctional tachycardia or AV node reentry. A concealed nodoventricular bypass tract can be demonstrated by advancement, delay, or termination to the subsequent His activation after a His-refractory PVC is given. However, bundle branch reentry (BBR) may also terminate with a PVC that renders the right bundle branch refractory. An HV during tachycardia similar to that of sinus rhythm can be seen with both orthodromic reentry and BBR, although functional prolongation of HV is more commonly seen during BBR. Therefore, a concealed nodoventricular bypass tract with antegrade left bundle branch block pattern cannot be differentiated from BBR based on the present information.

Question 2

Which subsequent maneuver is most specific for diagnosis?

A) Ventricular overdrive pacing

B) Atrial overdrive pacing

C) Adenosine

D) Left bundle recording

Figure 2.X.3

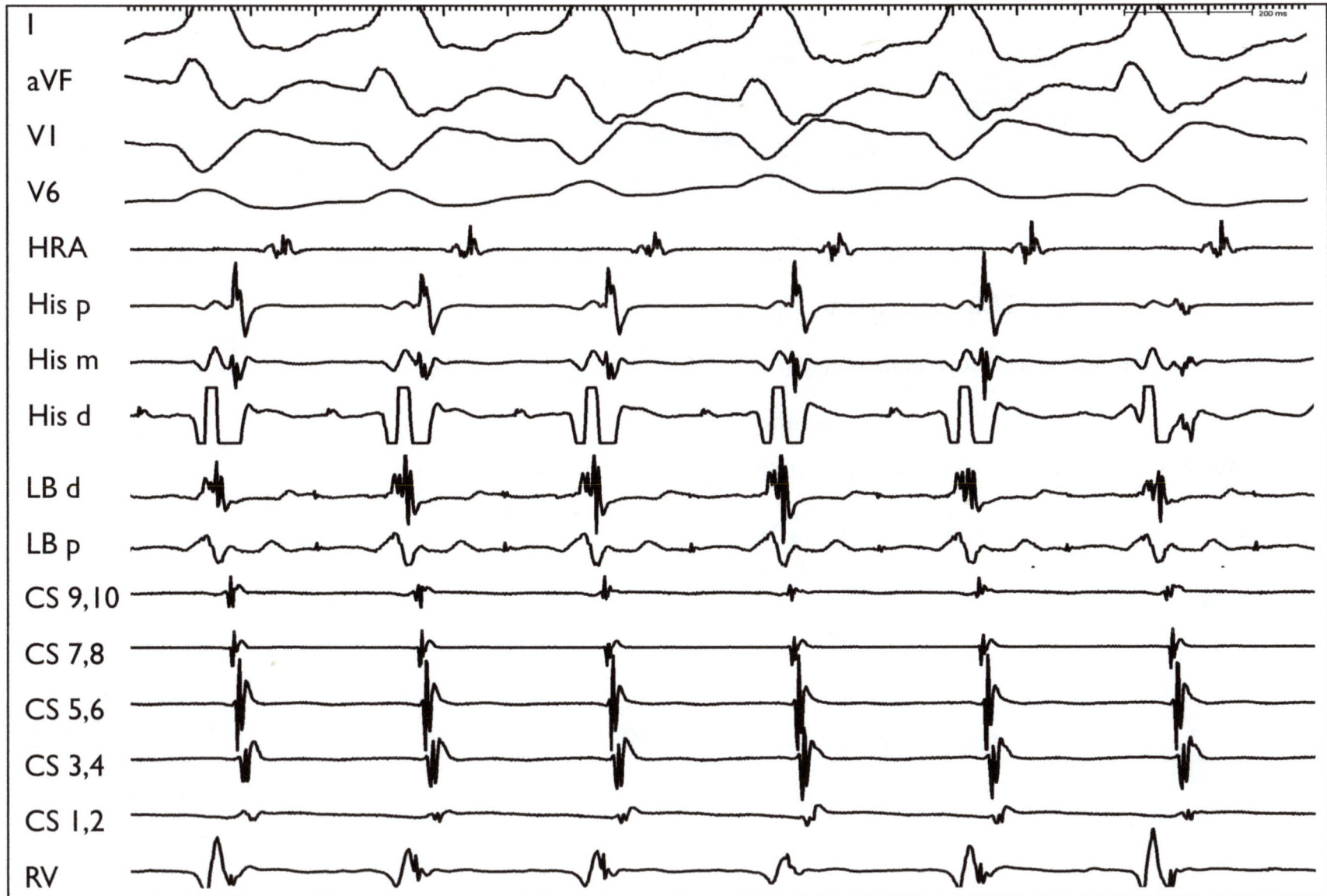

Figure 2.X.4

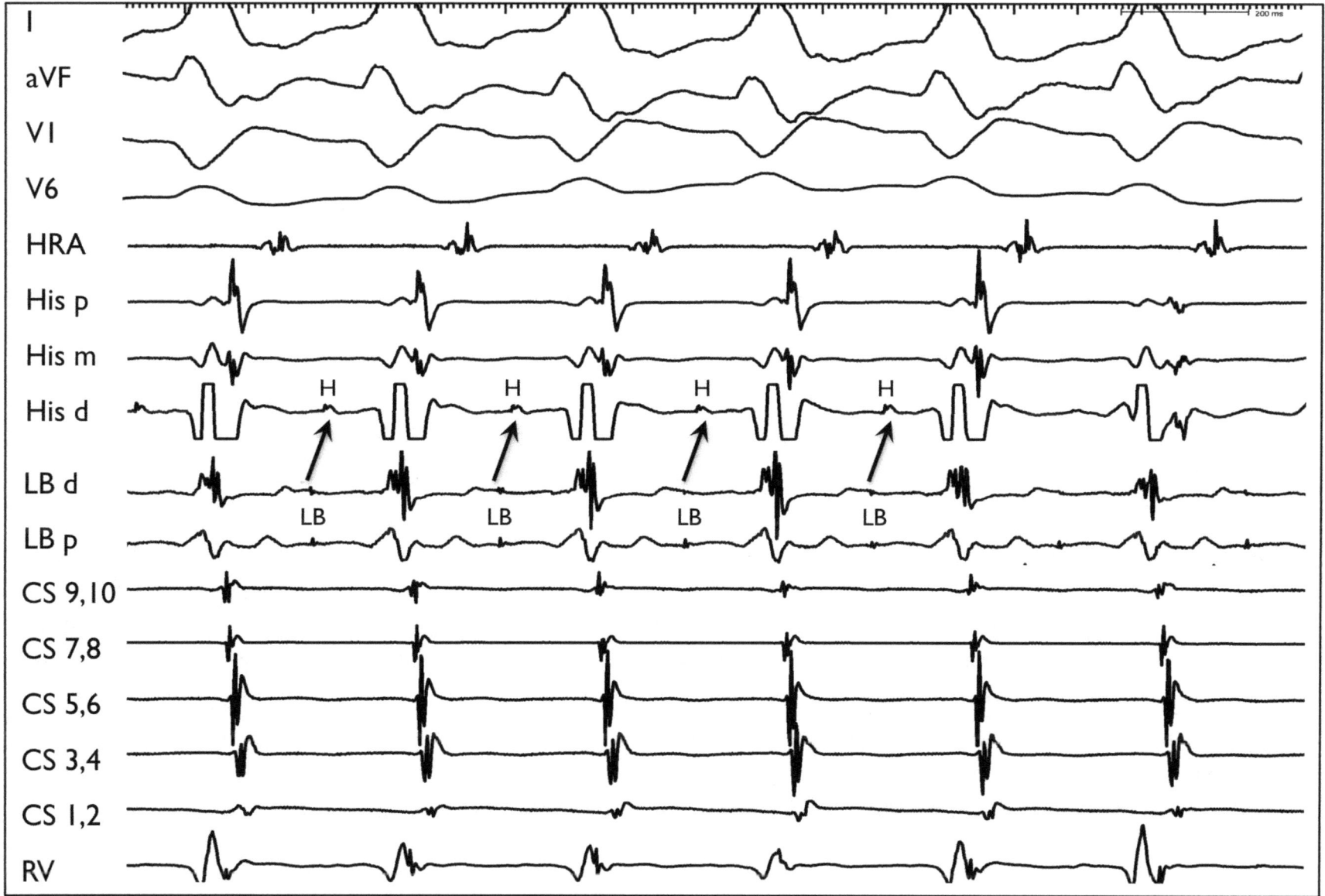

*A*nswer 2

The correct answer is **D**. Recording of a left bundle potential confirms the diagnosis of BBR.

Ventricular overdrive pacing is expected to yield a PPI similar to the tachycardia with overt fusion for both orthodromic reentry using a concealed nodoventricular bypass tract and BBR. Atrial overdrive pacing is also expected to result in similarly concealed entrainment as both tachycardias utilize the conduction system as the antegrade limb.

Adenosine is not expected to interrupt BBR as the circuit is entirely infranodal. Termination of tachycardia with adenosine is more supportive of orthodromic reentry, although fast pathway AV node resistance to adenosine has been reported. The recording of a left bundle potential that precedes the His bundle activation is diagnostic of retrograde His activation from the left bundle, which is pathognomonic for left-bundle type BBR.

References

1. Akhtar M, Gilbert C, Wolf FG, Schmidt DH. Reentry within the His-Purkinje system. Elucidation of reentrant circuit using right bundle branch and His bundle recordings. *Circulation*. 1978;58(2):295–304.

2. Caceres J, Jazayeri M, McKinnie J, Avitall B, Denker ST, Tchou P, Akhtar M. Sustained bundle branch reentry as a mechanism of clinical tachycardia. *Circulation*. 1989;79(2):256–270.

3. Volkmann H, Kühnert H, Dannberg G, Heinke M. Bundle branch reentrant tachycardia treated by transvenous catheter ablation of the right bundle branch. *Pacing Clin Electrophysiol*. 1989;12(1):258–261.

Question

An 18-year-old man with a 5-year history of recurrent palpitations is brought to the electrophysiology laboratory. The following tracing is recorded. The patient's preprocedure ECG is normal.

What is the most likely diagnosis?

A) Ventricular tachycardia

B) AV node reentry with aberrancy

C) ORT with aberrancy

D) Atriofascicular Mahaim tachycardia

E) Duodromic tachycardia with atriofascicular Mahaim and left-sided pathway

Figure 2.Y.1

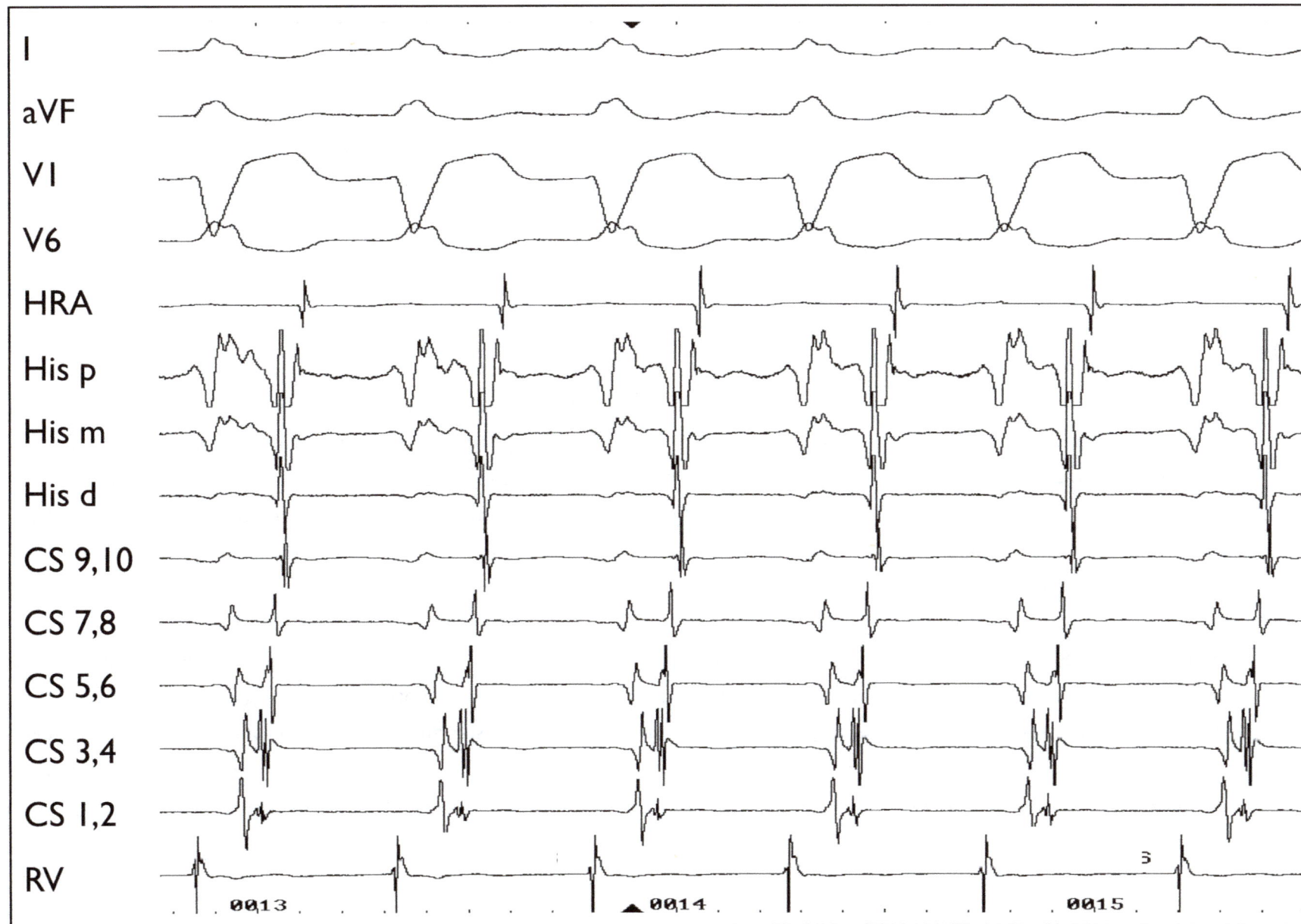

Answer

The correct answer is **E. A duodromic pathway-to-pathway tachycardia is seen**.

A left bundle branch, wide complex tachycardia is seen, which may represent VT or SVT with aberration or preexcitation. Importantly, a His is not seen during tachycardia, which excludes any SVT with aberrancy. The atrial activation is eccentric with distal to proximal CS activation, which demonstrates the presence of a left lateral pathway. This activation would be highly atypical for AV node reentry. As the surface could be explained by VT or Mahaim tachycardia, the presence of left lateral atrial activation excludes them as the most likely diagnosis. The likelihood of having both a VT and a retrograde accessory pathway is less than

having two pathways, as demonstrated by premature atrial and ventricular stimulation. The LBBB morphology shown in the tracings (Figure 2.Y.1 and 2.Y.2) is highly atypical for a VT with the sharp downslope seen in V_1 and V_6 and much more consistent with a pathway that inserts directly into the specialized conduction system.

A premature ventricular beat advances the atrial activation, which demonstrates presence and participation of left-sided retrograde pathway.

A premature atrial beat advances the ventricle, which demonstrate the presence and participation of an atriofascicular pathway.

Figure 2.Y.2

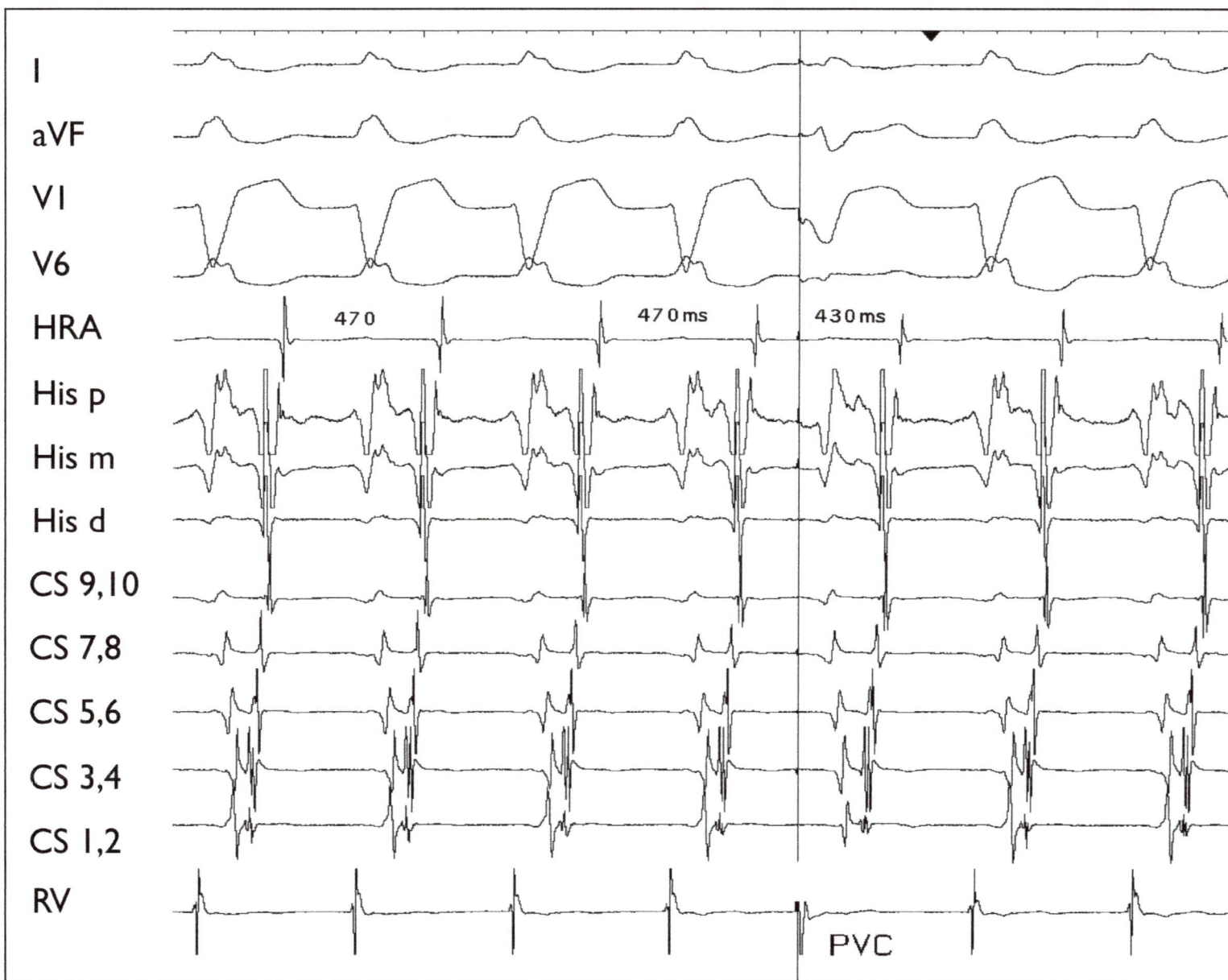

Figure 2.Y.3

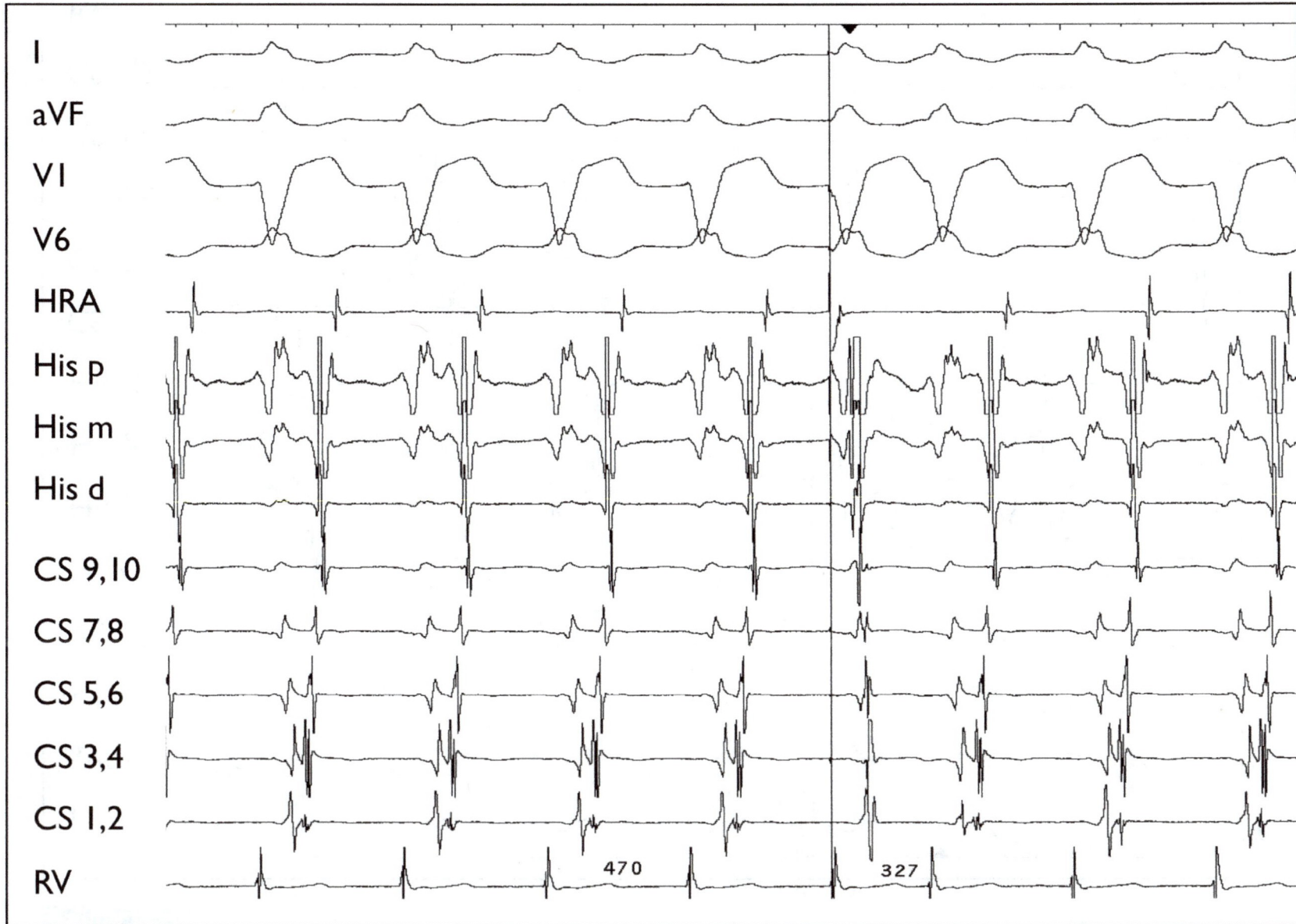

Figure 2.Y.4

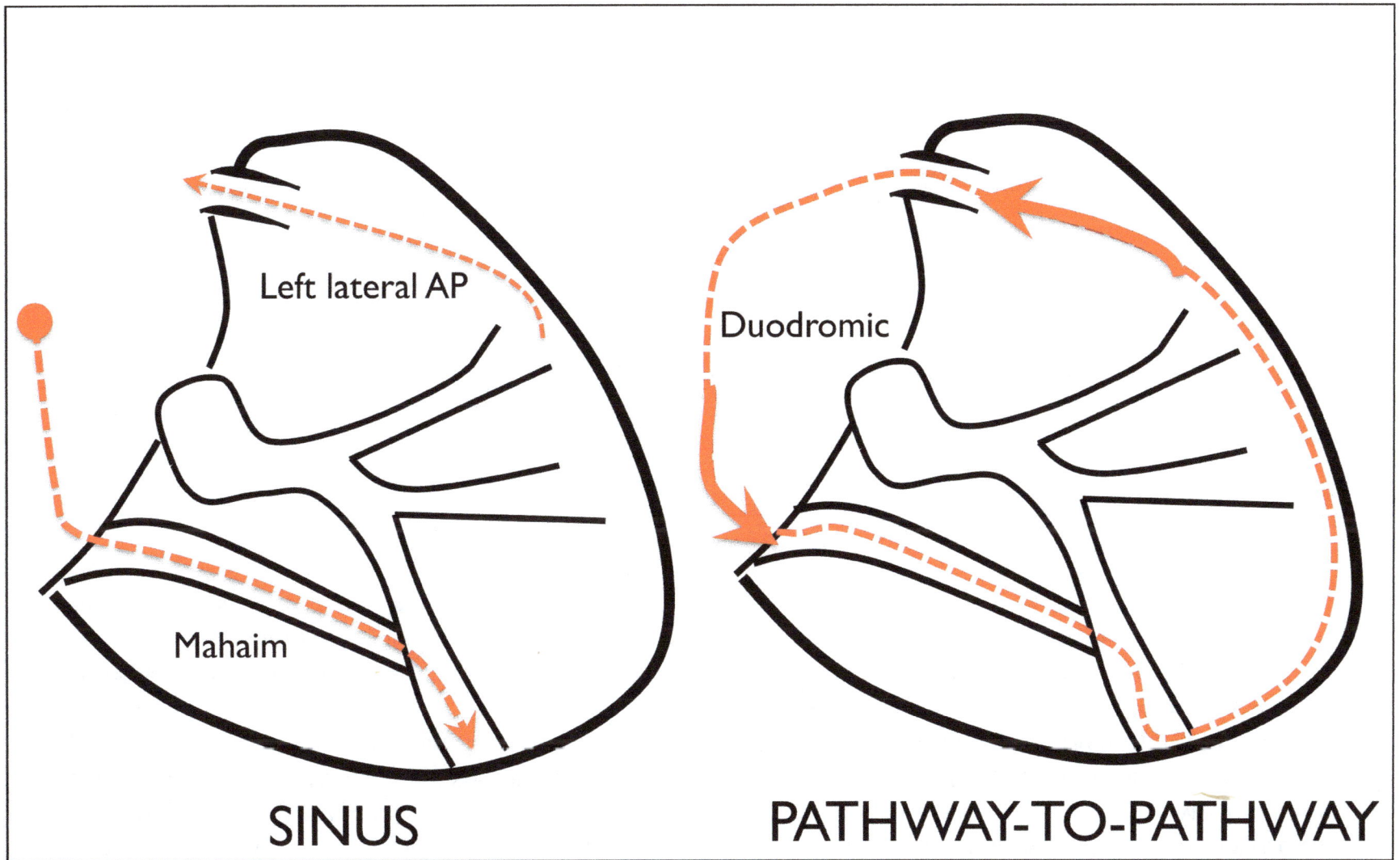

Left lateral AP

Mahaim

SINUS

Duodromic

PATHWAY-TO-PATHWAY

References

1. Vaseghi M, Shannon KM, Wetzel GT, Shivkumar K. Reentry around the heart. *Heart Rhythm*. 2007;4(2):236–238.

2. Gallagher JJ, Smith WM, Kasell JH, Benson DW, Sterba R, Grant AO. Role of Mahaim fibers in cardiac arrhythmias in man. *Circulation*. 1981;64:176–189.

3. Tchou P, Lehmann MH, Jazayeri, M, Akhtar M. Atriofascicular connection or a nodoventricular Mahaim fiber? Electrophysiologic elucidation of the pathway and associated reentrant circuit. *Circulation*. 1988;77:837–848.

4. Ellenbogen KA, Ramirez NM, Packer DL, O'Callaghan WG, Greer GS, Sintetos AL, et al. Accessory nodoventricular (Mahaim) fibers: a clinical review. *Pacing Clin Electrophysiol*. 1986;9:868–884.

5. Klein GJ, Guiraudon GM, Kerr CR, Sharma AD, Yee R, Szabo T, et al. "Nodoventricular" accessory pathway: evidence for a distinct accessory atrioventricular pathway with atrioventricular node-like properties. *J Am Coll Cardiol*. 1988;11:1035–1040.

PART 3

Atrial Fibrillation (AF)

Case 3.A

Question

A 67-year-old man underwent catheter ablation for drug-refractory atrial fibrillation.

Following circumferential ablation around both sets of pulmonary veins, pacing was performed from the circular mapping catheter to assess for exit block. The pacing output is decreased over the course of the recording. Catheter position is shown in the RAO and LAO projections.

What should be done next?

A) Additional ablation to isolate the left pulmonary veins

B) Additional ablation to isolate the right pulmonary veins

C) Additional ablation within the left atrial appendage

D) No further ablation is needed

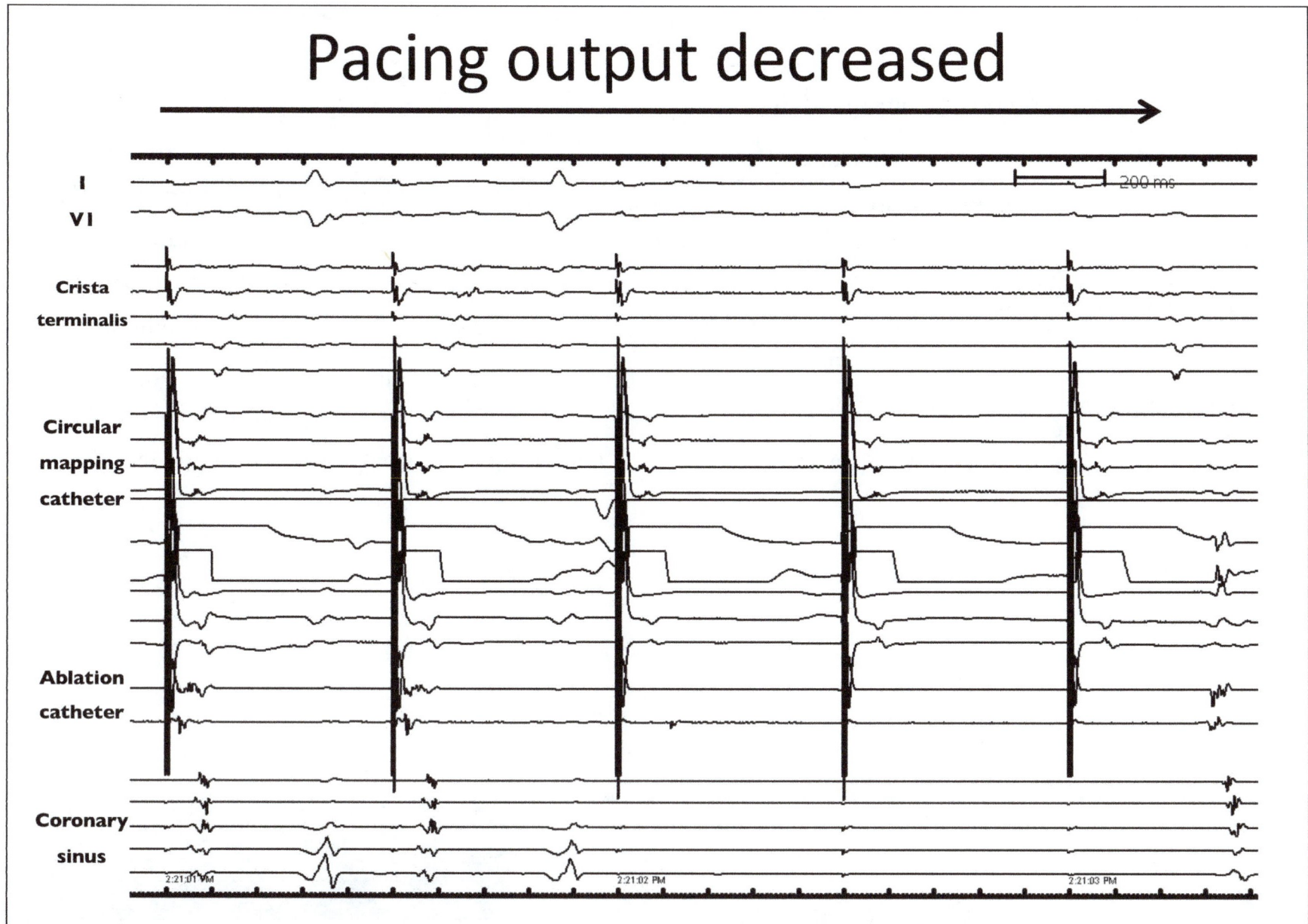

Figure 3.A.1

Figure 3.A.2

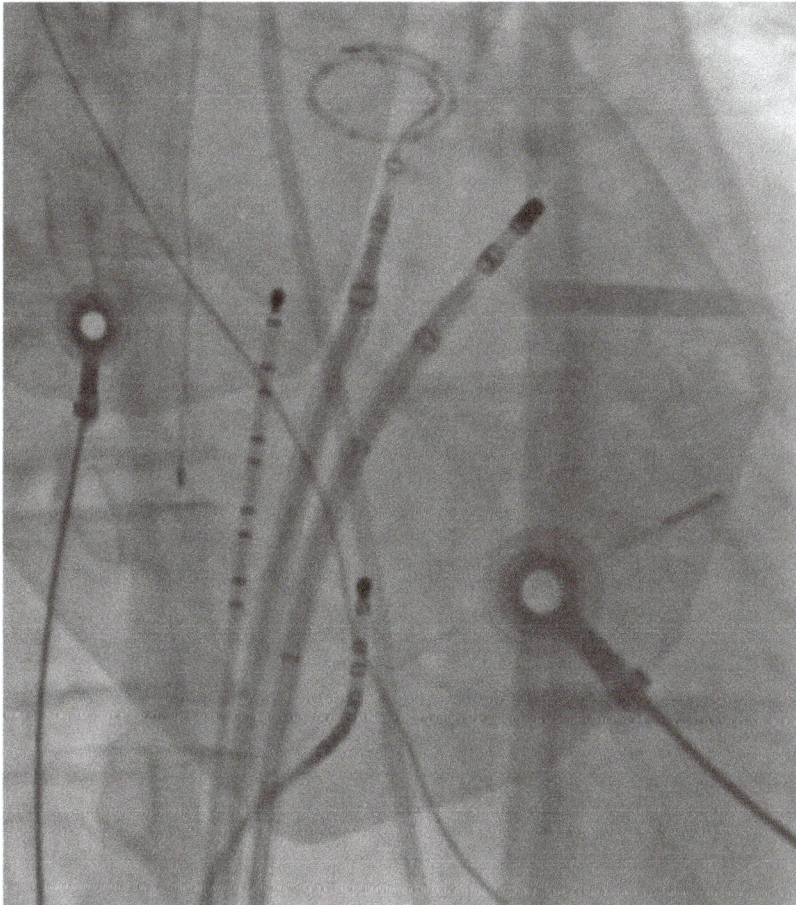 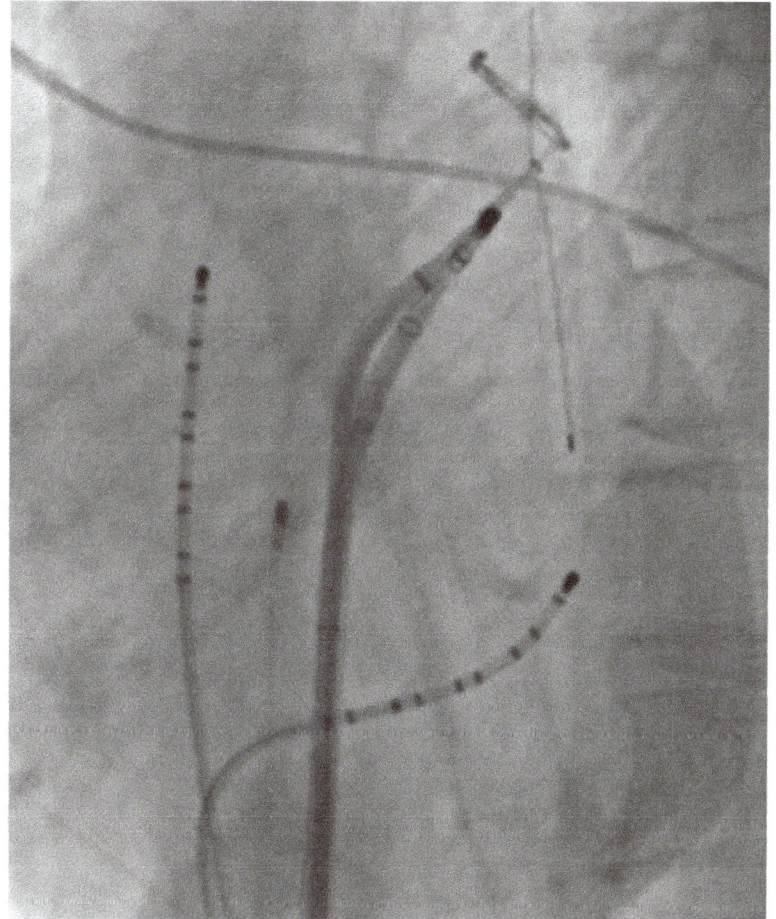

Answer

The correct answer is **D**. The circular mapping catheter is positioned in the left superior pulmonary vein and the ablation catheter in the left atrial appendage. Pacing is performed from the circular mapping catheter. Initially, the left atrial appendage is captured directly, as suggested by immediate activation recorded by the ablation catheter. As the pacing output is decreased, capture of the pulmonary vein is preserved (arrows), while far-field capture of the left atrial appendage (stars) is lost.

Thus, exit block is present in the left pulmonary veins, and **further ablation is not needed**. No conclusion can be drawn about the right pulmonary veins with this catheter position. No evidence is provided of triggers from the left atrial appendage.

Far-field capture of the left atrial appendage is not uncommon when pacing the anterior aspect of the left superior pulmonary veins. Similarly, far-field capture of the superior vena cava can occur when pacing deep within the right superior pulmonary vein. When far-field capture is suspected, pacing at lower output should be performed. If pulmonary vein capture is preserved while atrial capture is lost, exit block is truly present, and further ablation should not be delivered.

References

1. Gerstenfeld EP, Dixit S, Callans D, Rho R, Rajawat Y, Zado E, et al. Utility of exit block for identifying electrical isolation of the pulmonary veins. *J Cardiovasc Electrophysiol.* 2002;13:971–979.
2. Vijayaraman P, Dandamudi G, Naperkowski A, Oren J, Storm R, Ellenbogen KA. Assessment of exit block following pulmonary vein isolation: far-field capture masquerading as entrance without exit block. *Heart Rhythm.* 2012;9:1653–1659.

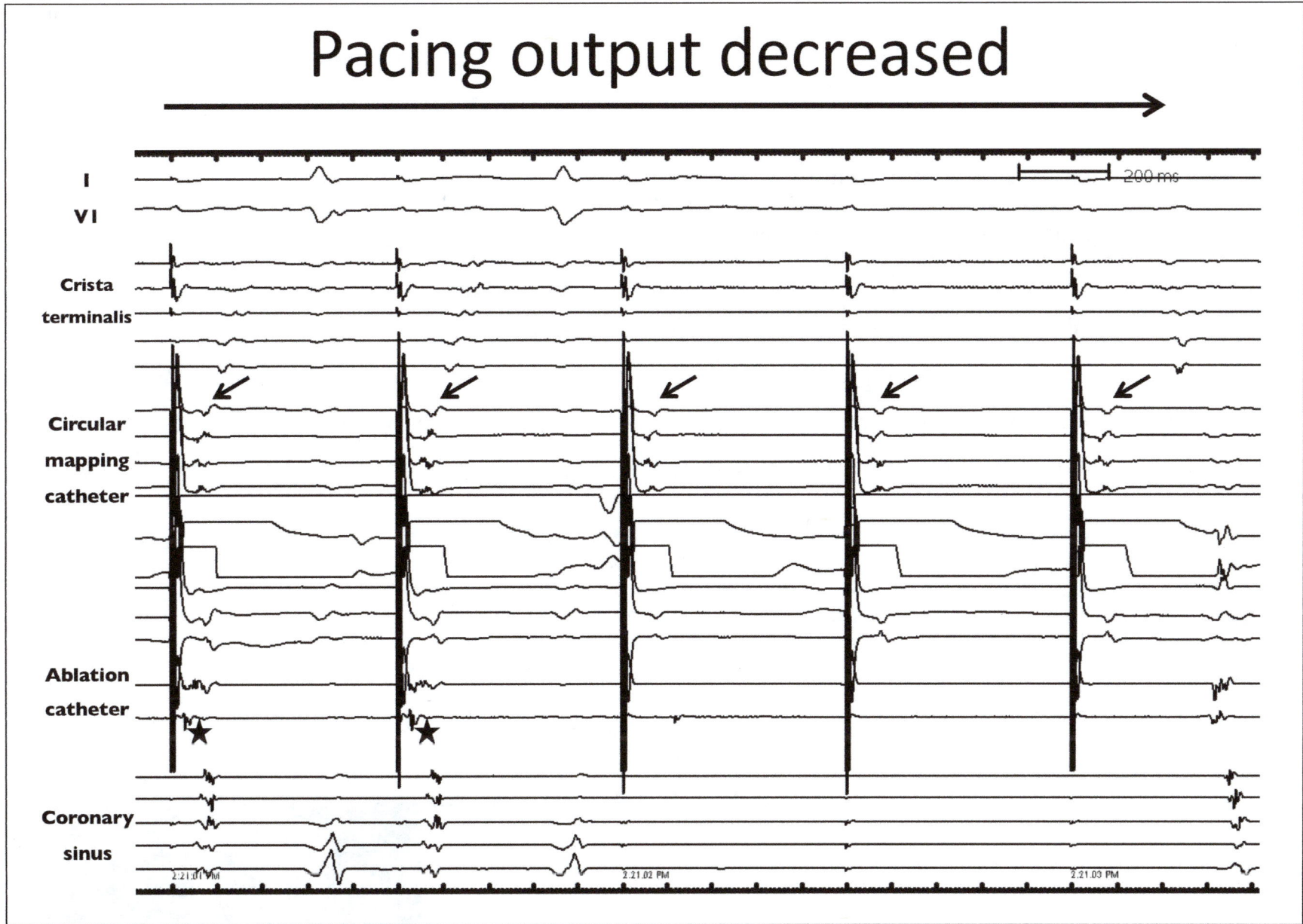

Figure 3.A.3

Case 3.B

Question

A 52-year-old man undergoes pulmonary vein isolation because of symptomatic, drug-refractory atrial fibrillation. A circular mapping catheter is positioned along the antrum of the left superior pulmonary vein (LSPV), where wide-area circumferential ablation is begun. The following tracing is recorded after the 17th radiofrequency (RF) lesion around the vein.

What is the next best option?

A) Position the ablation catheter on the antrum of the LSPV closest to the third ring electrode and deliver RF energy

B) Position the ablation catheter along the antrum of the LSPV closest to the proximal ring electrode and deliver RF energy

C) Pace the left atrial appendage (LAA) to determine if the signals seen on the circular mapping catheter are far-field arising from the LAA

D) Pace within the LSPV to see if exit block exists

Figure 3.B.1

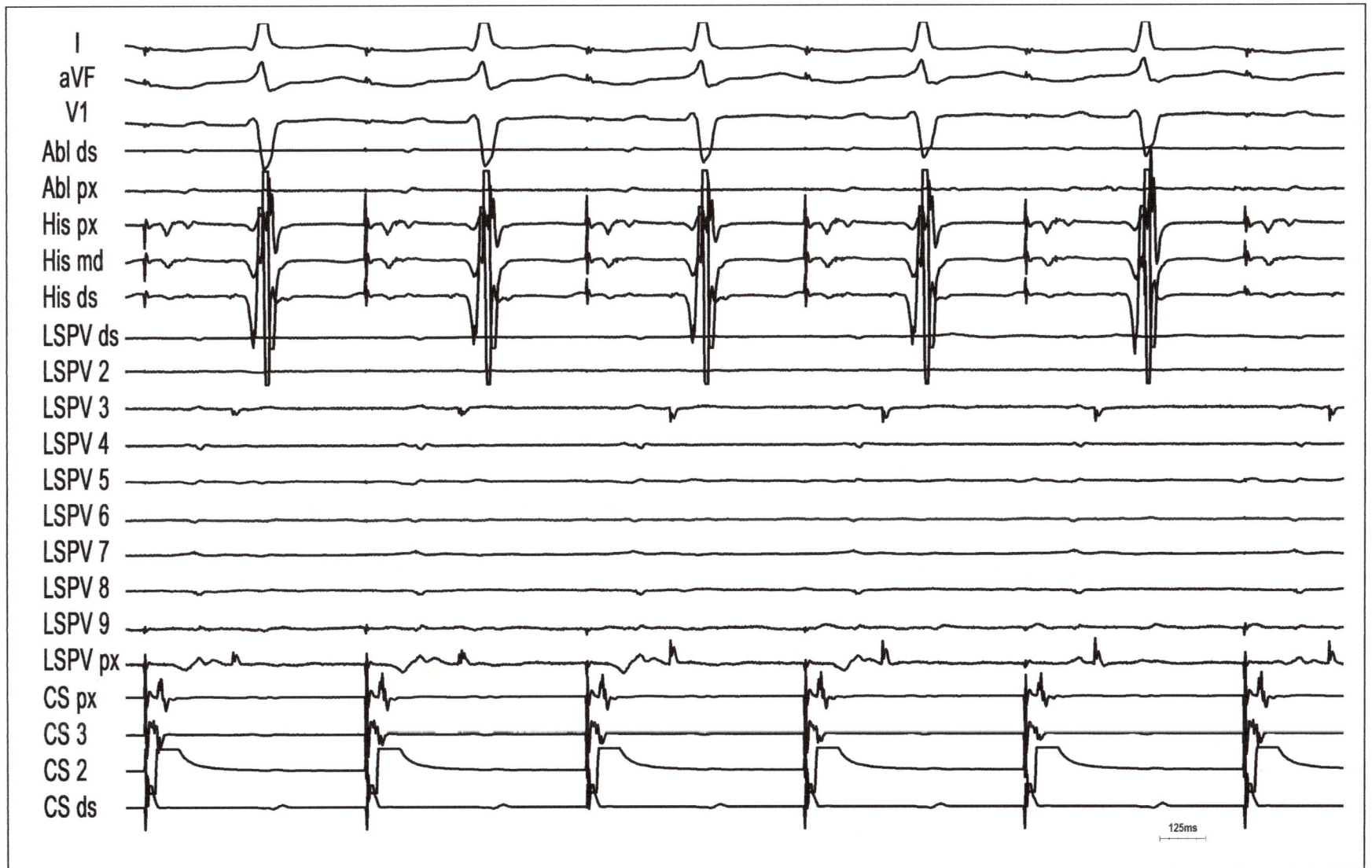

125ms

Answer

The correct answer is **D**. After RF delivery, the circular mapping catheter records low-amplitude atrial electrograms and absence of pulmonary vein potentials on all electrodes except two (proximal, third) both of which record high-frequency signals (arrows) that might represent residual pulmonary vein conduction. Aside from pulmonary vein potentials, another source of signals on a mapping catheter in the LSPV are far-field atrial electrograms originating from the LAA, particularly on the electrodes closest to the LAA. These can be differentiated from true pulmonary vein potentials by directly capturing the LAA. Close inspection of these signals on the proximal and third-ring electrode, however, show that not only are they completely simultaneous and "mirror images" of each other but also demonstrate variability in timing with the truly captured atrial electrograms. This indicates that they are actually recording artifacts mimicking pulmonary vein potentials resulting from intermittent beat-to-beat contact between these two adjacent electrodes. Since these high-frequency signals are neither atrial nor pulmonary vein in origin, and that entrance block into the LSPV is otherwise present, the next best option is to confirm coexistent exit block and then move on to the next vein.

Figure 3.B.2

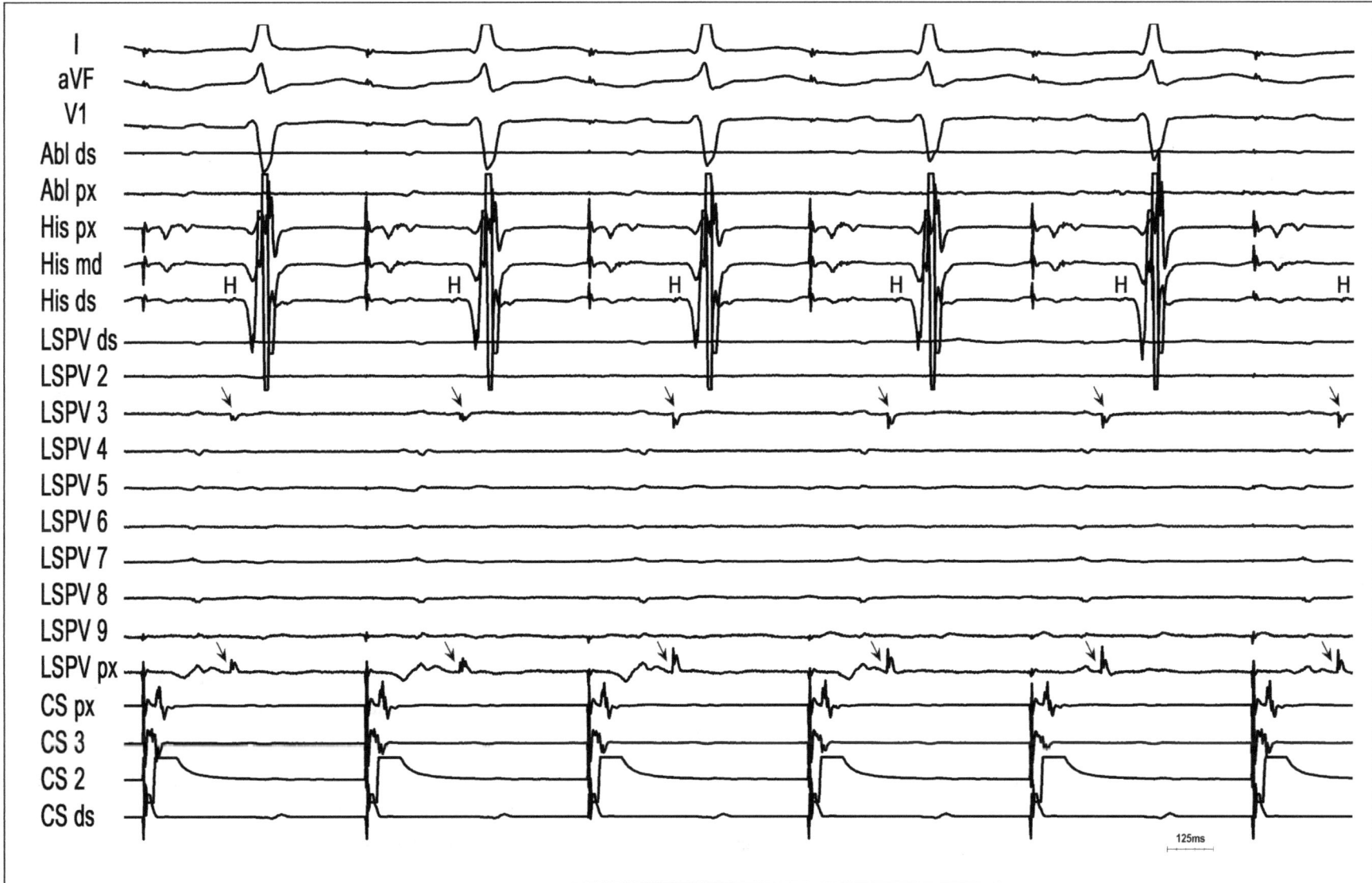

References

1. Haïssaguerre M, Jaïs P, Shah DC, et al. Spontaneous initiation of atrial fibrillation by ectopic beats originating in the pulmonary veins. *N Engl J Med*. 1998;339:659–666.

2. Lemoa K, Oral H, Chugh A, et al. Pulmonary vein isolation as an endpoint for left atrial circumferential ablation of atrial fibrillation. *J Am Coll Cardiol*. 2005;46:1060–1066.

3. Shah D, Haïssaguerre M, Jaïs P, Hocini M, Yamane T, Macle L, et al. Left atrial appendage activity masquerading as pulmonary vein potentials. *Circulation*. 2002;105:2821–2825.

Case 3.C

Question 1

An 80-year-old man without history of arrhythmia undergoes mapping of atrial flutter. Entrainment mapping is performed from different anatomic sites.

Which region should be targeted with ablation?

A) Cavotricuspid isthmus

B) Mitral isthmus

C) Left superior pulmonary vein

D) Left side of septum

E) Left atrial roof

Figure 3.C.1

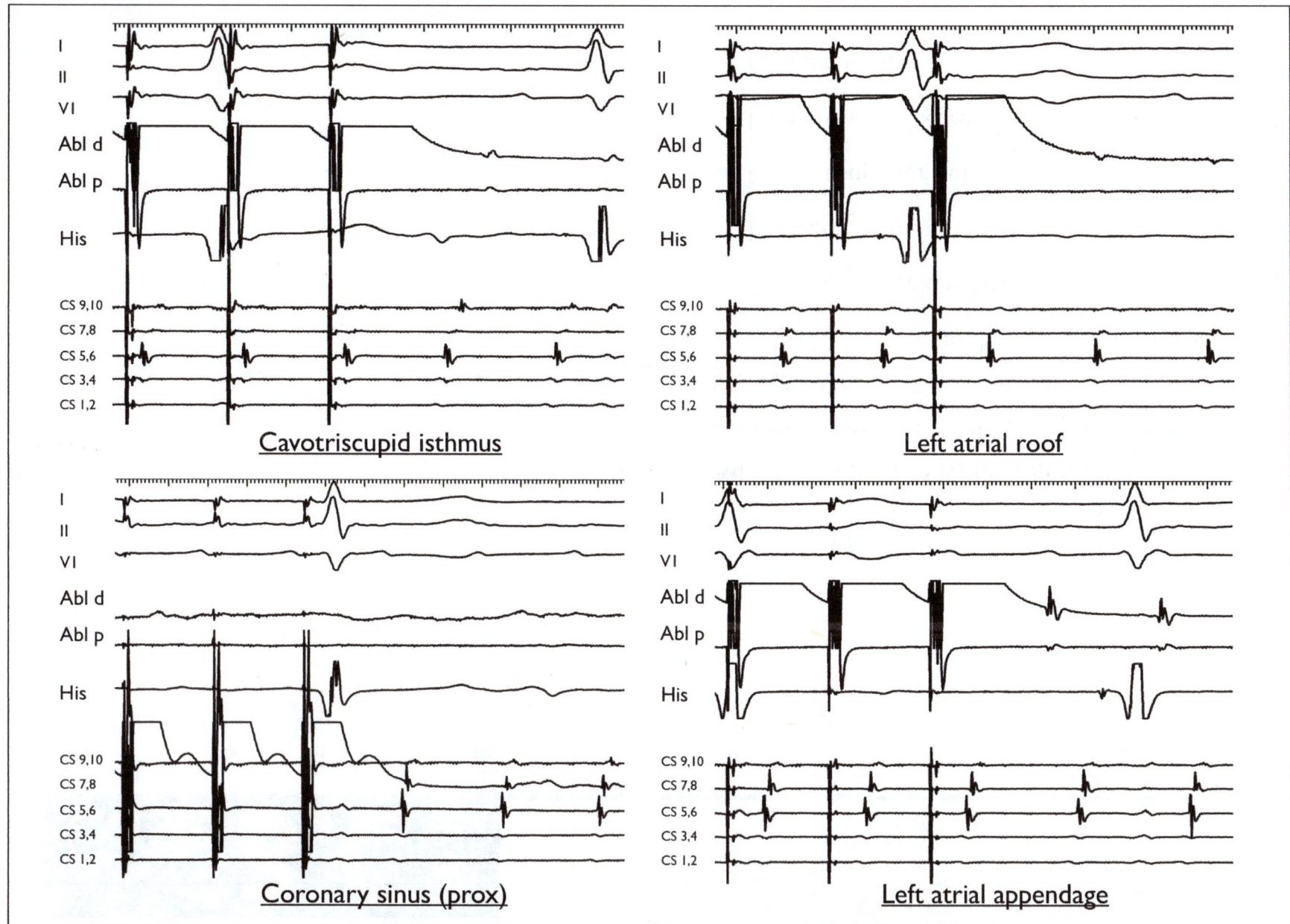

Cavotriscupid isthmus

Left atrial roof

Coronary sinus (prox)

Left atrial appendage

Figure 3.C.2

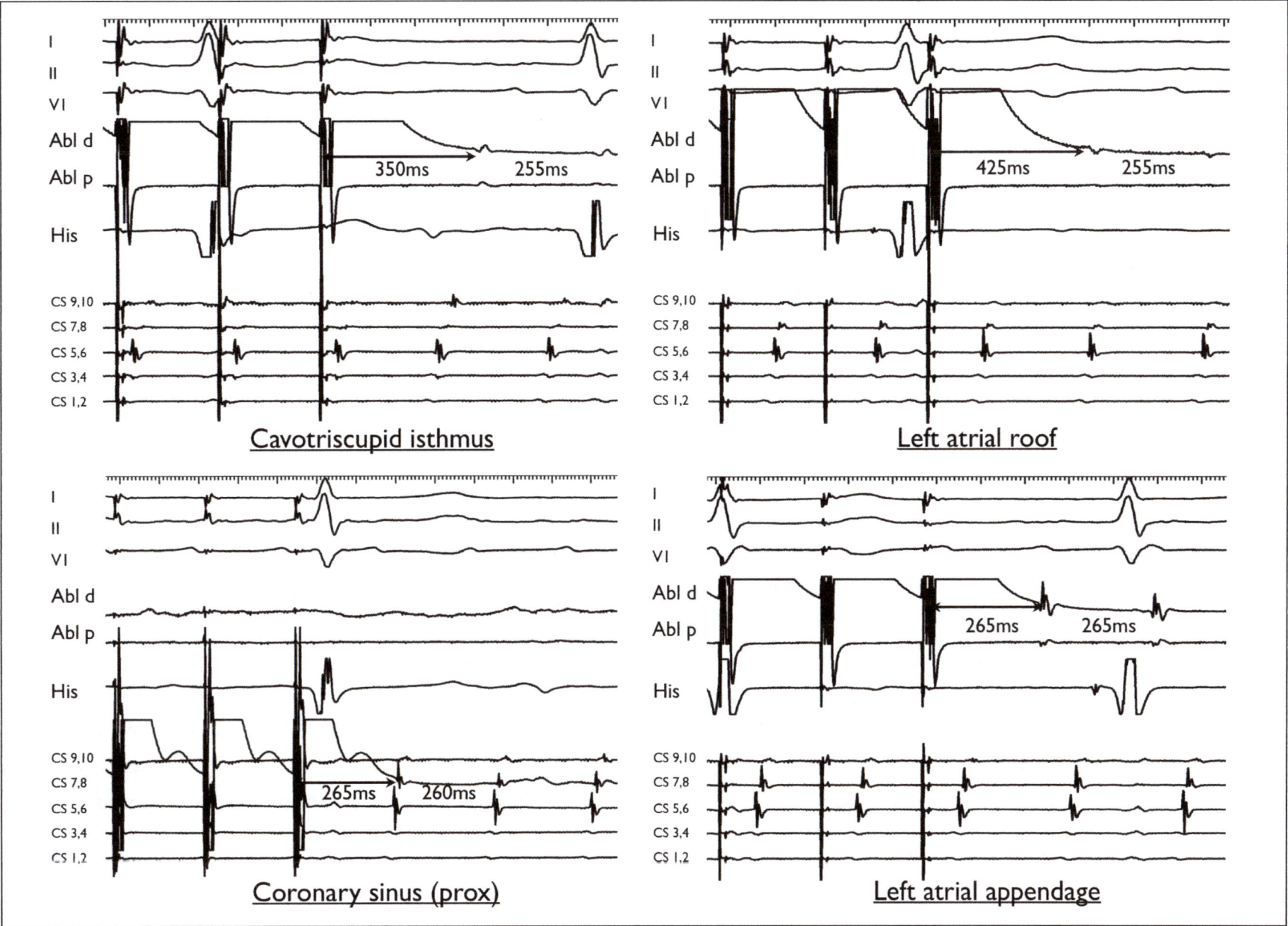

Cavotriscupid isthmus

Left atrial roof

Coronary sinus (prox)

Left atrial appendage

Answer 1

The correct answer is **B. Mitral isthmus flutter is suggested by entrainment mapping.**

The flutter waves on the surface leads are not typical of cavotricuspid isthmus flutter. In the setting of atrial fibrosis (seen in this patient) and prior ablation, surface characteristics are less diagnostic. Distal-to-proximal coronary sinus activation is suggestive of clockwise mitral annular flutter. Roof flutter typically results in fusion of wavefronts in the coronary sinus. The coronary sinus activation pattern is unlikely in a septal flutter and can be seen in typical flutter from Bachmann bundle activation of the left atrium.

Entrainment shows long postpacing intervals from the cavotriscuspid isthmus and left atrial roof, which suggests that the circuit is remote from these anatomic regions. Entrainment with short PPI from the proximal coronary sinus and left atrial appendage, which is in close proximity to the anterolateral mitral annulus, is highly suggestive of mitral isthmus flutter. Inferior and anterior ablation lines connecting the mitral annulus to the left inferior or right superior pulmonary vein can result in block across the mitral isthmus. Note the annular signal of the entrainment response from the mitral isthmus.

Figure 3.C.3

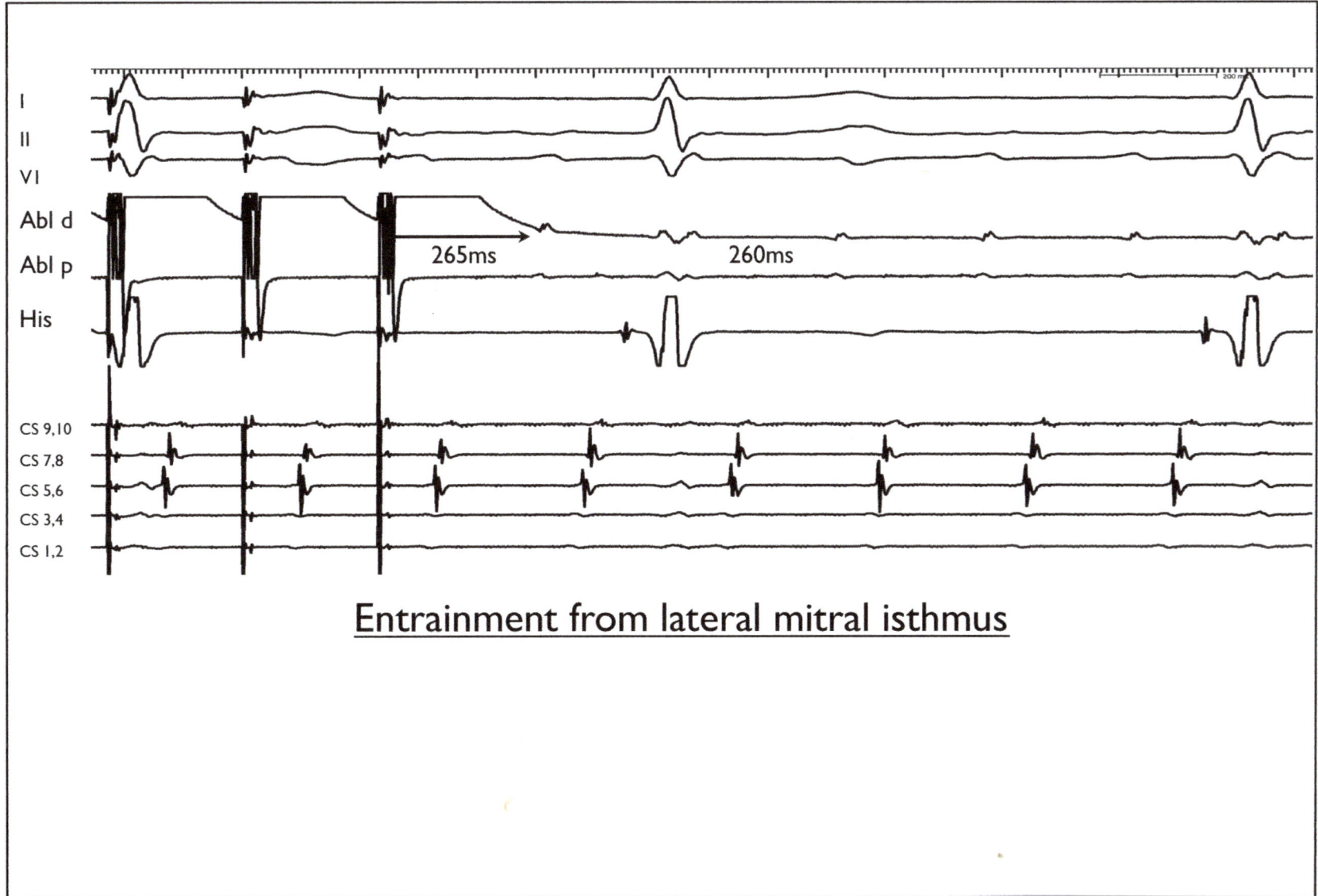

Entrainment from lateral mitral isthmus

Question 2

During ablation, the following phenomenon is seen. What should be the next step?

A) Discontinue radiofrequency application immediately and monitor AV conduction

B) Re-map atrial flutter

C) Check for mitral block

D) Continue ablation

Figure 3.C.4

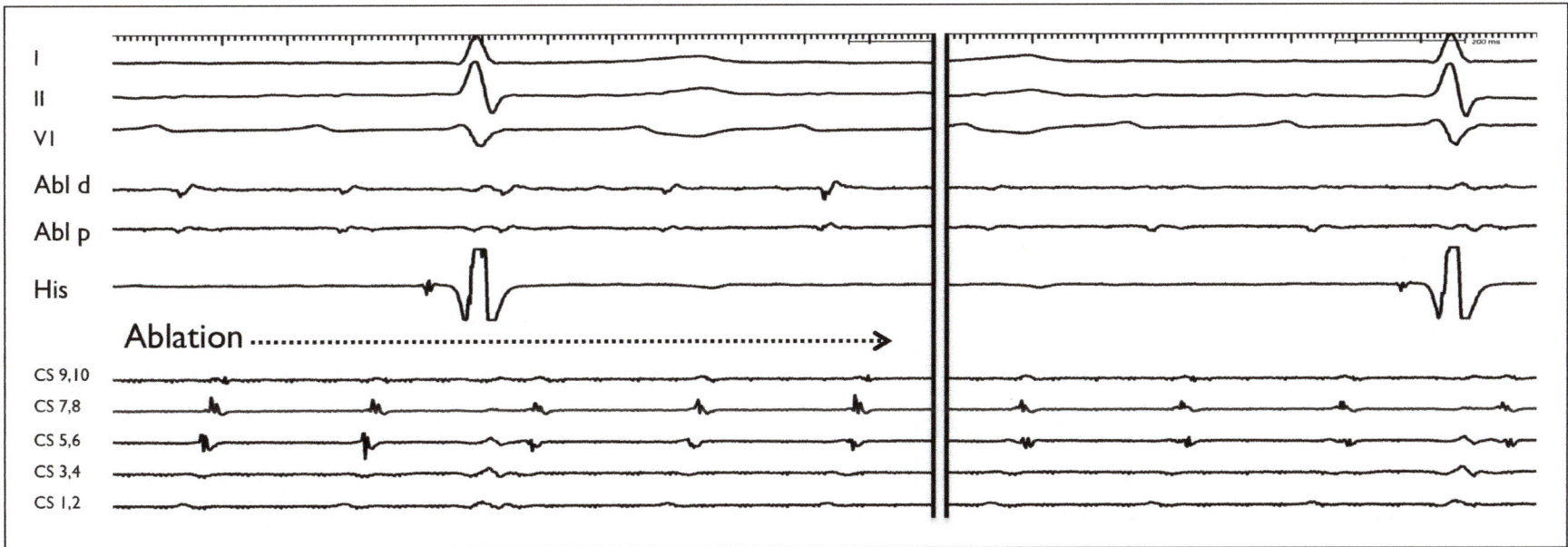

Answer 2

The correct answer is **D**. Ablation should be continued.

Ablation in the mitral isthmus is anatomically remote from the AV node and left sided His and unlikely to result in heart block. Additionally, the His catheter demonstrates 4:1 block at the level of the AV node. The tachycardia cycle length is unchanged (260 ms), although activation in the coronary sinus appears to be different from the initial flutter. This suggests a transition to a different flutter and/or the development of mitral block.

Coronary sinus (CS) electrograms represent a superimposition of far-field left atrial endocardial activation and near-field epicardial component. Closer examination of the electrograms in the CS demonstrate delay or block in the local CS musculature, which gives the appearance that activation is reversed.

The far-field left atrial component, which reflects the endocardial left atrial activation, still proceeds from distal to proximal, indicating that the same flutter continues. Misinterpretation of CS musculature as left atrial endocardial activation is a common pitfall when evaluating activation during flutter and mitral isthmus block.

Figure 3.C.5

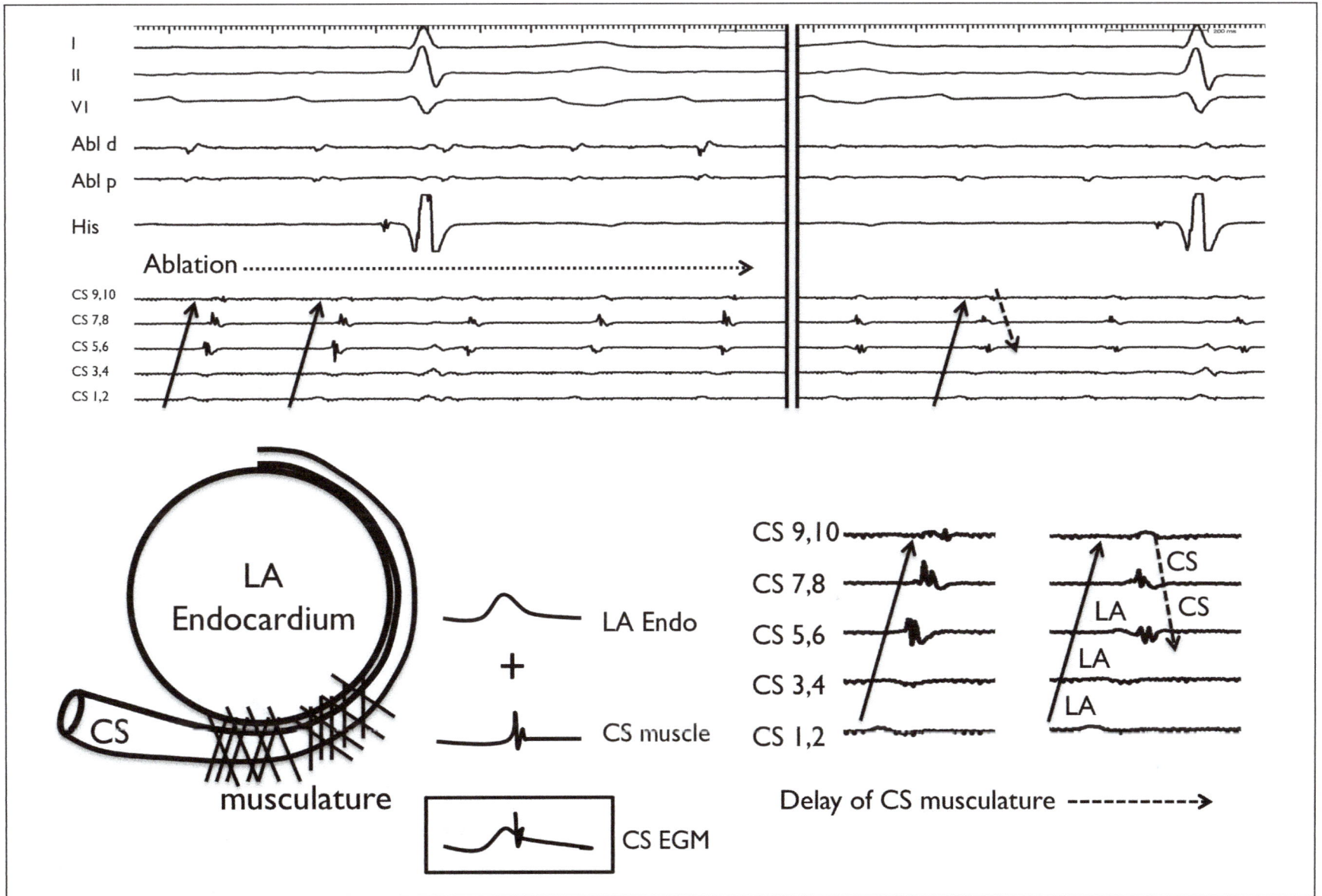

Figure 3.C.5

References

1. Miyazaki H, Stevenson WG, Stephenson K, Soejima K, Epstein LM. Entrainment mapping for rapid distinction of left and right atrial tachycardias. *Heart Rhythm*. 2006;3(5):516–523.

2. Pascale P, Shah AJ, Roten L, et al. Pattern and timing of the coronary sinus activation to guide rapid diagnosis of atrial tachycardia after atrial fibrillation ablation. *Circ Arrhythm Electrophysiol*. 2013;6(3):481–490.

3. Pascale P, Shah AJ, Roten L, et al. Disparate activation of the coronary sinus and inferior left atrium during atrial tachycardia after persistent atrial fibrillation ablation: prevalence, pitfalls, and impact on mapping. *J Cardiovasc Electrophysiol*. 2012;23(7):697–707.

Question

During RF ablation to isolate the pulmonary veins, the following bradyarrhythmia is observed.

Catheter position during the ablation lesion is shown in the RAO and LAO projections.

What is the likely mechanism of this brady-arrhythmia?

A) Thermal injury to the sinus node

B) Thermal injury to the compact AV node

C) Increased vagal tone secondary to ablation of a ganglionated plexus

D) Increased vagal tone secondary to injury of the phrenic nerve

E) Thermal injury to the sinus nodal artery

Figure 3.D.1

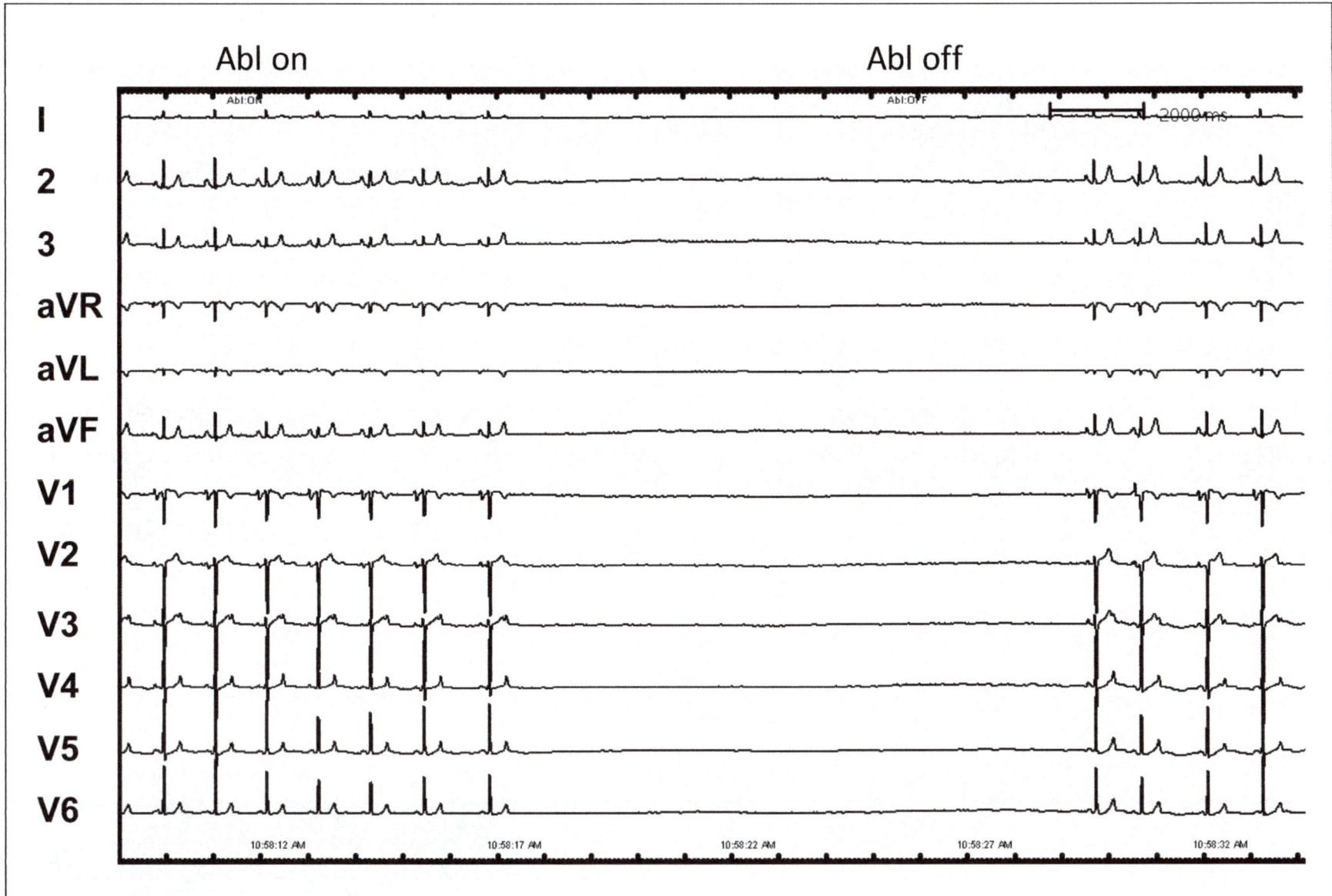

Figure 3.D.2

RAO

LAO

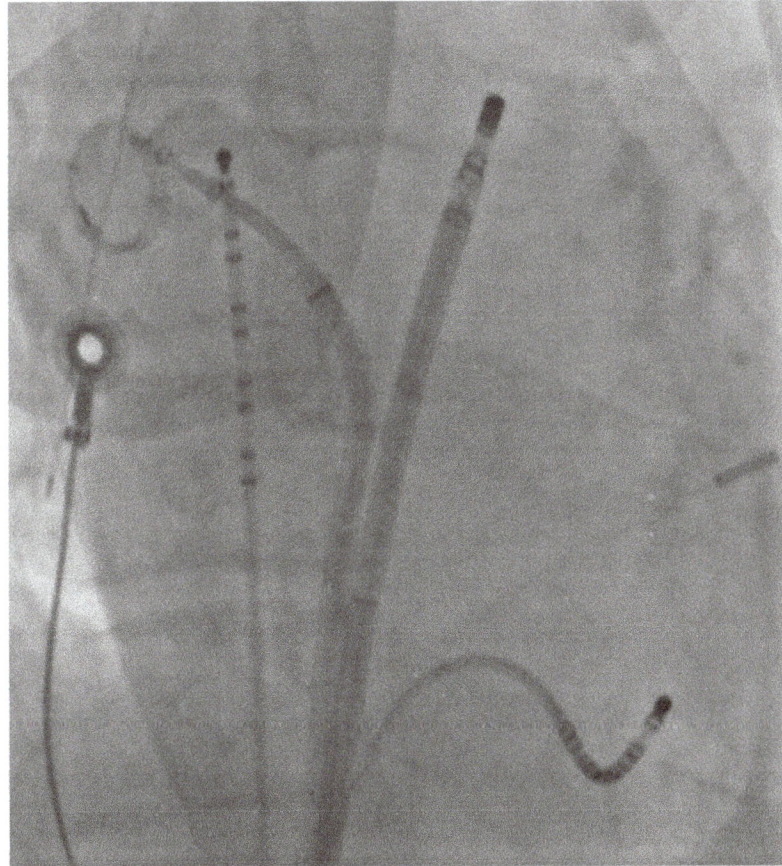
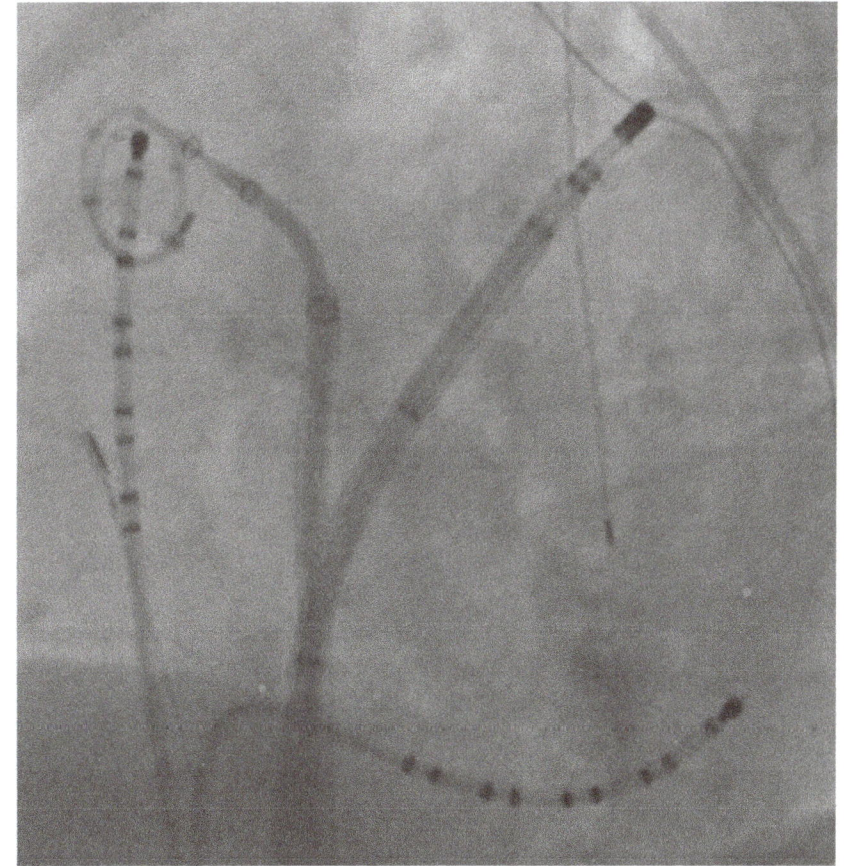

*A*nswer

The correct answer is **C**. During ablation, the sinus rate slows and then arrests, as evidenced by an absence of P waves. Several seconds after discontinuing ablation, the sinus node recovers. Injury to the compact AV node would cause AV block, rather than sinus arrest.

The ablation catheter is positioned at the top of the left superior pulmonary vein. Thus, thermal injury directly to the sinus node or to the sinus nodal artery are both unlikely. The sinus node is located at the superior aspect of the right atrium, at the junction with the superior vena cava. The sinus nodal artery can be injured when performing linear ablation from the right pulmonary veins to the septal mitral annulus ("anterior or septal line"), as is commonly done to treat mitral annular flutter. The right phrenic nerve can be injured when ablating along the septal aspect of the right pulmonary veins. Injury to the phrenic nerve causes diaphragmatic paralysis, not increased vagal tone.

Ganglionated plexi (GP) are frequently located around the pulmonary veins, including the roof. Some investigators advocate mapping and ablating GPs to improve outcomes following atrial fibrillation ablation. **When ablating a GP, changes in autonomic tone can cause sinus arrest, AV block, or vasodilation**.

References

1. Katritsis DG, Pokushalov E, Romanov A, Giazitzoglou E, Siontis GC, Po SS, et al. Autonomic denervation added to pulmonary vein isolation for paroxysmal atrial fibrillation: a randomized clinical trial. *J Am Coll Cardiol.* 2013;62:2318–2325.
2. Yokokawa M, Sundaram B, Oral H, Morady F, Chugh A. The course of the sinus node artery and its impact on achieving linear block at the left atrial roof in patients with persistent atrial fibrillation. *Heart Rhythm.* 2012;9:1395–1402.

Question

A 73-year-old man underwent catheter ablation for drug-refractory atrial fibrillation. Following circumferential ablation around both sets of pulmonary veins, the following electrograms were recorded.

Catheter position is shown in RAO and LAO projections.

What conclusion can be drawn regarding conduction between the pulmonary veins and left atrium?

A) Entrance block is present in the left pulmonary veins

B) Exit block is present in the left pulmonary veins

C) Entrance block is present in the right pulmonary veins

D) Exit block is present in the right pulmonary veins

E) Neither entrance nor exit block is present

Figure 3.E.1

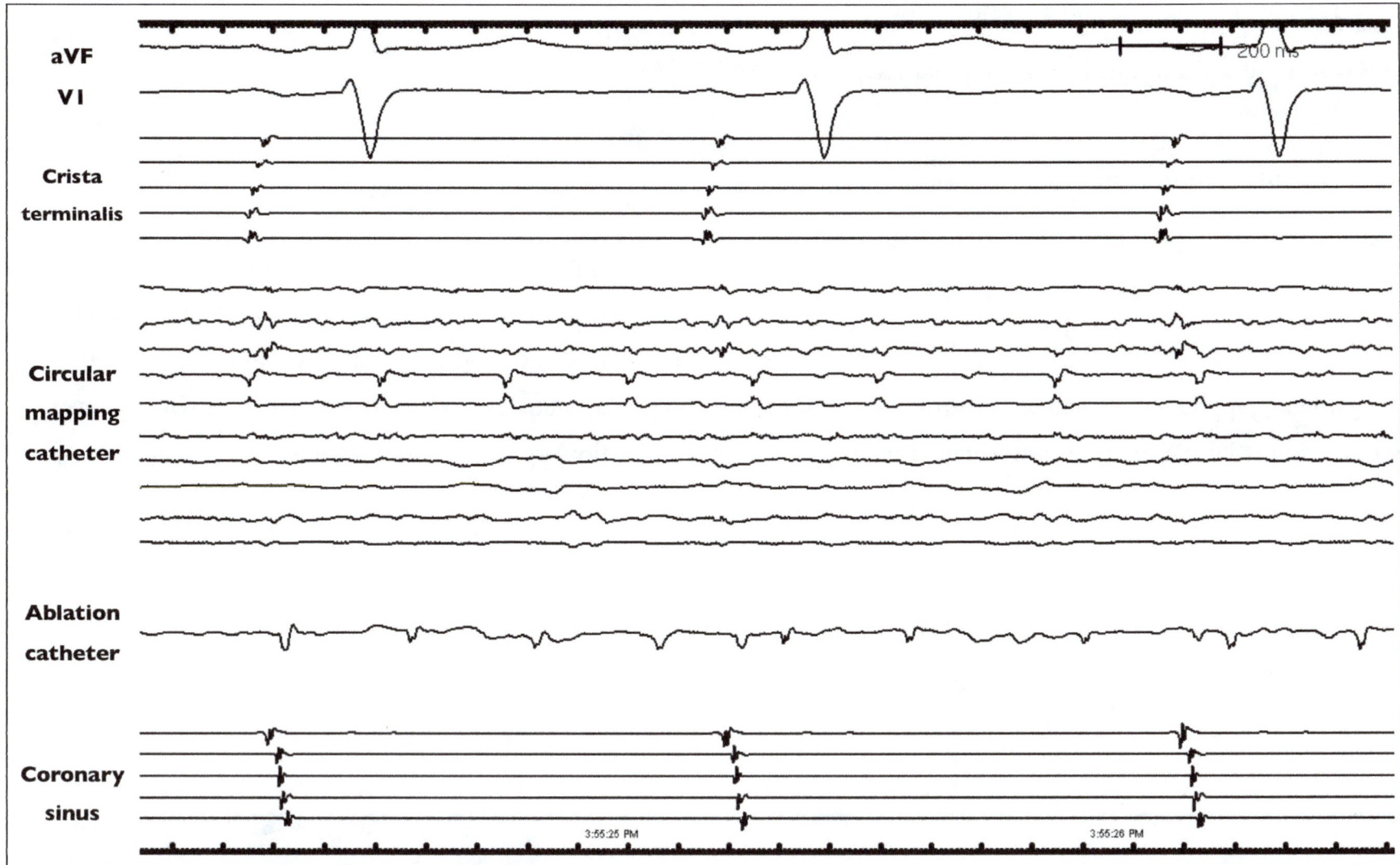

Figure 3.E.2

RAO

LAO

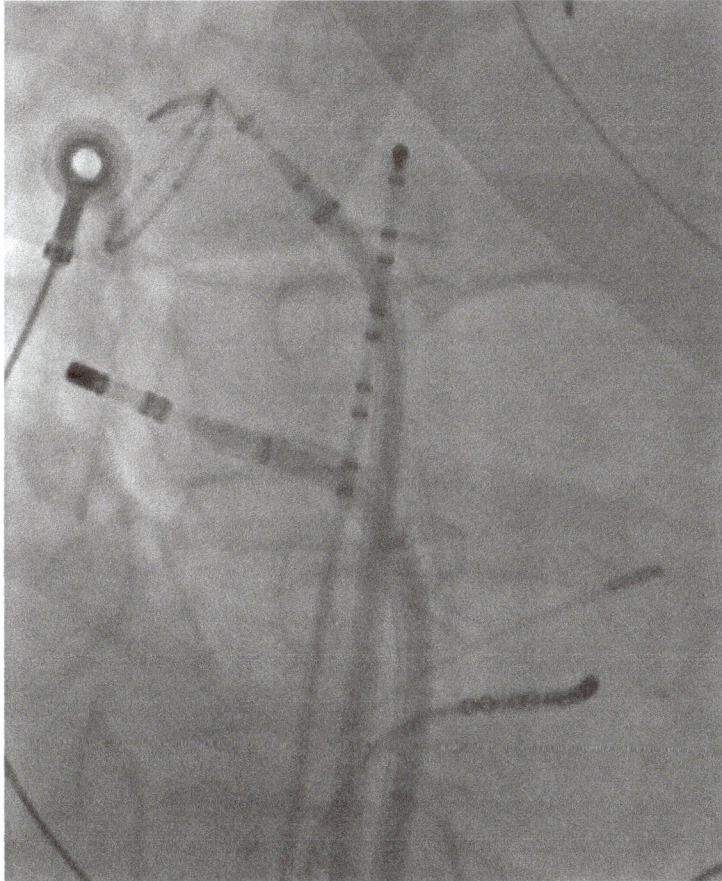
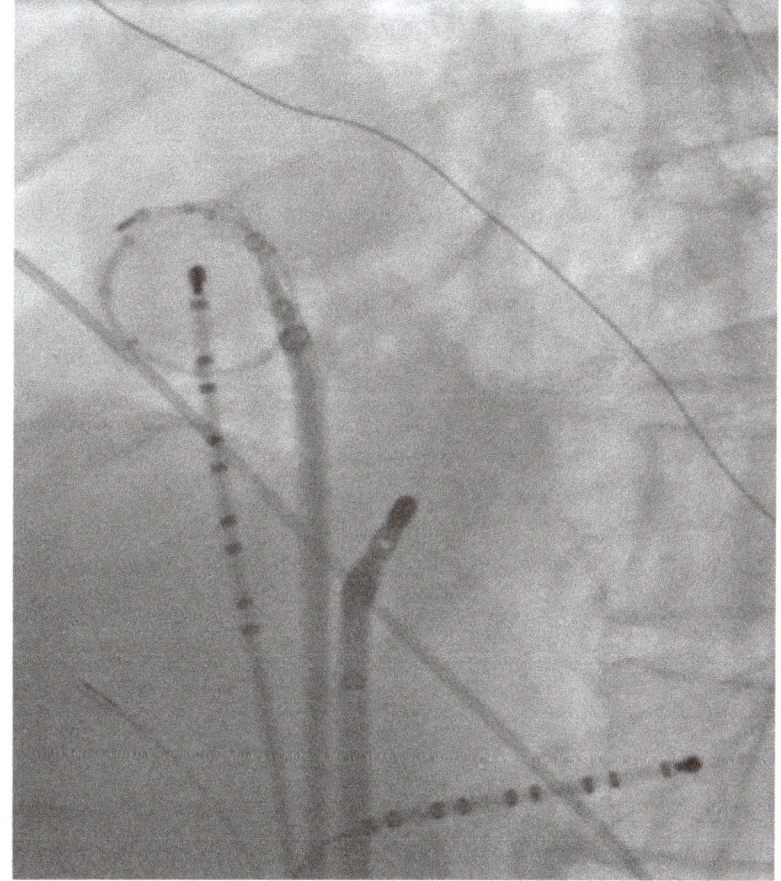

Answer

The correct answer is **D**. The circular mapping catheter is positioned in the right superior pulmonary vein and the ablation catheter in the right inferior pulmonary vein. While the pulmonary veins are in atrial fibrillation, the atria remain in sinus rhythm, as reflected by the surface electrocardiogram, as well as recordings from the coronary sinus and crista terminalis. **Exit block is present, as the rapid depolarizations within the right pulmonary veins do not conduct to the atrium**. Entrance conduction cannot be assessed while the right pulmonary veins are fibrillating.

Shown for comparison are the circular mapping catheter in the left superior pulmonary vein and the ablation catheter in the left inferior pulmonary vein.

Figure 3.E.3

RAO

LAO

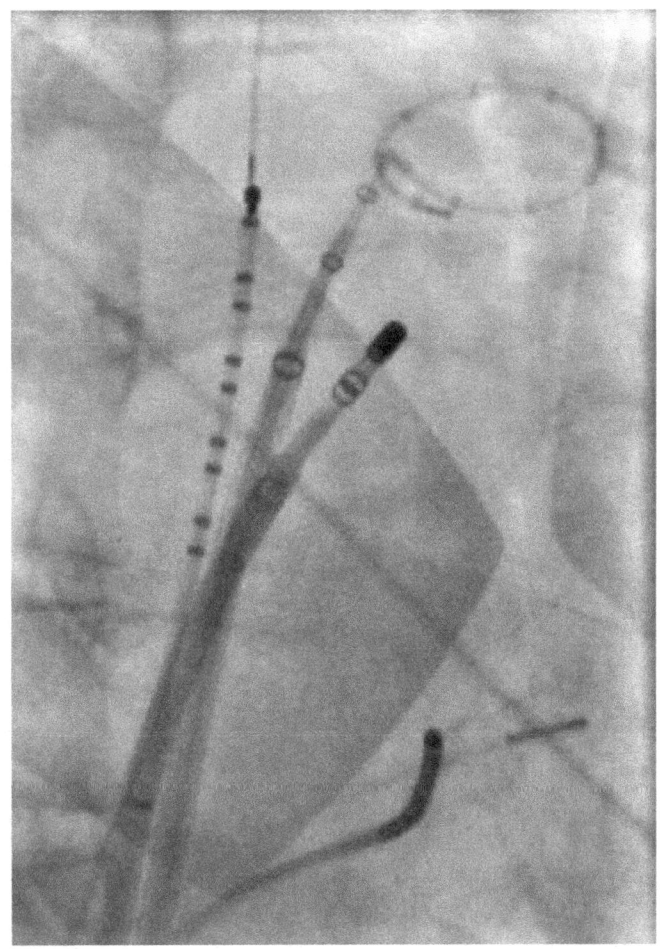
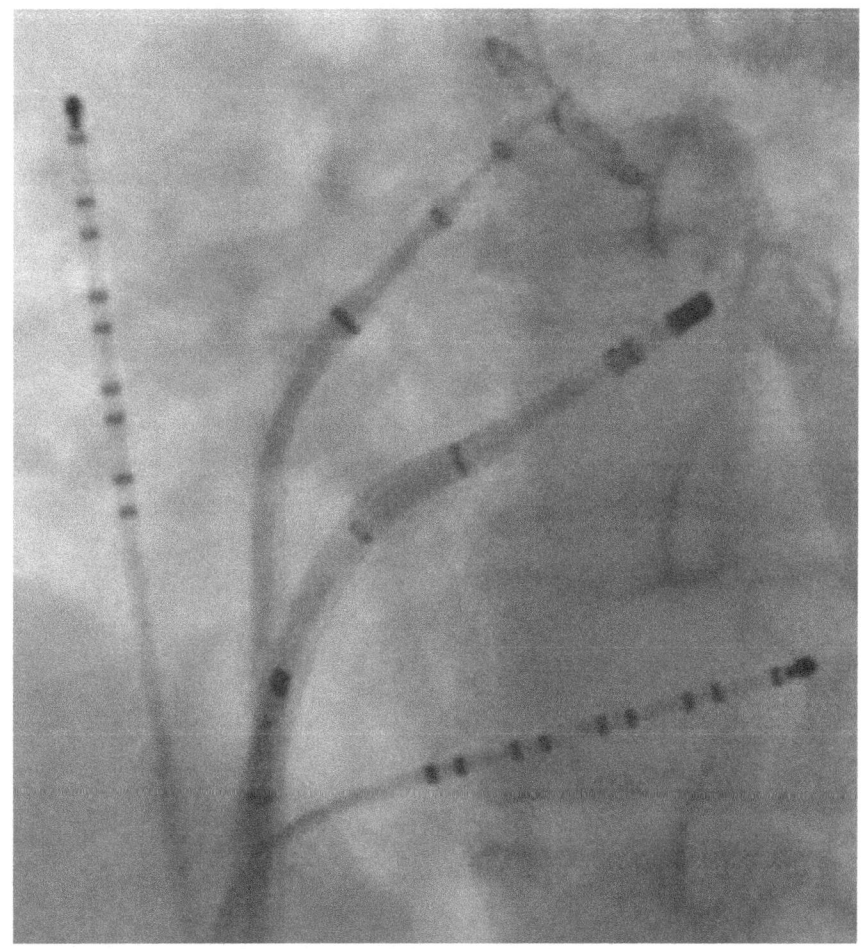

Reference

1. Gerstenfeld EP, Dixit S, Callans D, Rho R, Rajawat Y, Zado E, et al. Utility of exit block for identifying electrical isolation of the pulmonary veins. *J Cardiovasc Electrophysiol*. 2002;13:971–979.

PART 4

Ventricular Tachycardia (VT)

Question

A 70-year-old man presented with recurrent ventricular tachycardia. Entrainment mapping was performed from the LV.

Where is the ablation catheter located?

A) Outer loop

B) Inner blind loop

C) Isthmus entrance site

D) Isthmus exit site

Figure 4.A.1

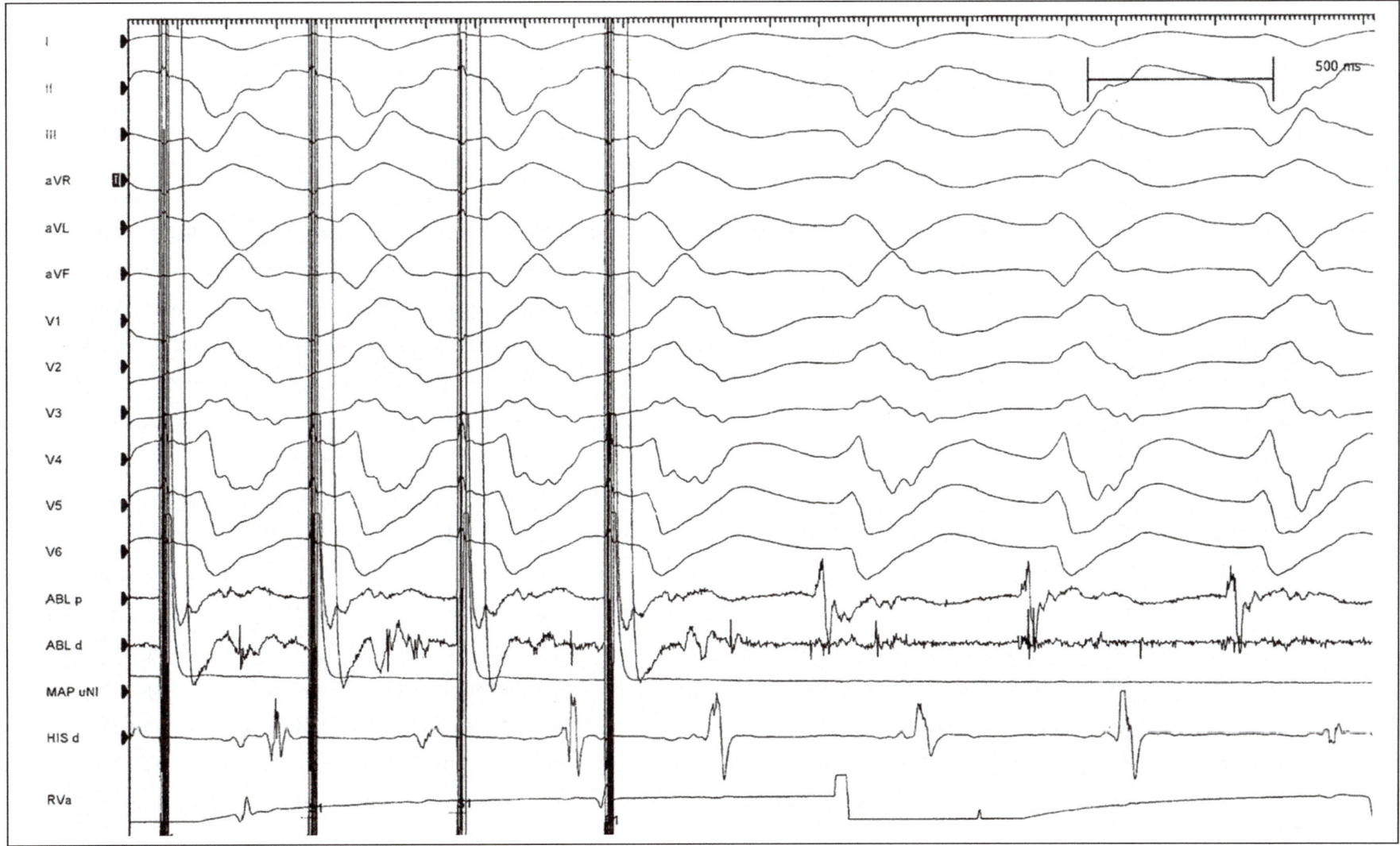

Figure 4.A.1

Answer

The correct answer is **D**. The tachycardia cycle length (565 ms) is accelerated to the pacing cycle length (400 ms), and the tachycardia resumes after termination of pacing. Typically, however, during entrainment maneuvers, it is best to pace 10 to 30 ms faster than the tachycardia cycle length.

In this case, the paced QRS morphology is nearly identical to the tachycardia QRS morphology complex (the initial R wave of tachycardia complexes in V_4 are taller and sharper than paced complexes; the initial R wave of tachycardia complexes in V_5 are taller than paced complexes). Presence of concealed entrainment indicates that the pacing site is within the tachycardia circuit and rules out a remote site of pacing or outer loop site.

Measurement of the postpacing interval is often difficult because of low voltage in the area of scarring. In this case, a larger electrogram is the far-field activation (marked by ★), and the small potential indicated by an arrow is the near-field (local) potential.

The near-field electrogram can be discerned because it should be captured during pacing and thus brought very close to the stimulus, or in many cases is not seen due to the high output of the pacing stimulus. The sharp potential marked by the dot is dissociated from the tachycardia. The postpacing interval is equal to the tachycardia cycle length; therefore, the pacing site is within the isthmus or in the inner loop. Identical stimulus to QRS and electrogram to QRS duration measured on the ablation catheter rules out a blind loop or adjacent bystander site.

The location of the pacing site within the isthmus can be determined by the time taken for the stimulus to exit the isthmus (indicated by the QRS). The proportion of the stimulus to QRS duration in relation to tachycardia cycle length (100 : 560) is less than 30%, which confirms that the pacing site is near the exit of the isthmus. Ablation at this site led to termination within 2 seconds of RF application.

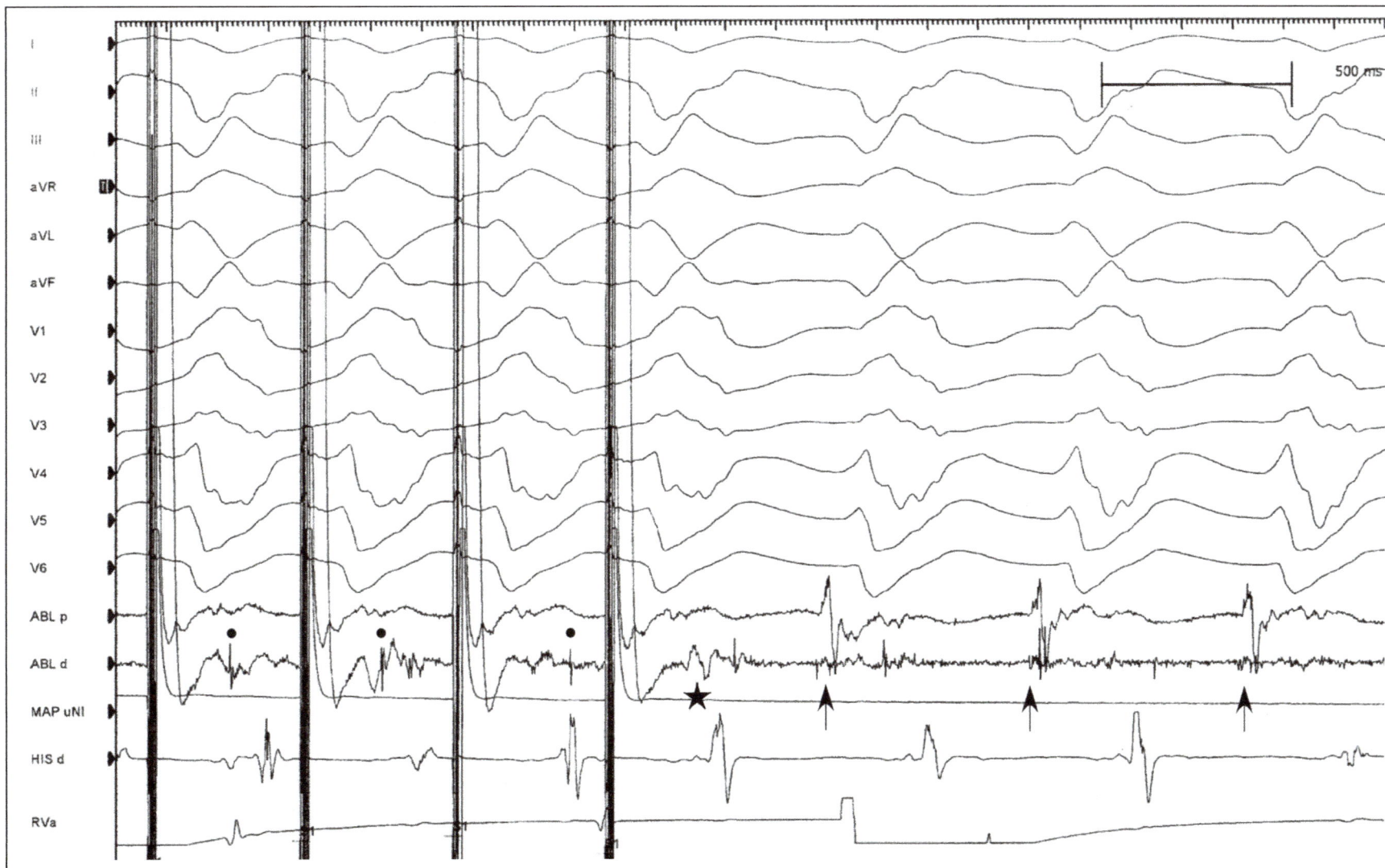

Figure 4.A.2

References

1. Stevenson WG, Khan H, Sager P, et al. Identification of reentry circuit sites during catheter mapping and radiofrequency ablation of ventricular tachycardia late after myocardial infarction. *Circulation.* 1993;88:1647–1670.

2. Stevenson WG, Sager PT, Friedman PL. Entrainment techniques for mapping atrial and ventricular tachycardias. *J Cardiovasc Electrophysiol.* 1995;6:201–216.

Question

A 50-year-old man with history of remote myocardial infarction presented with the following ventricular tachycardia.

Based on the ECG morphology, where is the VT most likely to be exiting?

A) A

B) B

C) C

D) D

Figure 4.B.1

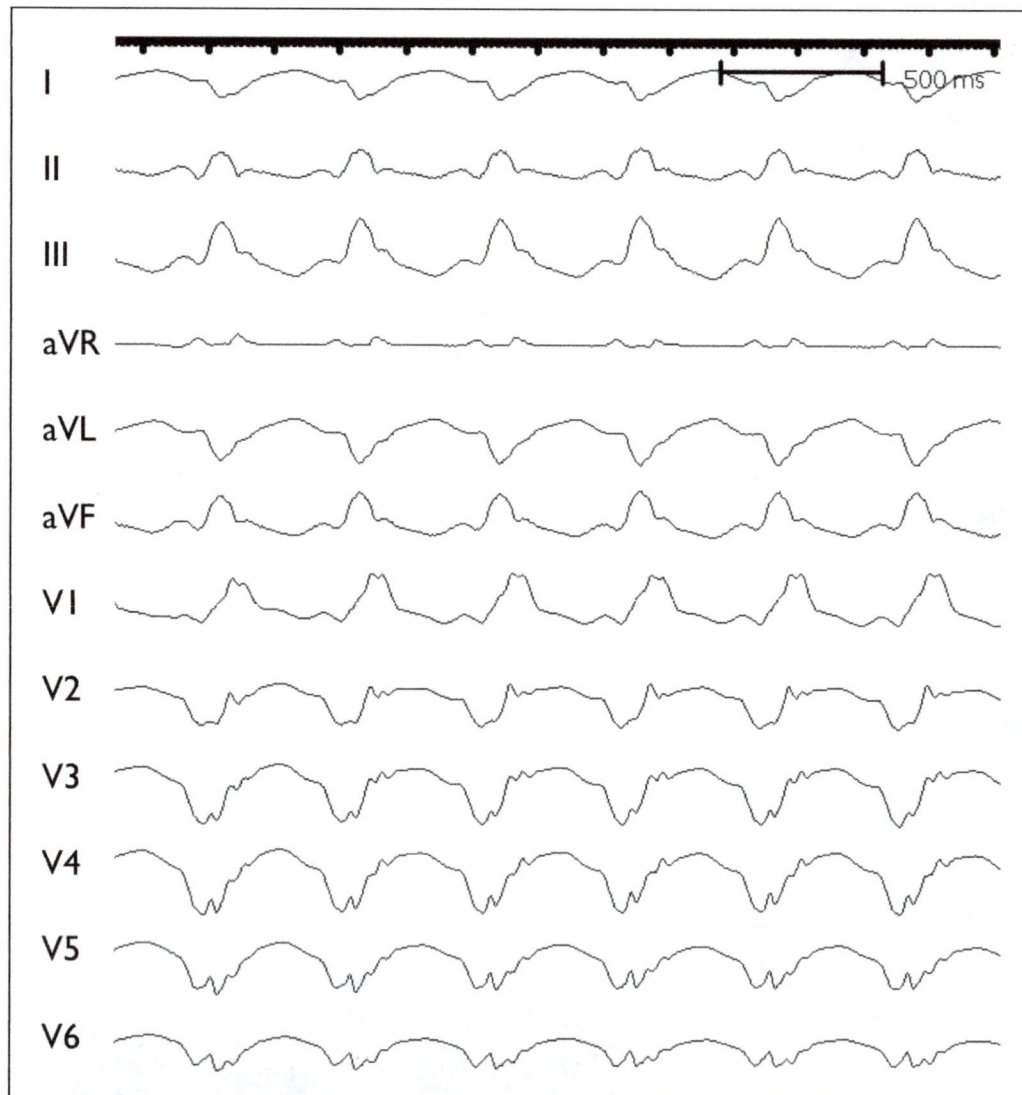

Figure 4.B.2

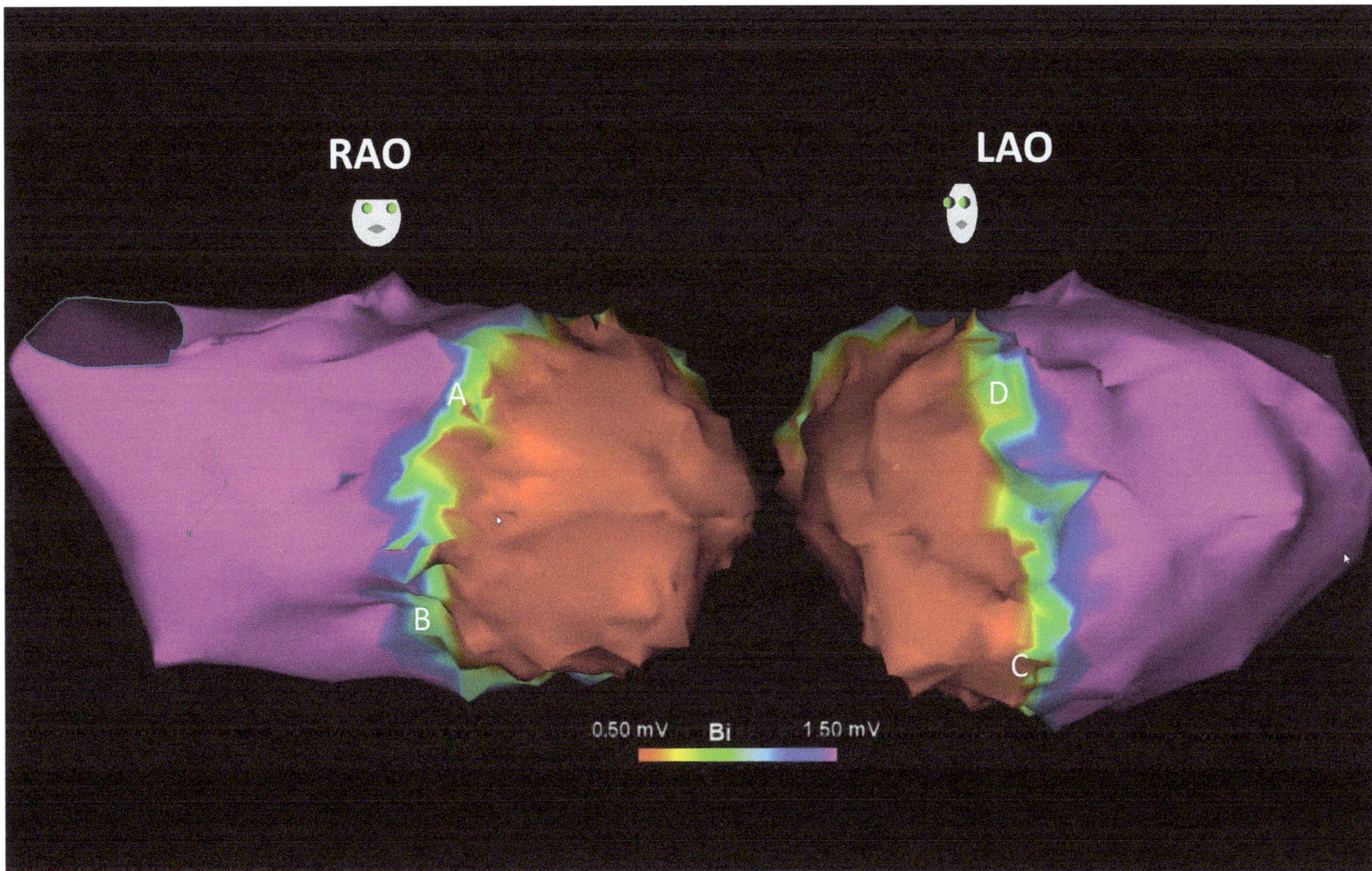

Answer

The correct answer is **D**. The voltage map demonstrates a large, anteroapical scar, consistent with occlusion of the left anterior descending coronary artery. The VT has a right bundle configuration in lead V_1 with a right inferior axis, suggestive of **exit along the anterolateral aspect of the scar**. Even though the VT is exiting the scar relatively basally, the precordial transition is very early, given absence of healthy myocardium apical to the exit site.

This is confirmed by the minimal positive forces throughout the precordium during atrial paced rhythm.

VT exiting from the septal side of the scar (A and B) would have a left bundle configuration in lead V_1 and positivity in lead I. VT exiting from the inferolateral aspect of the scar (C) would be superiorly directed.

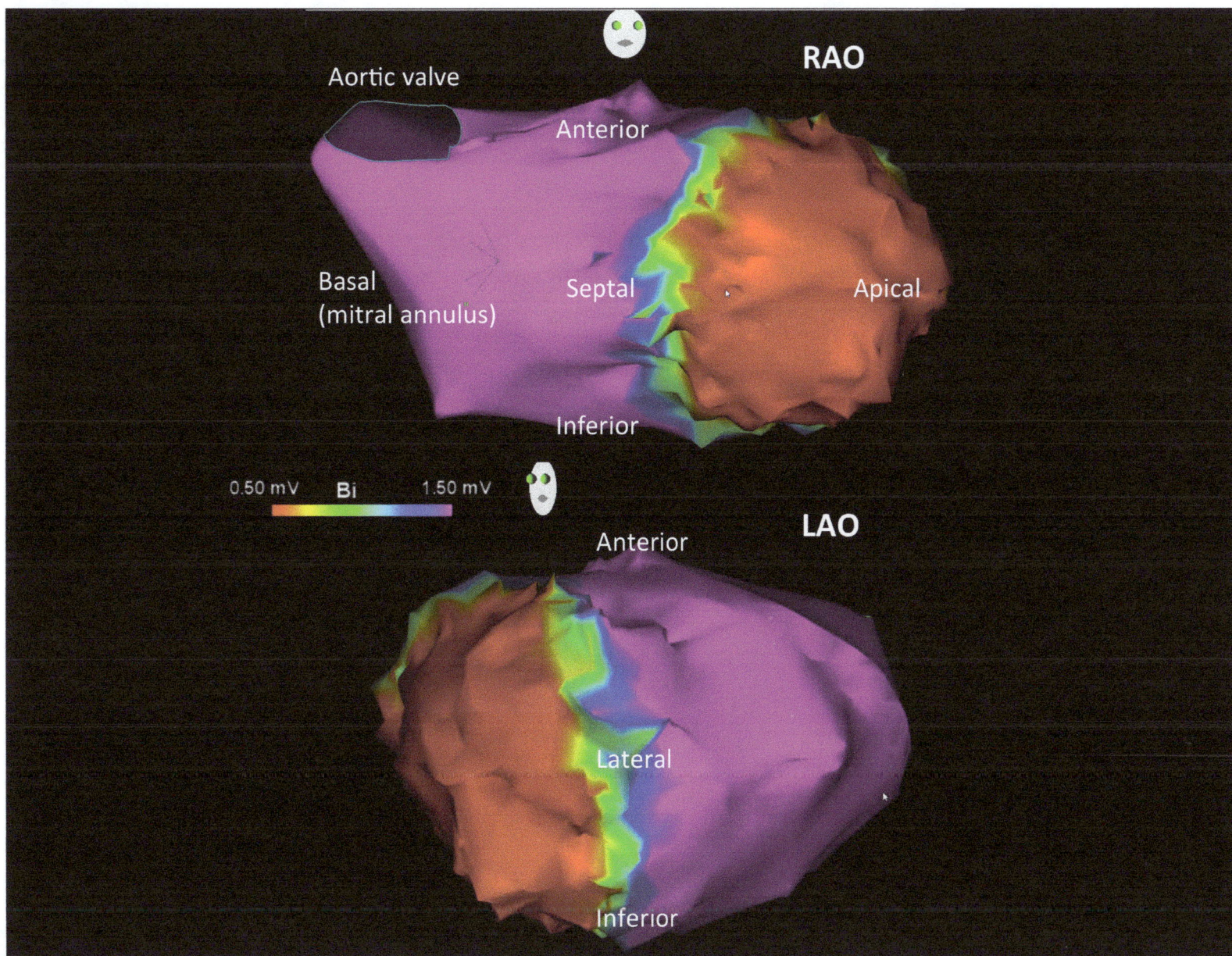

Figure 4.B.3

Figure 4.B.4

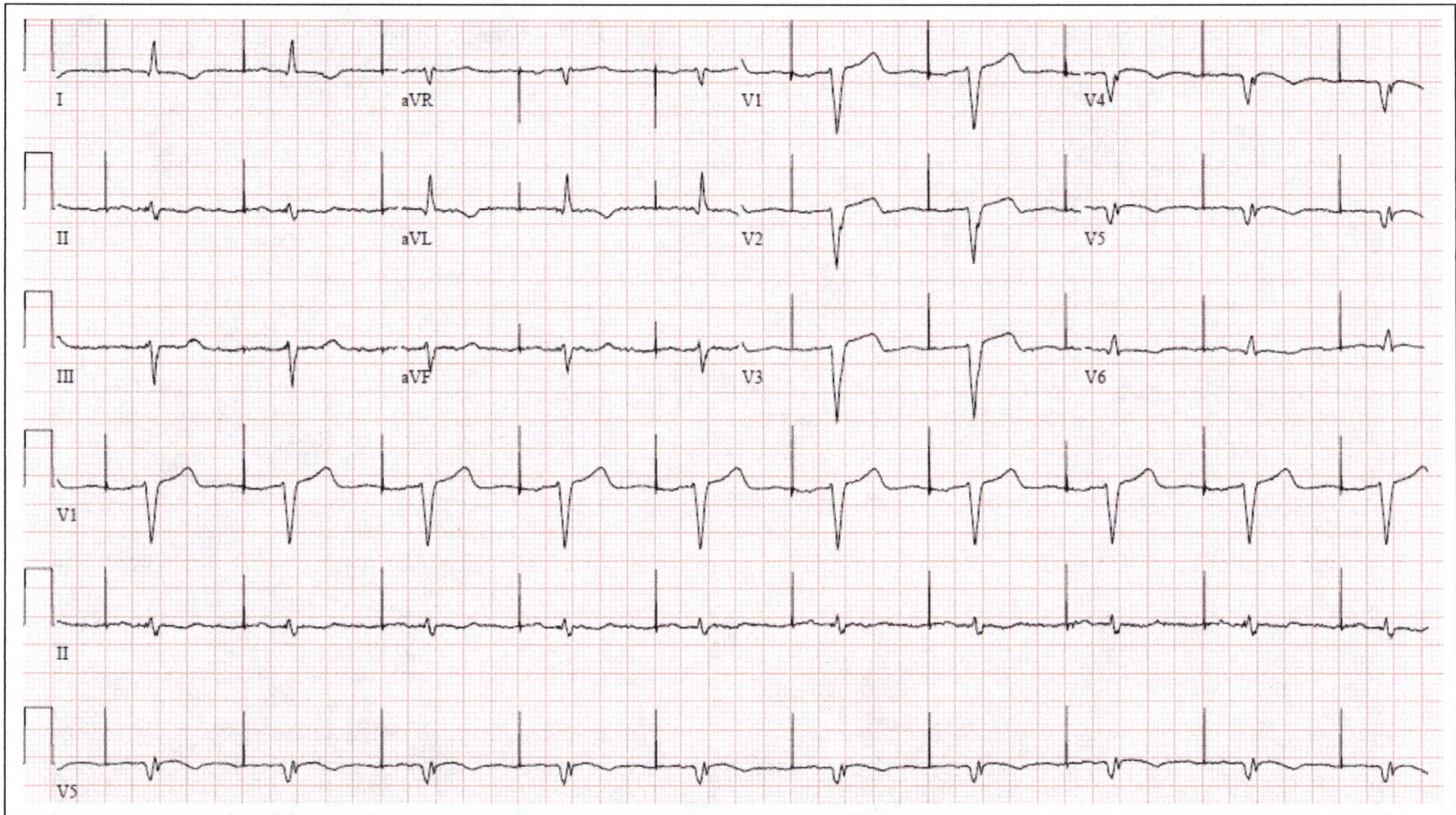

Reference

1. Miller JM, Marchlinski FE, Buxton AE, Josephson ME. Relationship between the 12-lead electrocardiogram during ventricular tachycardia and endocardial site of origin in patients with coronary artery disease. *Circulation*. 1988;77:759–766.

Question

What is the most likely substrate in this patient with four ventricular tachycardia morphologies?

A) Arrhythmogenic right ventricular cardiomyopathy

B) Anterior myocardial infarction

C) Idiopathic

D) Nonischemic left ventricular cardiomyopathy with basal lateral predominance

E) Nonischemic left ventricular cardiomyopathy with septal predominance

Figure 4.C.1

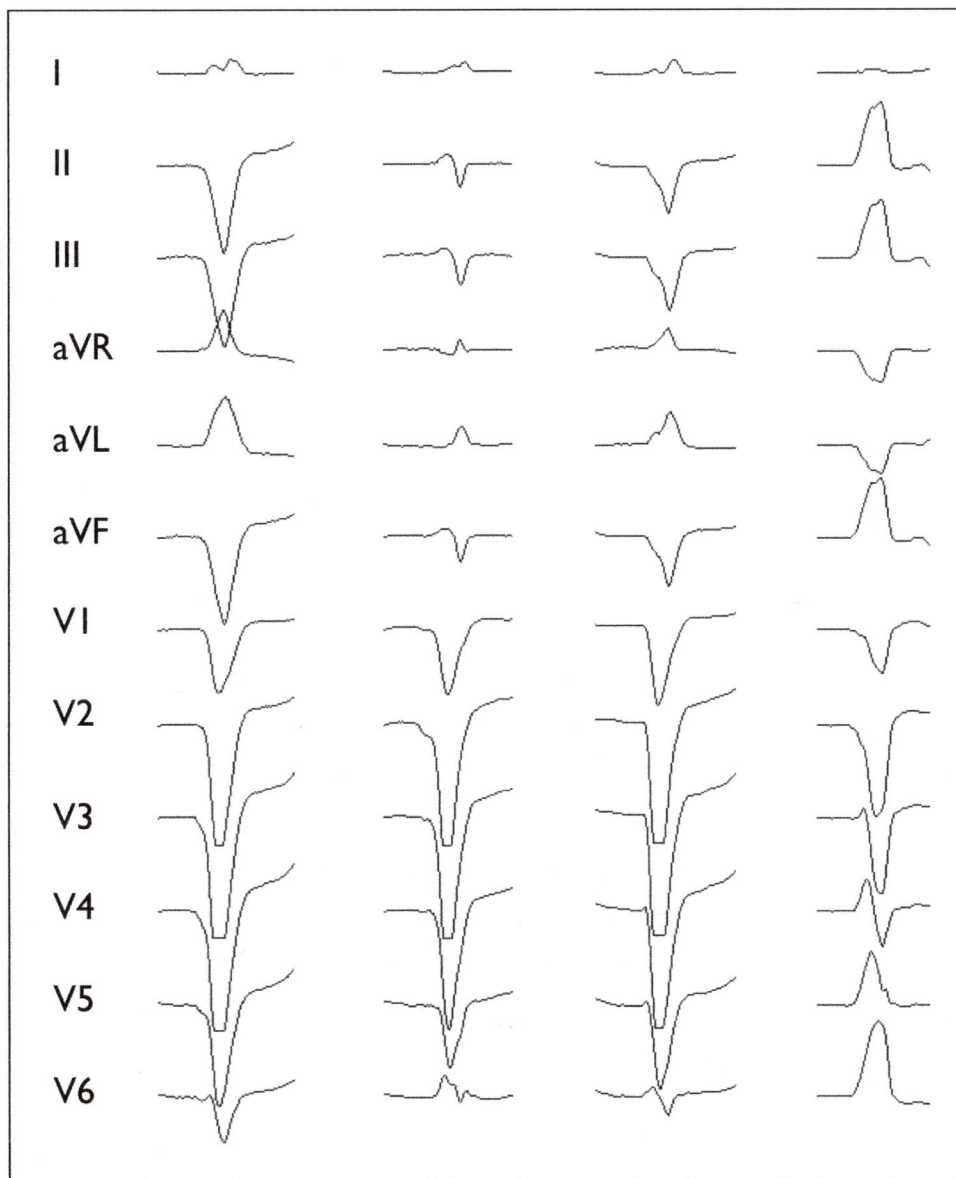

I
II
III
aVR
aVL
aVF
V1
V2
V3
V4
V5
V6

*A*nswer

The correct answer is **A**. All four ventricular tachycardia morphologies have a left bundle configuration in lead V_1, with late precordial transition, ranging from V_5 to negative concordance, consistent with RV free wall exit sites. The first three morphologies are superiorly directed and the fourth is inferiorly directed. While the fourth VT in isolation could be an idiopathic RVOT tachycardia, patients with idiopathic VT usually have a single morphology only. **Multiple morphologies raise suspicion for a scar-based substrate**. Further, RVOT VT in the setting of ARVC tends to be wider, more notched, and with later precordial transition than idiopathic RVOT VT.

VTs in the setting of anterior myocardial infarction have a right or left bundle configuration in lead V_1, with the axis depending on which portion of the scar they exit from. VTs originating from basal lateral scar have a right bundle configuration in lead V_1 with late precordial transition and rightward axis. VTs originating from septal scar can exit along the right or left ventricular septum, but rarely the RV free wall.

References

1. Hoffmayer KS, Machado ON, Marcus GM, et al. Electrocardiographic comparison of ventricular arrhythmias in patients with arrhythmogenic right ventricular cardiomyopathy and right ventricular outflow tract tachycardia. *J Am Coll Cardiol.* 2011;58(8):831–838.

2. Marchlinski FE, Zado E, Dixit S, Gerstenfeld E, Callans DJ, Hsia H, et al. Electroanatomic substrate and outcome of catheter ablative therapy for ventricular tachycardia in setting of right ventricular cardiomyopathy. *Circulation.* 2004;110:2293–2298.

Question

What is the most likely site of PVC origin?

A) Free wall right ventricular outflow tract

B) Septal right ventricular outflow tract

C) Right coronary cusp

D) Left coronary cusp

E) Aortomitral continuity

Figure 4.D.1

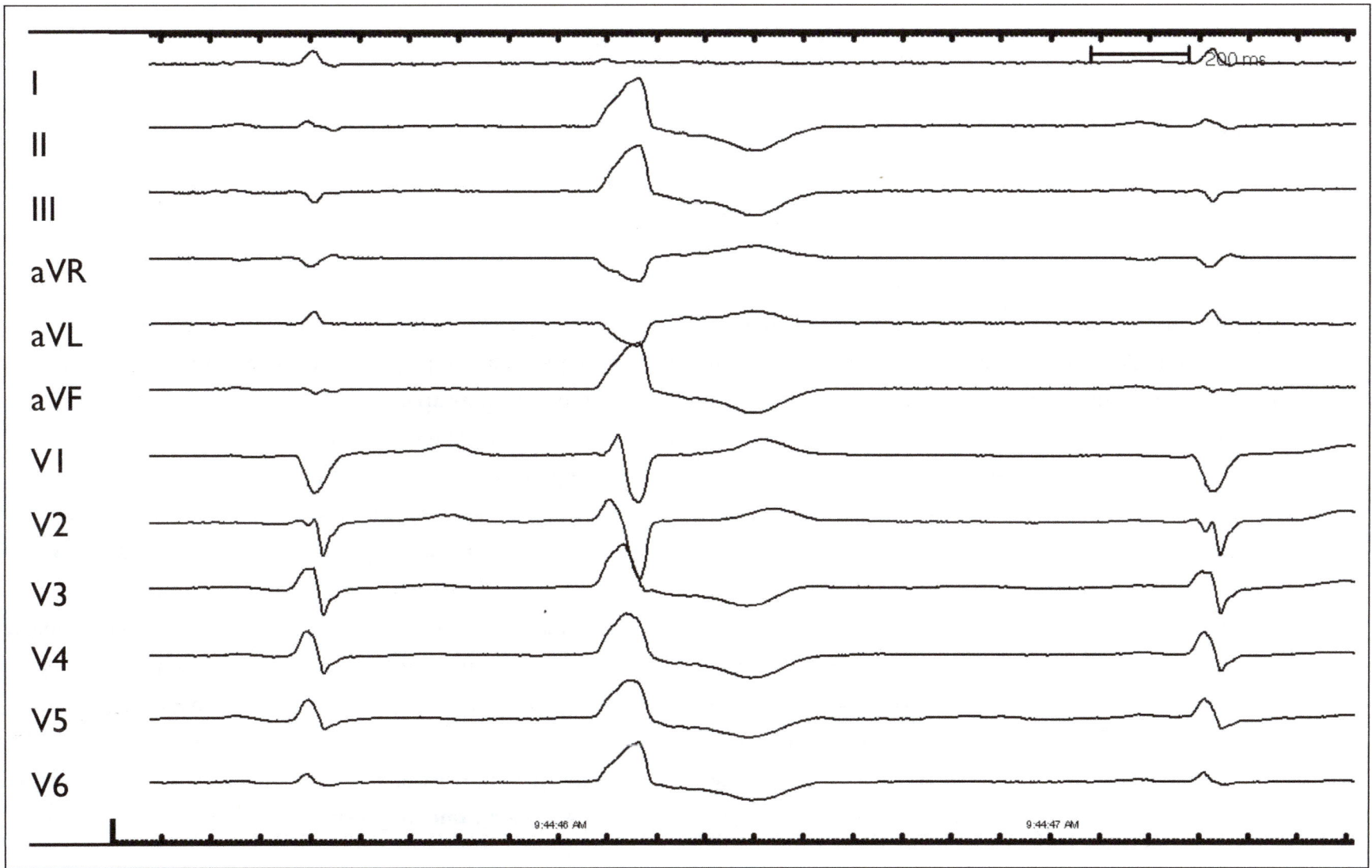

Answer

The correct answer is **C. The PVC has a left bundle configuration in lead V$_1$, with an inferior axis, consistent with an outflow tract site of origin**.

As this CT image demonstrates, the free wall of the right ventricular outflow tract lies immediately beneath the sternum and precordial ECG leads. Therefore, an activation wavefront originating from the free wall of the right ventricular outflow tract moves away from the precordial leads, generating negativity in lead V$_1$ with a late precordial transition. As one moves posteriorly within the chest, from the septal right ventricular outflow tract to the right coronary cusp, left coronary cusp, aortomitral continuity, and superior mitral annulus, the activation wavefront shifts progressively toward the precordial ECG leads, generating greater degrees of positivity in lead V$_1$ and earlier precordial transitions.

This PVC transitions at lead V$_3$. Outflow tract PVCs that transition at V$_4$ or later originate from the right ventricular outflow tract. Outflow tract PVCs that transition at or before V$_2$ originate from the left ventricular outflow tract. PVCs that transition at V$_3$ can originate from the septal right ventricular outflow tract or right coronary cusp. Adjusting the PVC precordial transition for the sinus rhythm precordial transition by calculating the V$_2$ transition ratio can help distinguish right from left ventricular outflow tract sites of origin.

PVCs with a V$_2$ transition ratio >0.6 almost always originate from the left ventricular outflow tract. The V$_2$ transition ratio for this PVC is 1.7. Interestingly, the V$_3$ transition ratio is less useful for making this distinction. Activation mapping of both outflow tracts confirmed a right coronary cusp site of origin, and ablation here eliminated the PVC.

Figure 4.D.2

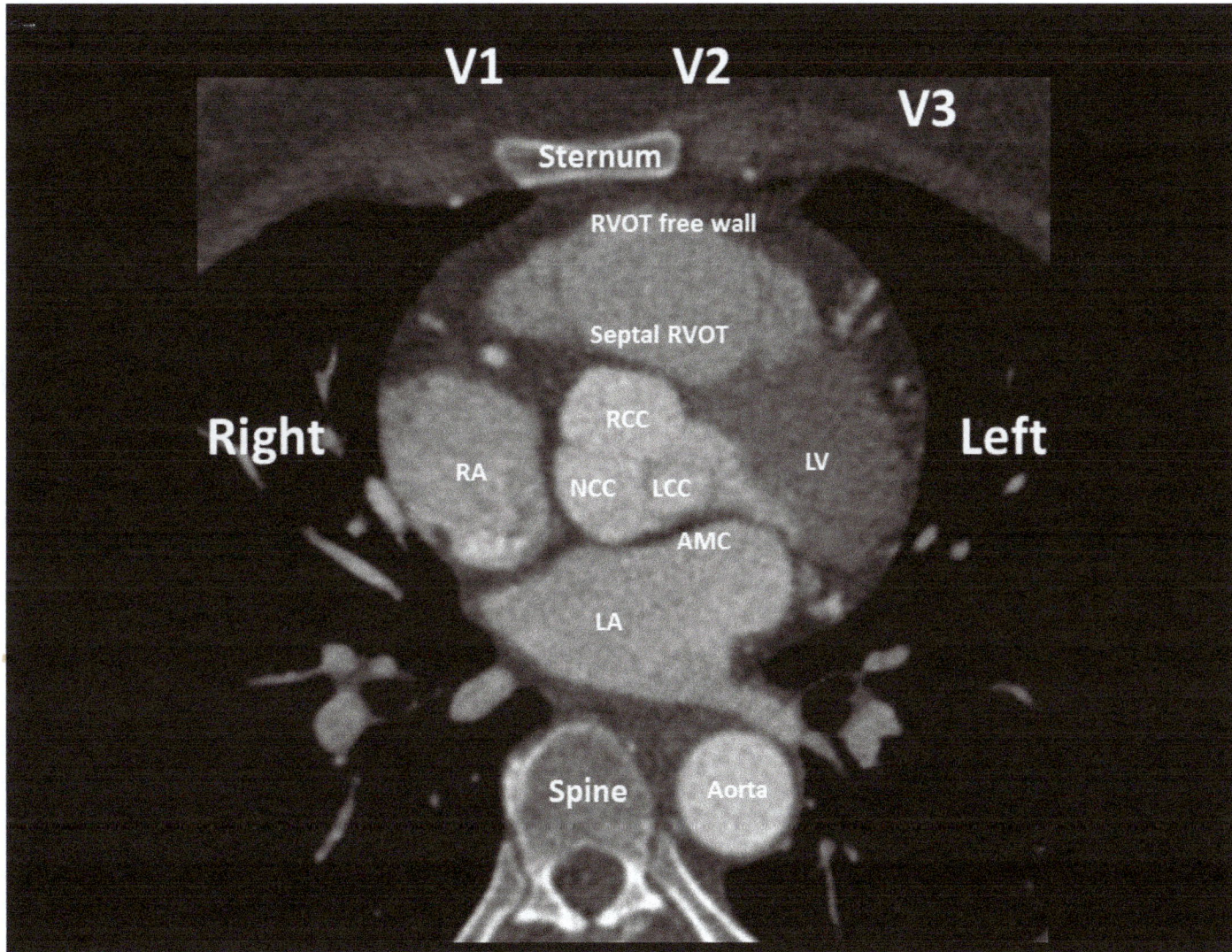

Source: Adapted from Liang JJ, Han, Y, Frankel DS. *Curr Treat Options Cardiovasc Med.* 2015 Feb: 17(2):363.

Figure 4.D.3

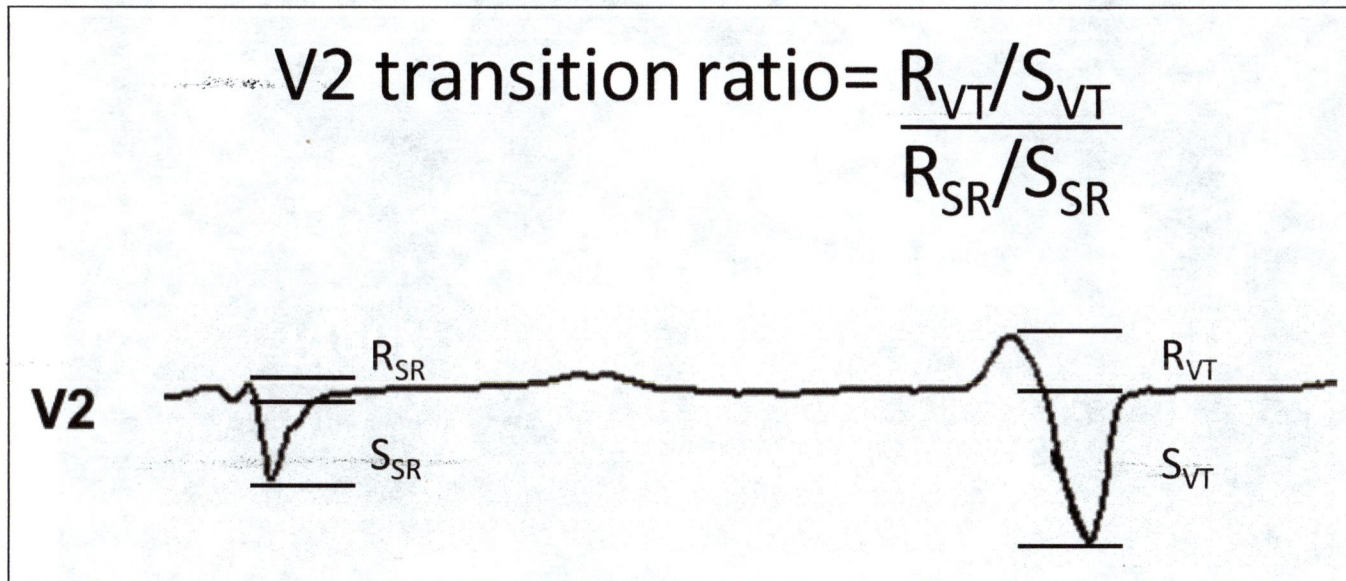

$$\text{V2 transition ratio} = \frac{R_{VT}/S_{VT}}{R_{SR}/S_{SR}}$$

Reference

1. Betensky BP, Park RE, Marchlinski FE, Hutchinson MD, Garcia FC, Dixit S, et al. The V(2) transition ratio: a new electrocardiographic criterion for distinguishing left from right ventricular outflow tract tachycardia origin. *J Am Coll Cardiol*. 2011;57:2255–2262.

Question

Pacing is delivered from the ablation catheter during ventricular tachycardia with the following response.

The ablation catheter is located in:

A) Adjacent bystander

B) Remote bystander

C) Outer loop

D) Isthmus

E) Exit

Figure 4.E.1

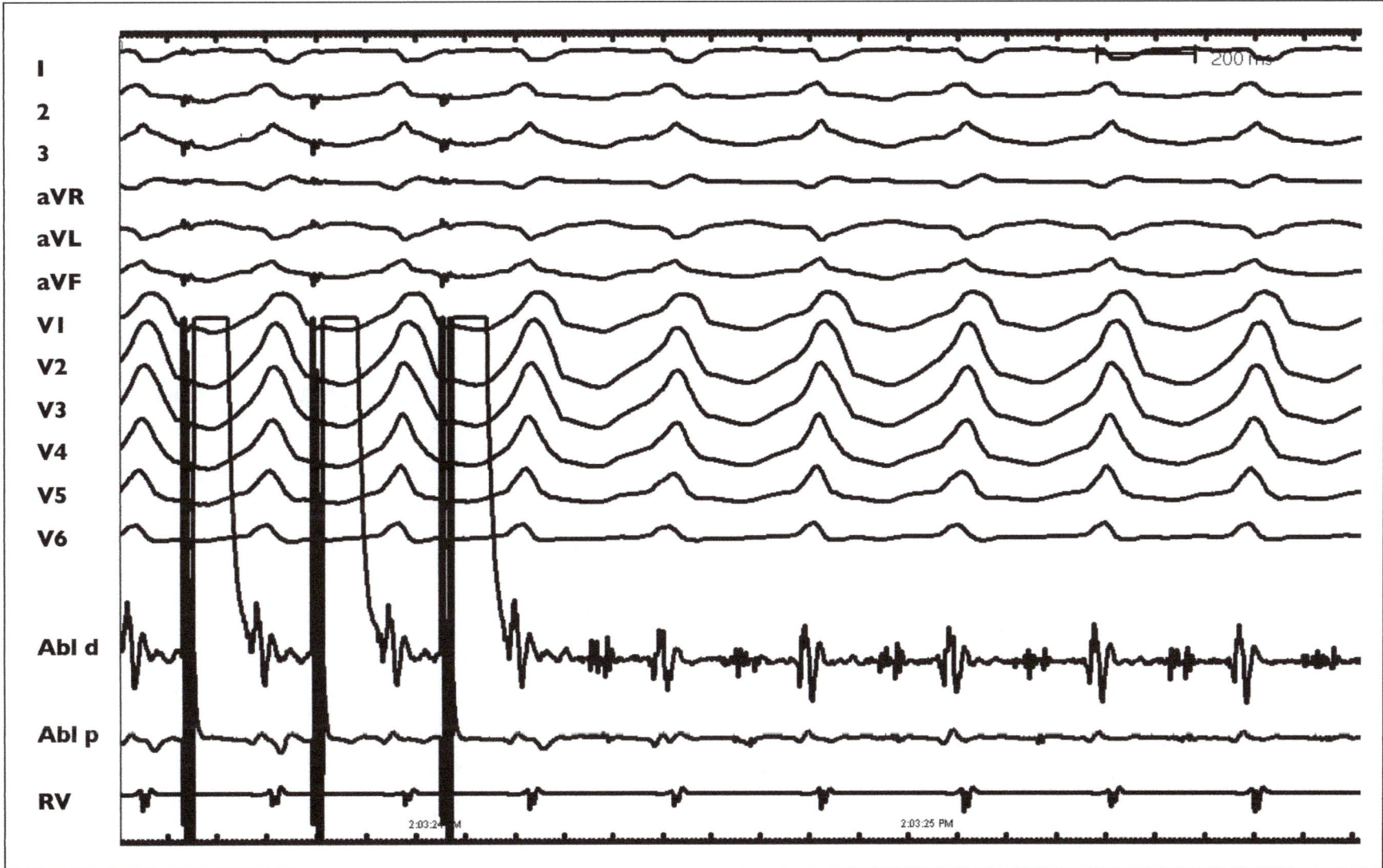

Answer

The correct answer is **D**. The paced QRS morphology is identical to the VT morphology, ruling out a remote bystander and an outer loop site. The postpacing interval is the same as the VT cycle length, ruling out remote and adjacent bystander sites. While the postpacing interval is long for both remote and adjacent bystander sites, manifest fusion is present at remote bystander sites, but not at adjacent bystander sites. The stimulus to QRS interval on the paced beat is 100 ms, which is 33% of the tachycardia cycle length. **Pacing at an isthmus site results in a stimulus to QRS interval between 30% and 70% of the tachycardia cycle length**. Pacing at an exit site results in a stimulus to QRS interval < 30% of the tachycardia cycle length. This is an excellent ablation site.

Reference

1. Stevenson WG, Khan H, Sager P, et al. Identification of reentry circuit sites during catheter mapping and radiofrequency ablation of ventricular tachycardia late after myocardial infarction. *Circulation*. 1993;88:1647–1670.

Figure 4.E.2

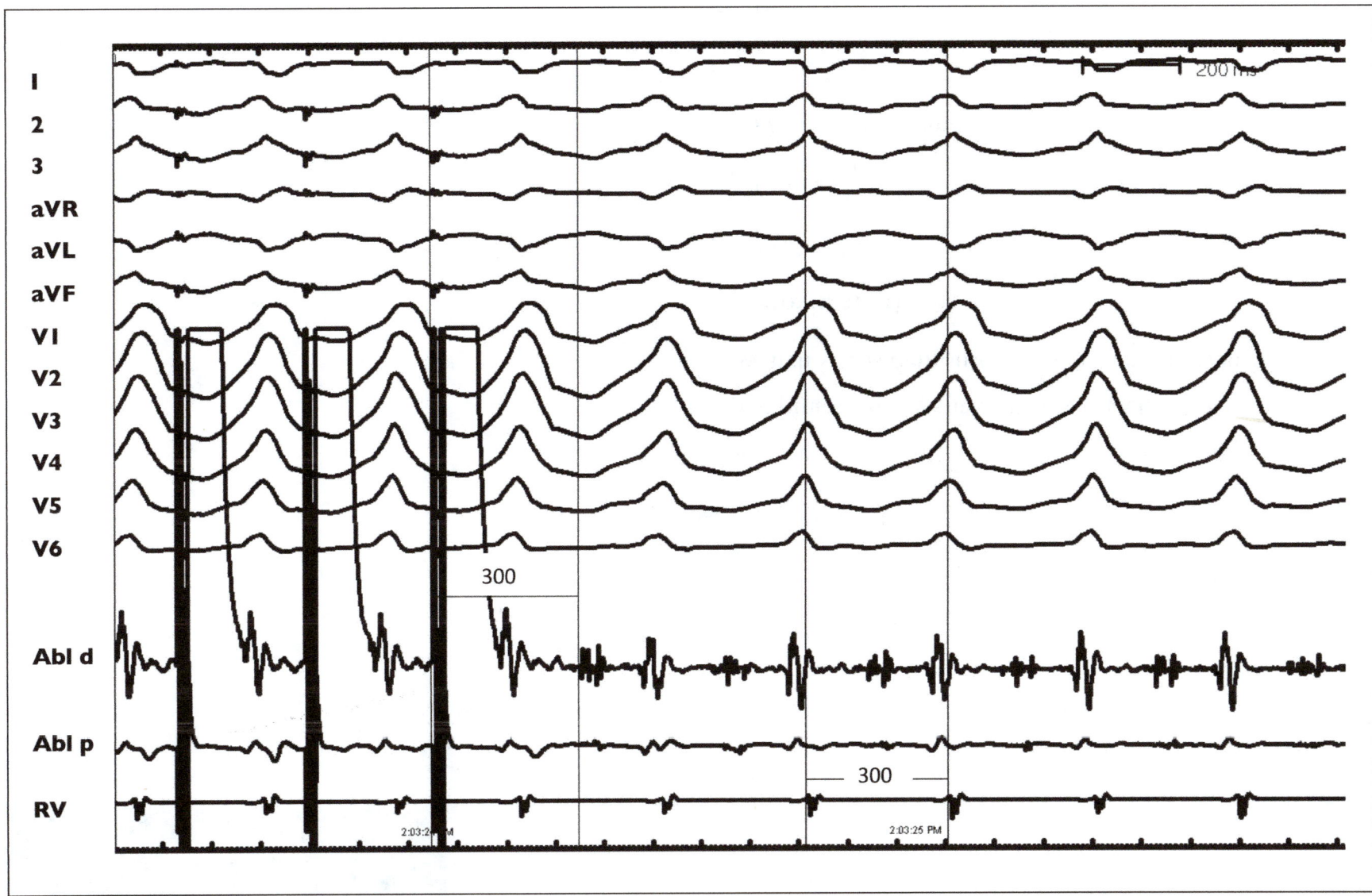

Question

A 75-year-old man with ischemic cardiomyopathy undergoes mapping of incessant ventricular tachycardia.

Which site is demonstrated with entrainment?

A) Proximal isthmus

B) Mid–isthmus

C) Outer loop

D) Dead–end bystander

E) Inner loop

F) Not captured

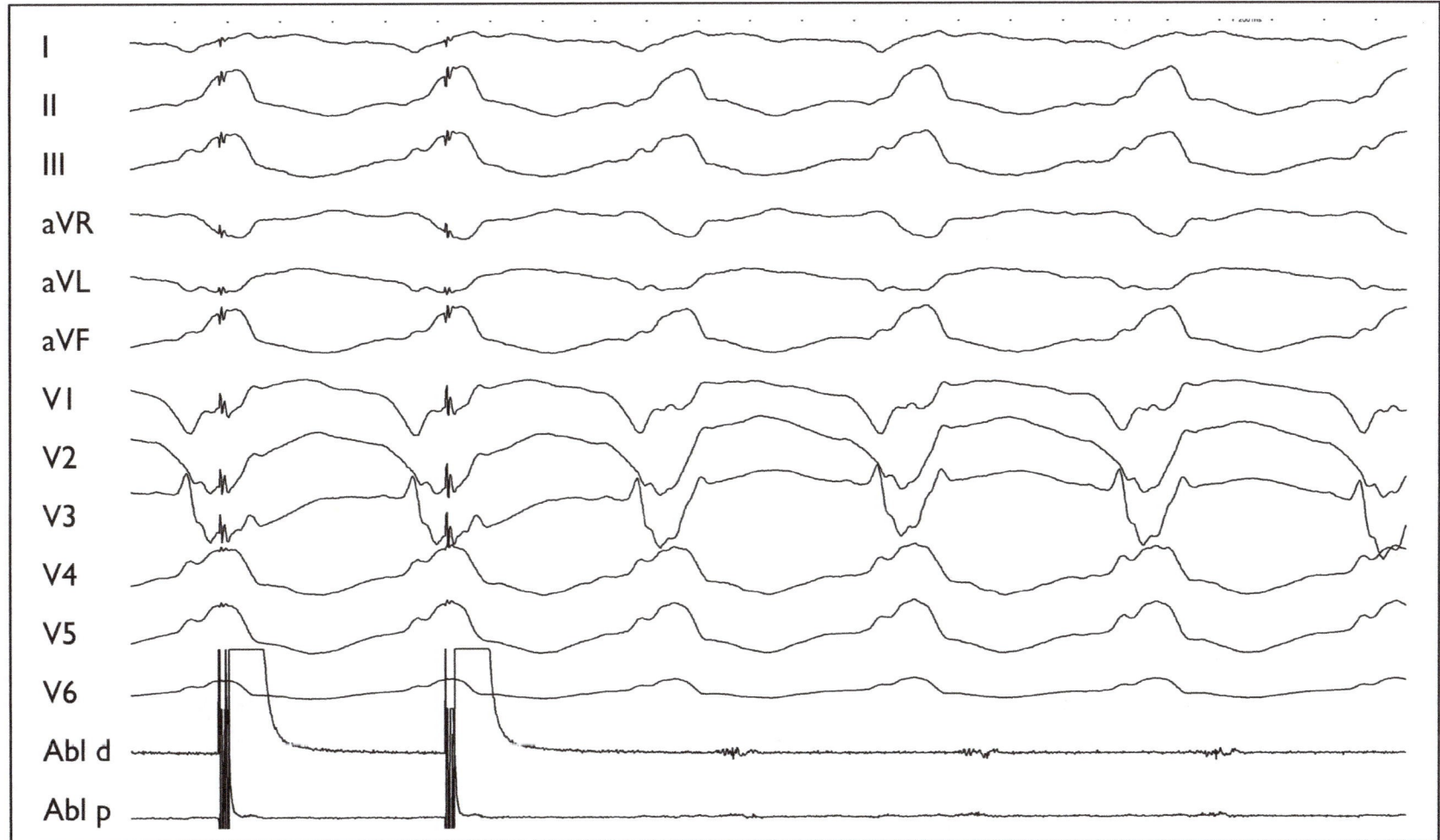

Figure 4.F.1

Answer

The correct answer is **D**. This demonstrates entrainment of a "dead-end" bystander.

Concealed fusion is present, indicating that the site of pacing is within or attached to the reentrant circuit. Outer loop sites demonstrate manifest fusion as the antidromic wavefront is not entirely bound within the circuit. Capture of the near-field component is consistent with acceleration of the RR intervals, and the postpacing interval is 60 ms longer than the TCL, which excludes a site within the circuit. The EGM-QRS (225 ms) is fixed and is 50% of the TCL, which also excludes proximal isthmus and inner loop sites (>70% TCL).

Most importantly, the S-QRS is longer than the EGM-QRS. The S-QRS (285 ms) exceeds the EGM-QRS (225 ms) by the same difference (60 ms) between the PPI and TCL (520 − 460 = 60 ms) in a dead-end bystander, as there is additional time required to "pace out of" and "sense into" the bystander.

Figure 4.F.2

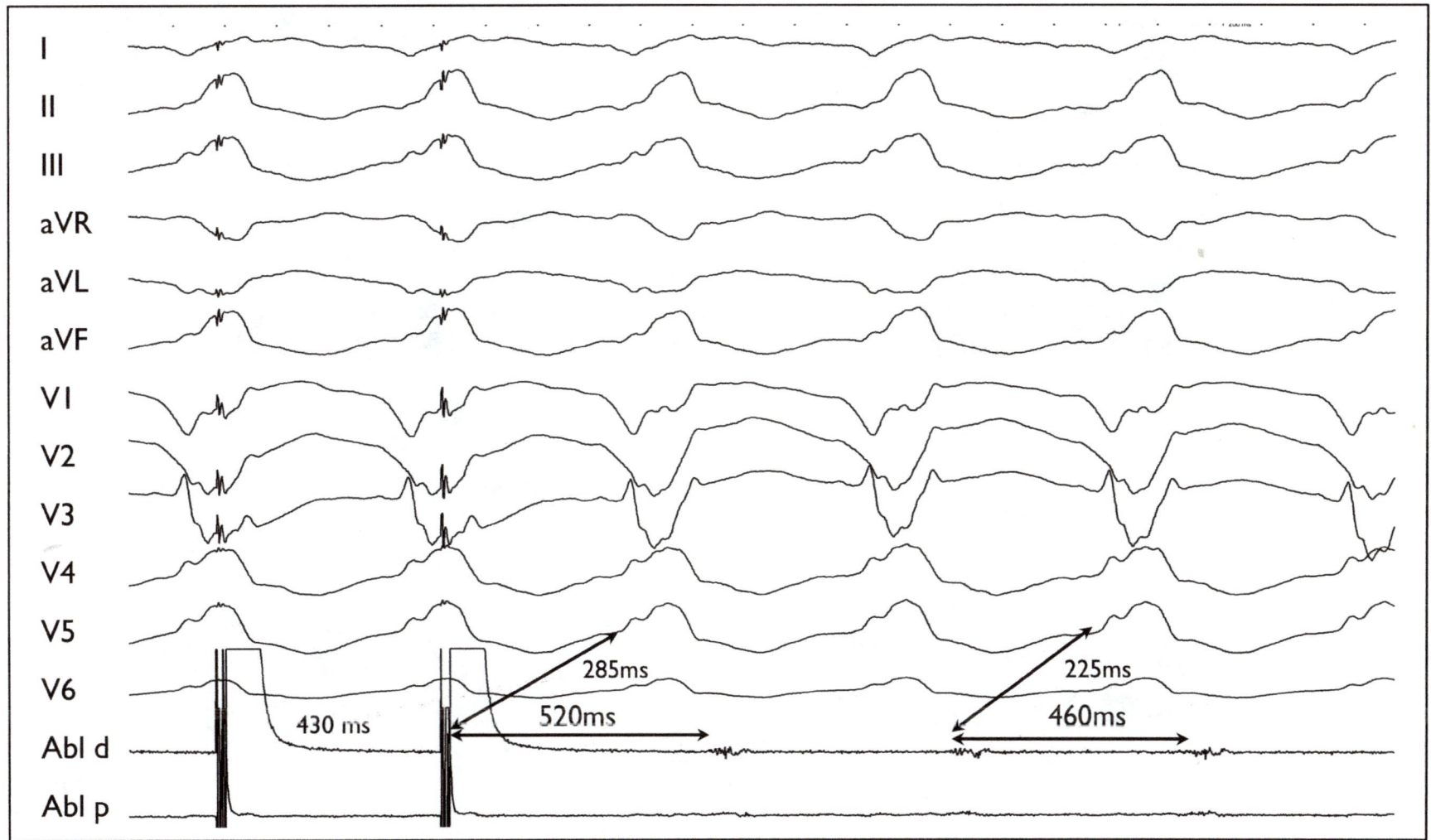

Figure 4.F.3

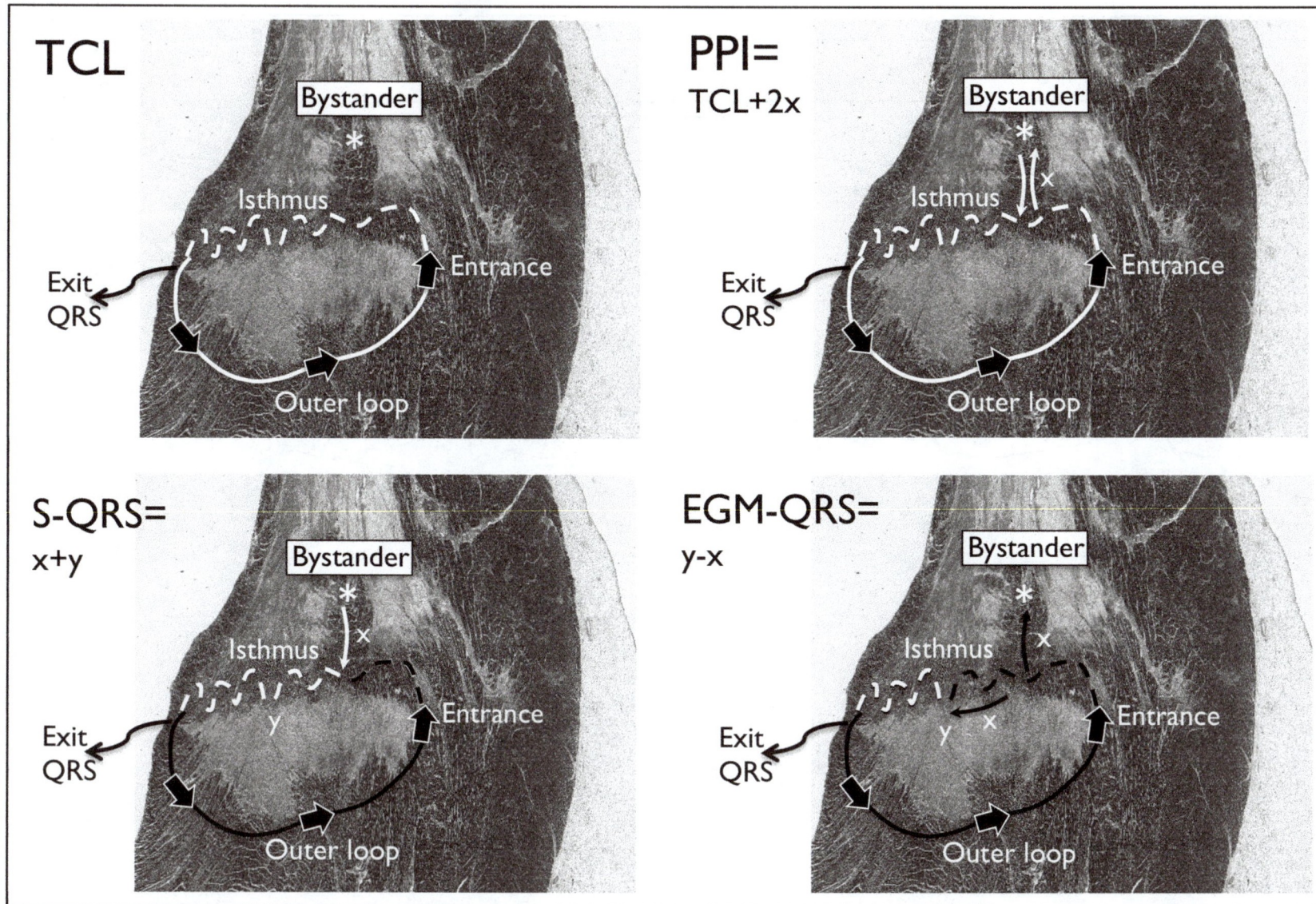

References

1. Stevenson WG, Khan H, Sager P, Saxon LA, Middlekauf HR, Natterson PD, Wiener I. Identification of reentry circuit sites during catheter mapping and radiofrequency ablation of ventricular tachycardia late after myocardial infarction. *Circulation*. 1993;88:1647–1670.

2. Almendral JM, Gottlieb CD, Rosenthal ME, Stamato NJ, Buxton AE, Marchlinski FE, et al. Entrainment of ventricular tachycardia: explanation for surface electrocardiographic phenomena by analysis of electrograms recorded within the tachycardia circuit. *Circulation*. 1988;77:569–580.

Question

What is the most likely site of PVC origin?

A) Right ventricular outflow tract

B) Left ventricular outflow tract

C) Posteromedial papillary muscle

D) Anterolateral papillary muscle

E) Moderator band

Figure 4.G.1

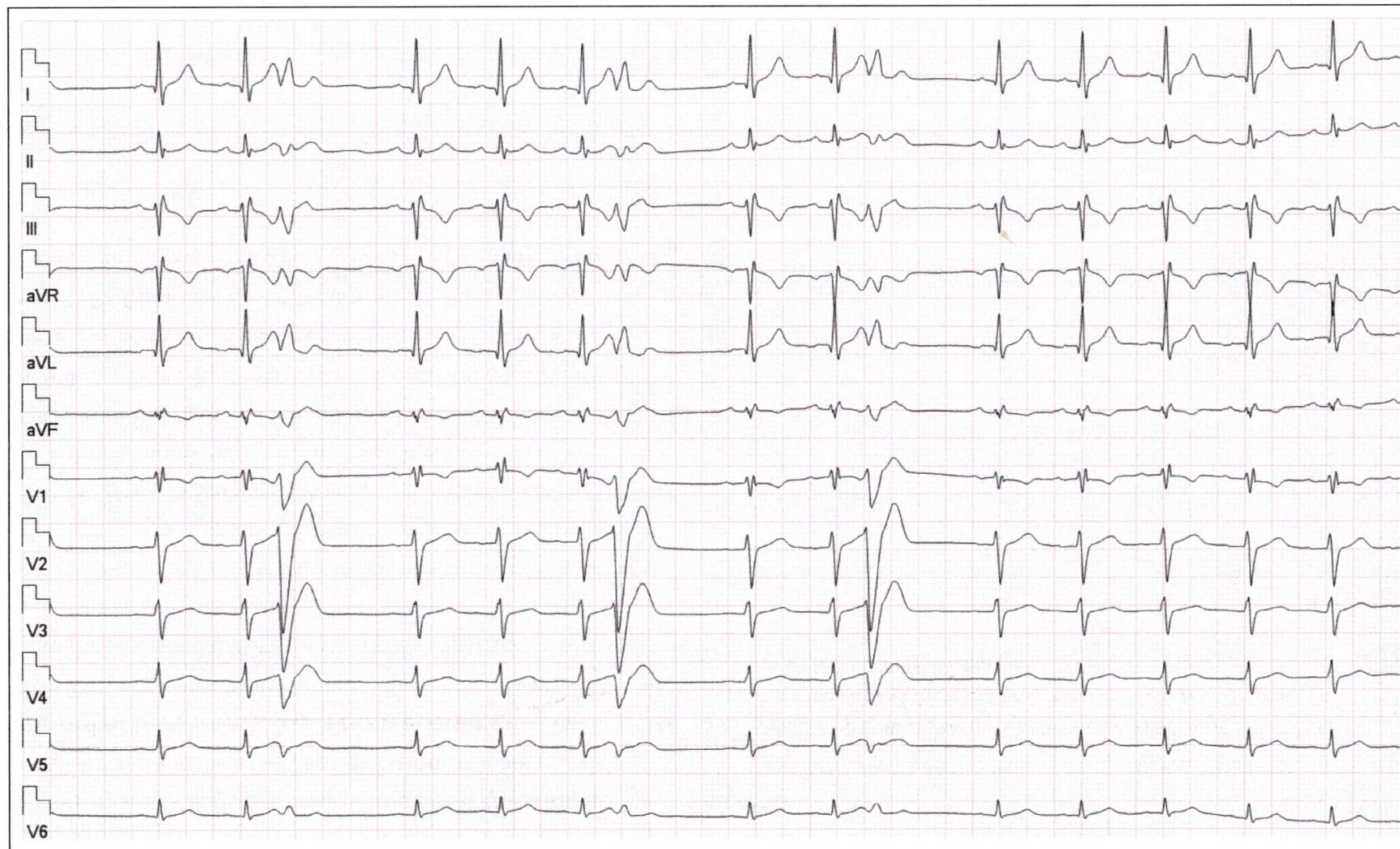

*A*nswer

The correct answer is **E. PVCs originating from the moderator band have a left bundle configuration in lead V$_1$, with late precordial transition ($\geq$V$_5$). The axis is superior and leftward.** The moderator band connects the interventricular septum to the anterior papillary muscle on the right ventricular free wall. It contains Purkinje fibers. PVCs from the moderator band are a common trigger for idiopathic ventricular fibrillation. Note the tight coupling interval in this example. Intracardiac echocardiography (ICE) is highly recommended for guiding catheter contact with this mobile, intracavitary structure.

PVCs from the right and left ventricular outflow tracts are inferiorly directed. Arrhythmias from the posteromedial papillary muscle have a right bundle configuration in lead V$_1$, with a superior axis. PVCs from the anterolateral papillary muscle also have a right bundle configuration in lead V$_1$, with a right inferior axis.

Reference

1. Sadek MM, Benhayon D, Sureddi R, et al. Idiopathic ventricular arrhythmias originating from the moderator band: electrocardiographic characteristics and treatment by catheter ablation. *Heart Rhythm.* 2015;12(1):67–75 (Epub 2014 Aug 23).

Figure 4.G.2

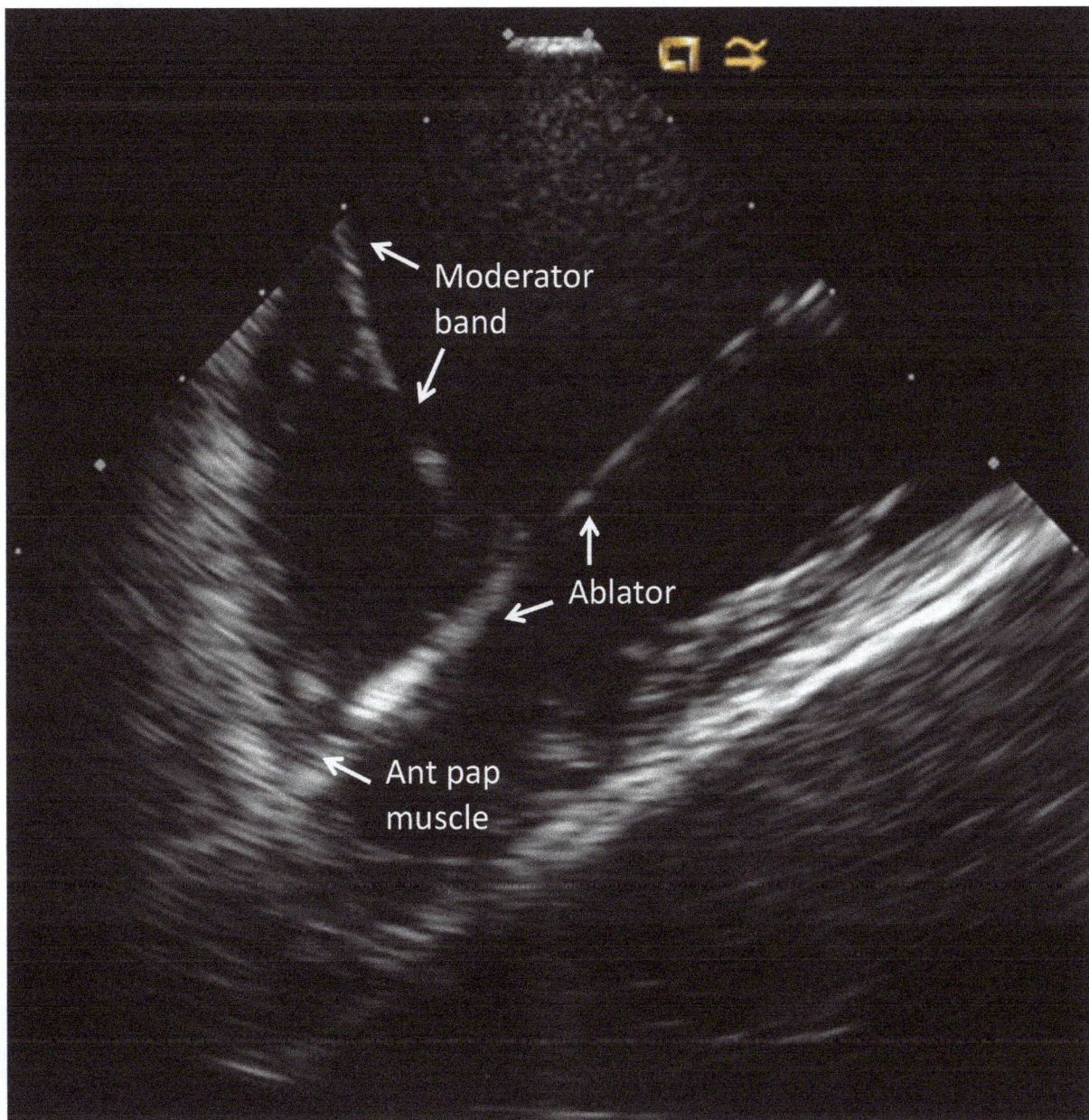

Question

Epicardial mapping was performed in a 45-year-old man with arrhythmogenic right ventricular cardiomyopathy.

Using a 2-mm spaced duodecapolar catheter, which bipole pair should be targeted for ablation during VT?

A) DD 1,2

B) DD 5,6

C) DD 7,8

D) DD 15,16

E) A critical site cannot be determine without entrainment

Figure 4.H.1

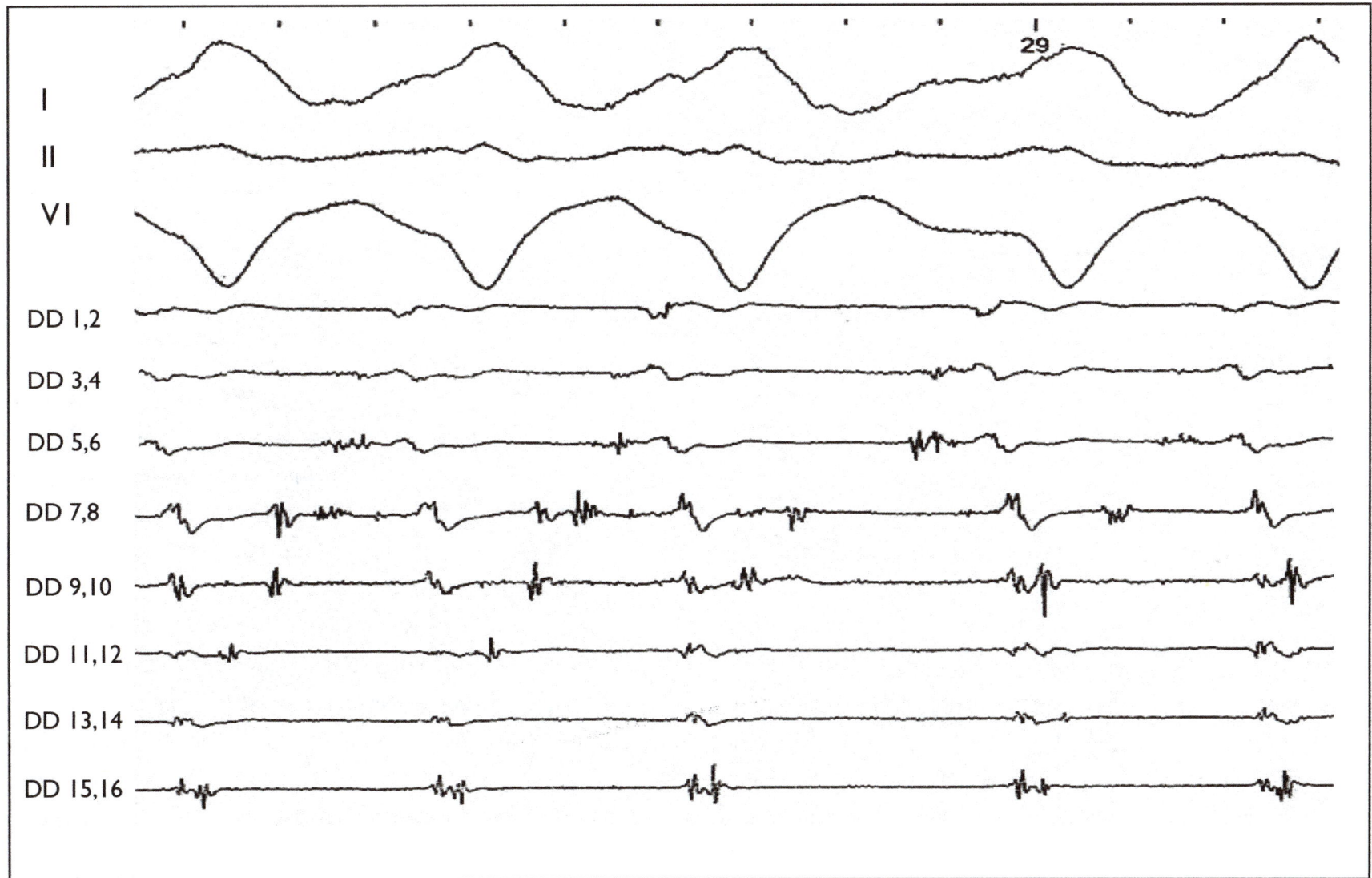

Answer

The correct answer is **C**. DD 7,8 represents the mid-isthmus of the reentrant circuit.

The use of a multipolar catheter allows for rapid activation mapping of VT originating from the epicardial RV free wall, which is a common scar location for ARVC. Diastolic activation is seen throughout the entire tachycardia cycle length, with entrance at DD 15,16 and exit at DD 1,2. The central isthmus comprises the middle of diastolic activation (30%–70% TCL). The first component of the fractionated electrogram on DD 7,8 has an EGM–QRS interval of 155 ms, which represents 56% of the TCL. The electrogram on bipolar 5,6 represents a location closer to the exit site (<30%) at 32% of the TCL.

Entrainment is not required to exclude a bystander site, as the delay seen between activation of DD 7,8 to DD 5,6 results in an oscillation of the ventricular tachycardia with a longer tachycardia cycle length on this beat. Ablation performed at this site, where intra-isthmus delay is demonstrated, resulted in rapid termination of VT within one second.

Reference

1. Stevenson WG, Khan H, Sager P, Saxon LA, Middlekauf HR, Natterson PD, Wiener I. Identification of reentry circuit sites during catheter mapping and radiofrequency ablation of ventricular tachycardia late after myocardial infarction. *Circulation*. 1993; 88:1647–1670.

Figure 4.H.2

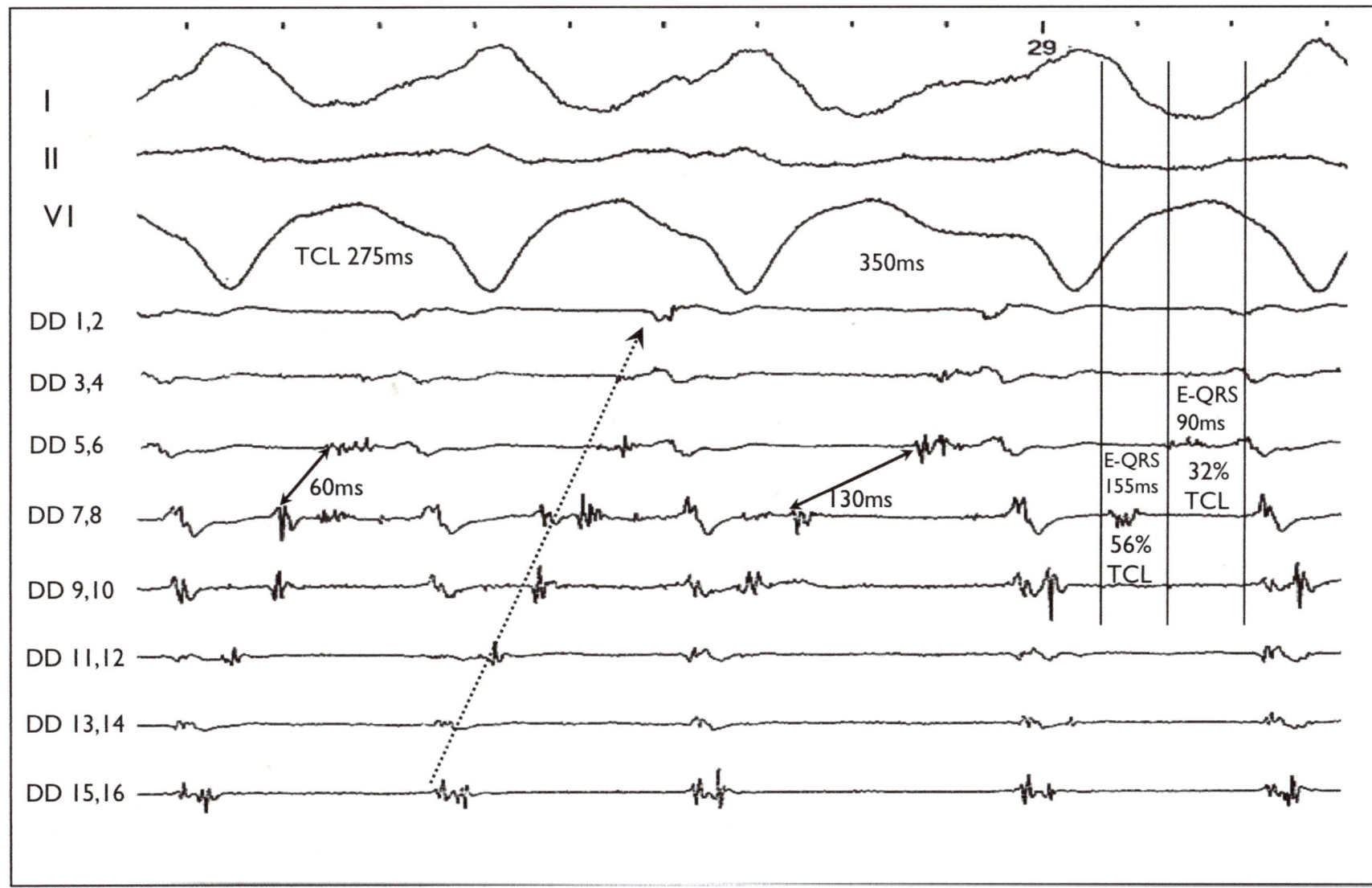

Question

The following tracing was recorded from a 20-year-old male college student after palpitations began while playing basketball. The tachycardia was terminated by verapamil in the emergency room.

The tracing shows:

A) AVNRT

B) AVRT

C) Ventricular tachycardia from the posterior papillary muscle

D) Fascicular VT

Figure 4.I.1

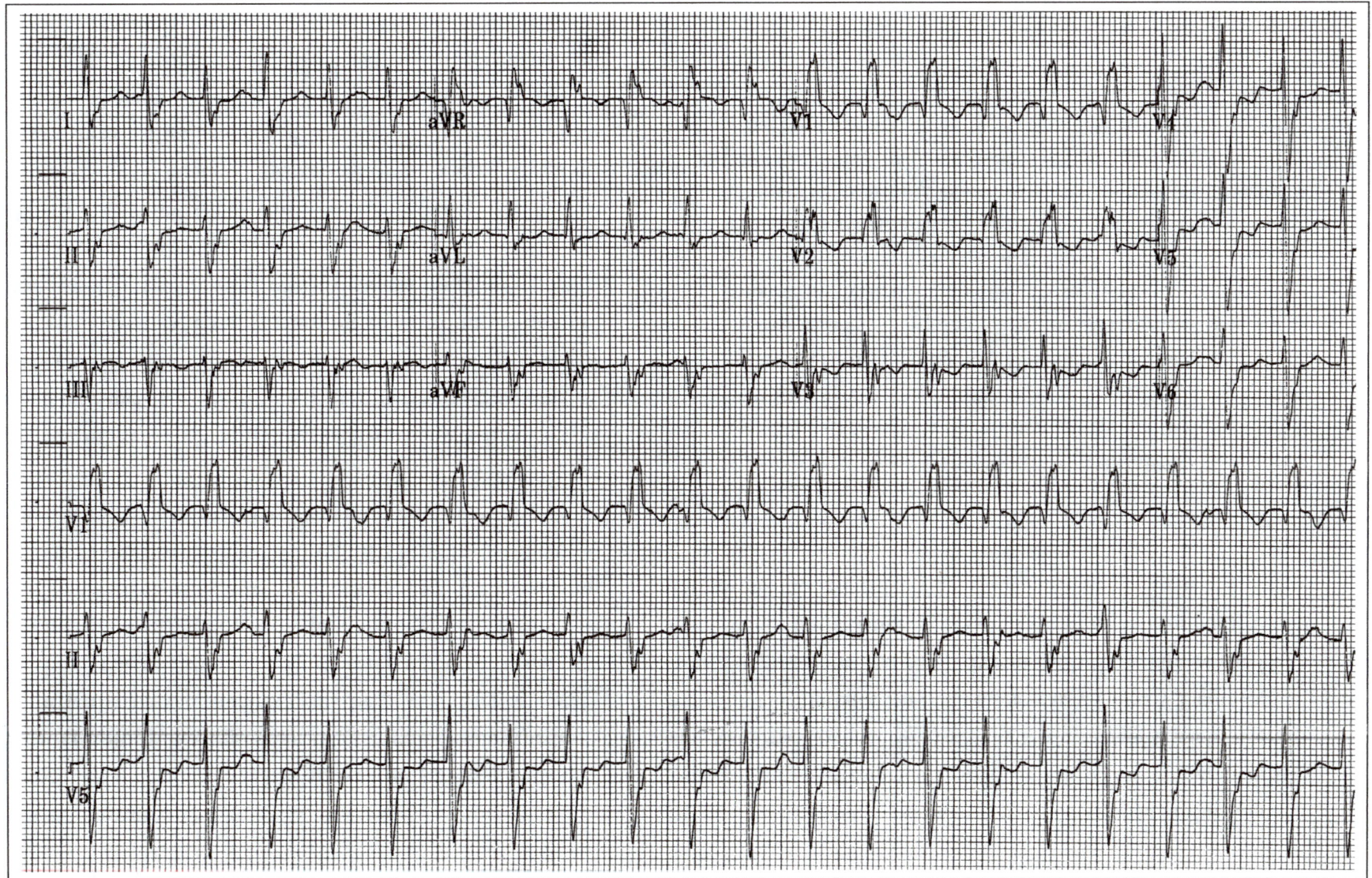

Answer

The correct answer is **D**. The ECG shows a wide complex tachycardia with left superior axis. **This activation pattern and/or QRS morphology is suggestive of fascicular tachycardia.**

Ventricular activation starts from the posteroinferior septal region giving rise to a short, inferiorly directed vector (small R wave in inferior leads) followed by predominant vector directed superiorly and leftward (S wave in inferior leads). VT originating from the left posterior fascicle resulting in a RBBB morphology associated with left superior axis is the most common form of fascicular VT.

Verapamil-sensitive ventricular tachycardia was first described by Zipes in 1979. This VT is sometimes referred to as "Belhassen's VT." The "relatively" narrow QRS during this VT makes it unlikely to be coming from the myocardium. The QRS duration was 135 ms. Presence of AV dissociation also supports the diagnosis of ventricular tachycardia.

This VT represents approximately 10% of idiopathic VTs. It is not commonly precipitated by exercise or emotional stress but may occur shortly after exercise. Adenosine has no effect on this arrhythmia. The circuit has been carefully studied and mapped by Nogami and colleagues. It is currently believed to involve the slow decremental conduction over the abnormal Purkinje network/adjacent ventricular myocardium as the antegrade limb and retrograde conduction over the left posterior fascicle. The main ECG difference between fascicular VT and VT coming from the posteromedial papillary muscle is the width of the QRS, being wider in the latter, generally a mean of 150 ms compared to 130 ms during fascicular VT.

References

1. Belhassen B, Rotmensch HH, Laniado S. Response of recurrent sustained ventricular tachycardia to verapamil. *Br Heart J.* 1981;46:679–682.
2. Nakagawa H, Beckman KJ, McClelland JH, et al. Radiofrequency catheter ablation of idiopathic left ventricular tachycardia guided by a Purkinje potential. *Circulation.* 1993;88:2607–2617.
3. Nogami A, Naito S, Tada H, et al. Demonstration of diastolic and presystolic Purkinje potentials as critical potentials in a macroreentry circuit of verapamil-sensitive idiopathic left ventricular tachycardia. *J Am Coll Cardiol.* 2000;36:811–823.
4. Zipes DP, Foster PR, Troup PJ, Pedersen DH. Atrial induction of ventricular tachycardia: reentry versus triggered automaticity. *Am J Cardiol.* 1979;44:1–8.

Figure 4.1.2

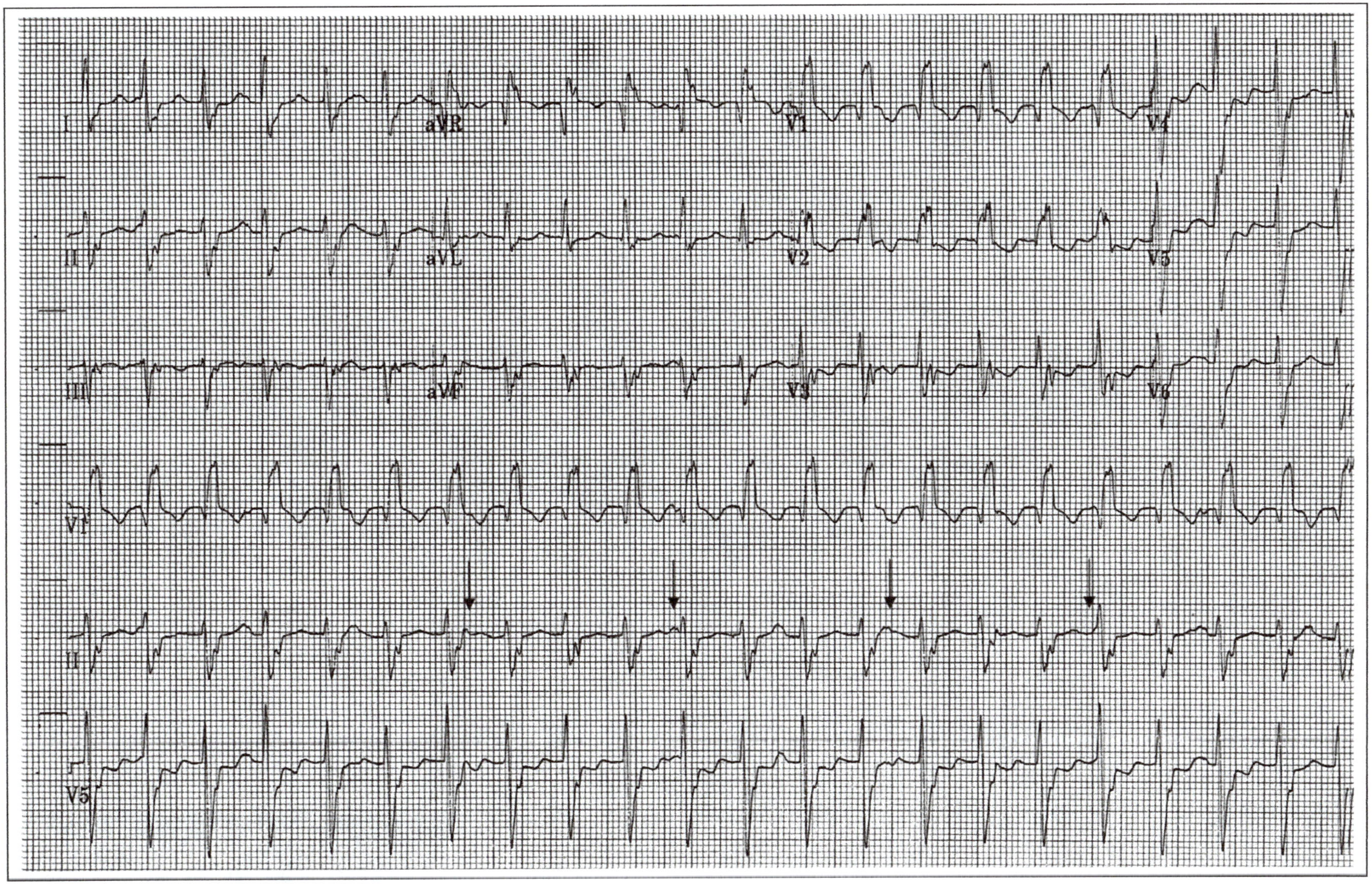

Question

A 63-year-old man with nonischemic cardiomyopathy undergoes mapping of ventricular tachycardia.

Which site is demonstrated with entrainment?

A) Distal isthmus (exit)

B) Mid–isthmus

C) Outer loop

D) Dead–end bystander

E) Remote bystander

Figure 4.J.1

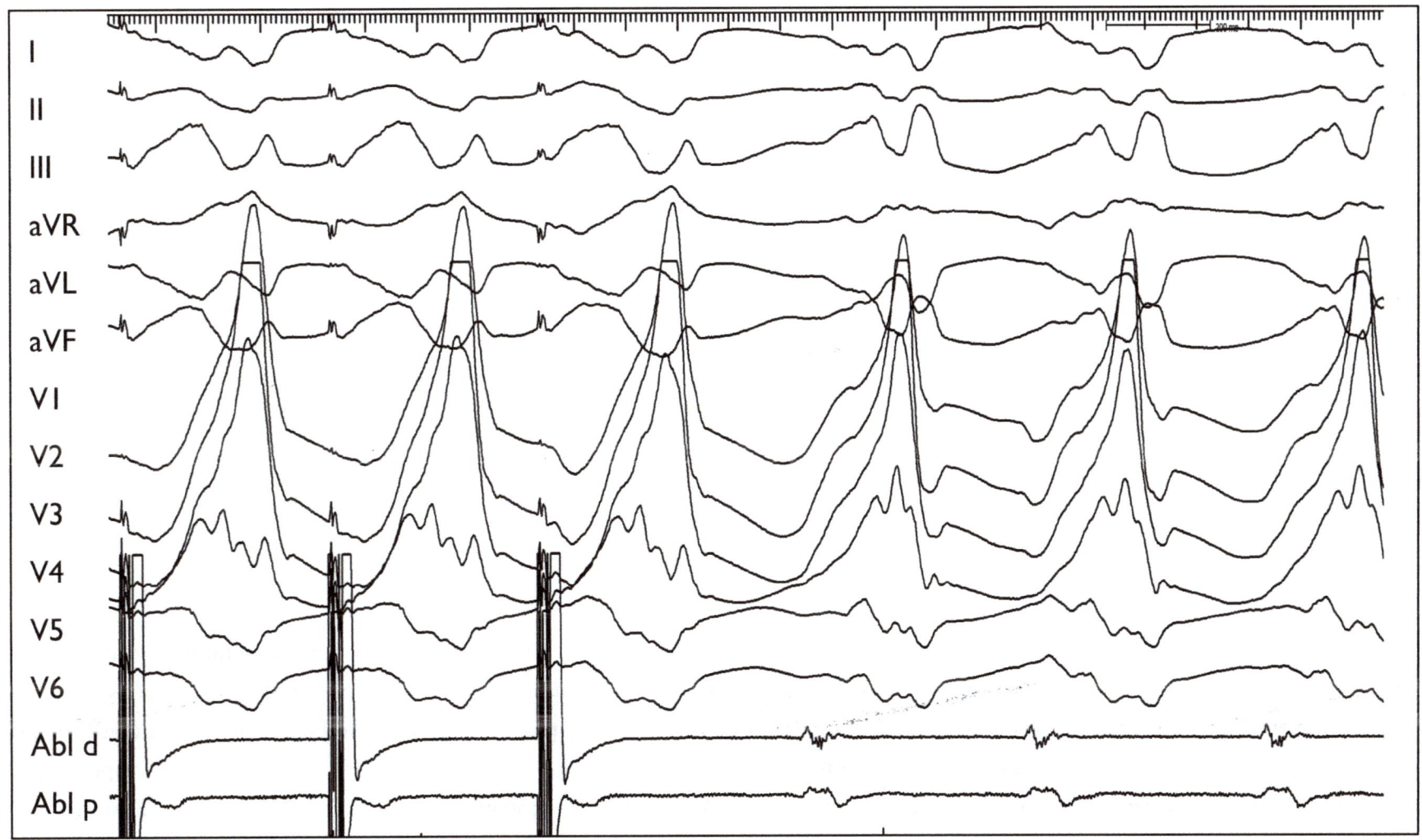

Answer

The correct answer is **E**. This demonstrates entrainment from a remote bystander.

Overt fusion is evident, excluding isthmus and "dead-end bystander" sites, both of which demonstrate concealed fusion. Although slight oscillation is seen after entrainment, the postpacing interval exceeds the longest tachycardia cycle length by 60 ms, which rules out an outer loop. Outer loop sites are in the circuit and demonstrate manifest fusion due to antidromic capture outside of the protected isthmus.

Figure 4.J.2

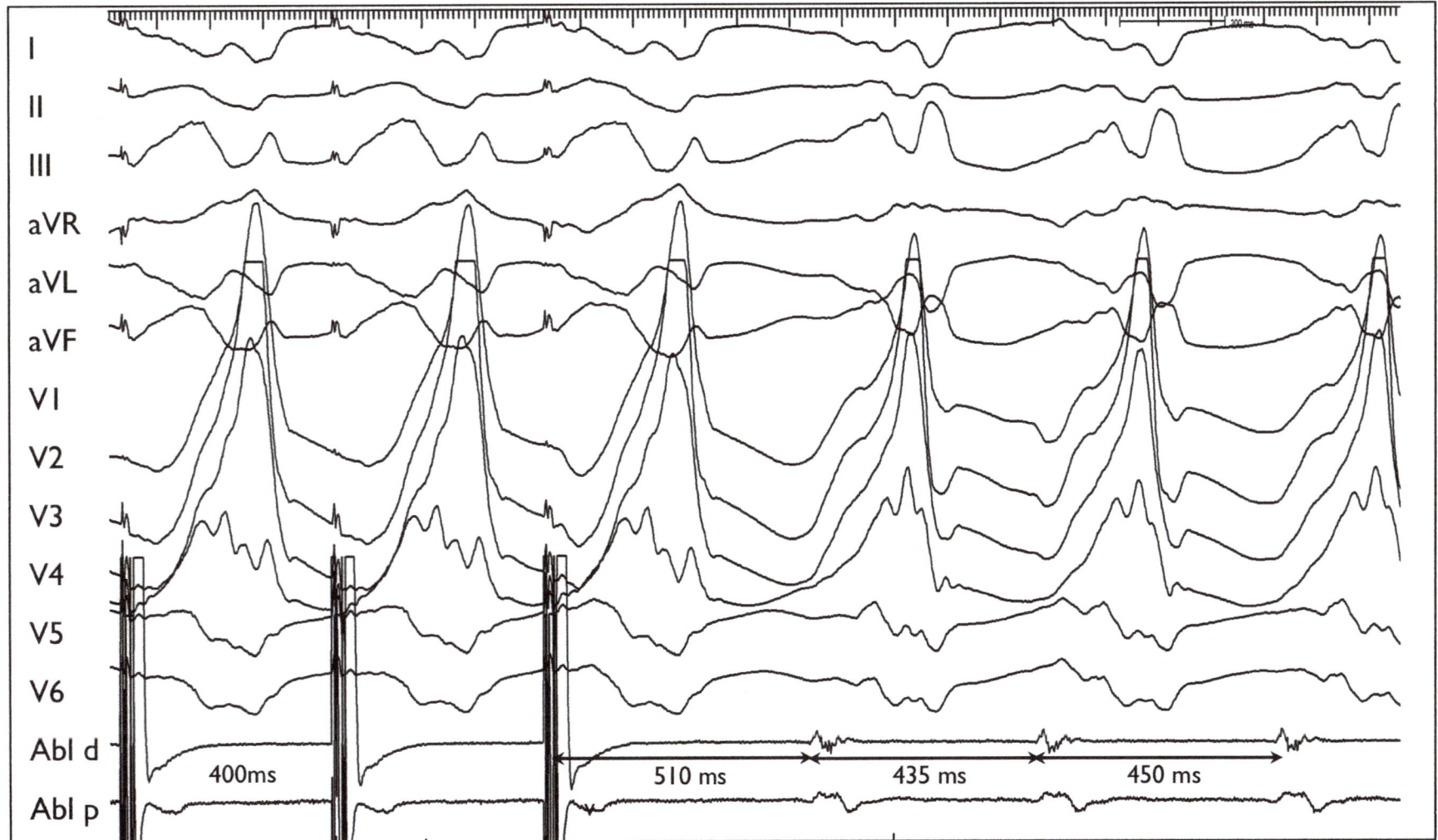

References

1. Stevenson WG, Khan H, Sager P, Saxon LA, Middlekauf HR, Natterson PD, Wiener I. Identification of reentry circuit sites during catheter mapping and radiofrequency ablation of ventricular tachycardia late after myocardial infarction. *Circulation*. 1993;88:1647–1670.

2. Almendral JM, Gottlieb CD, Rosenthal ME, Stamato NJ, Buxton AE, Marchlinski FE, et al. Entrainment of ventricular tachycardia: explanation for surface electrocardiographic phenomena by analysis of electrograms recorded within the tachycardia circuit. *Circulation*. 1988;77:569–580.

Question

Overdrive pacing of tachycardia is performed in a 65-year-old man with dilated cardiomyopathy from the basal lateral epicardium.

What is the mechanism of tachycardia?

A) Macroreentry

B) Focal

C) Microreentry

D) Cannot determine

Figure 4.K.1

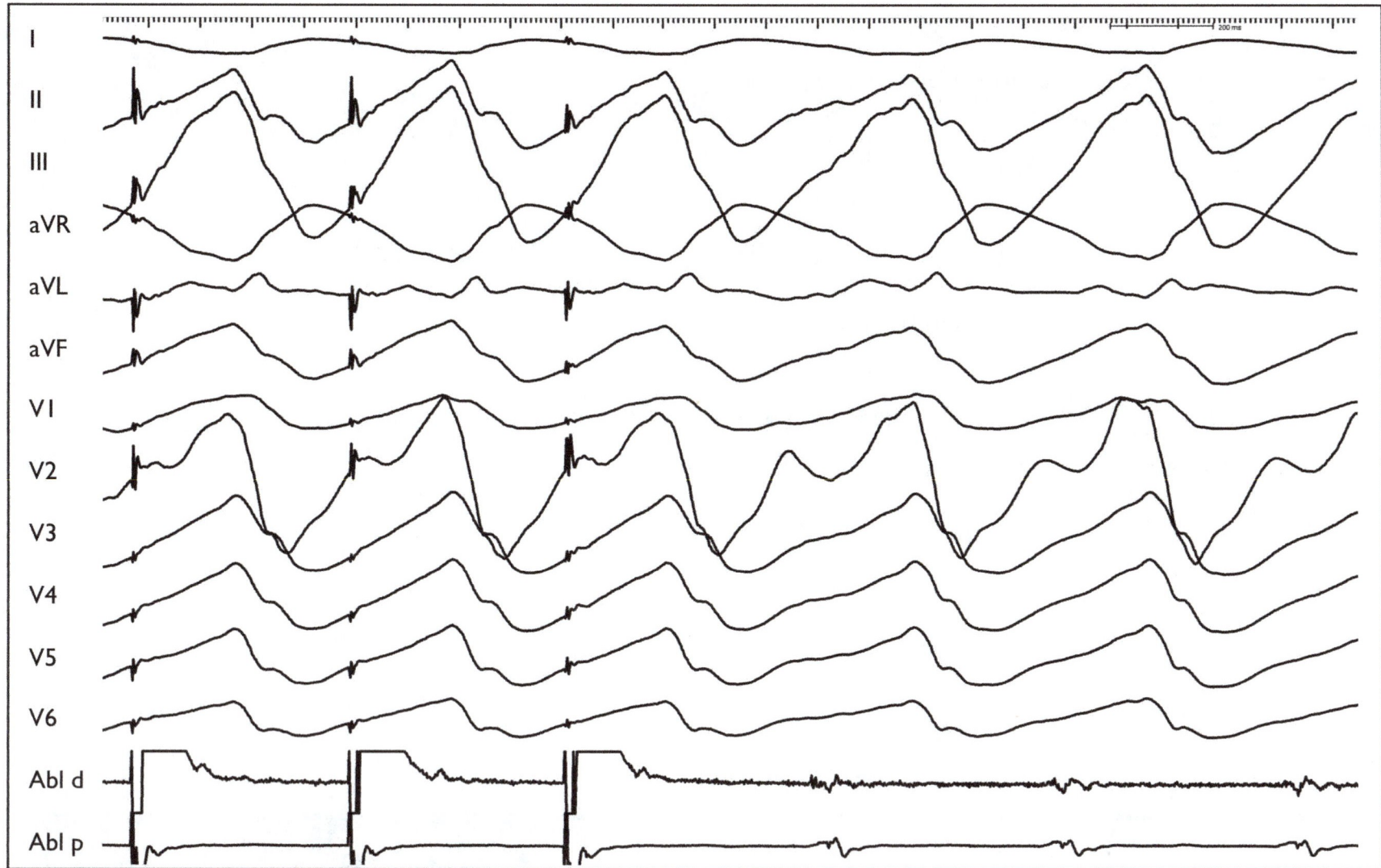

Figure 4.K.2

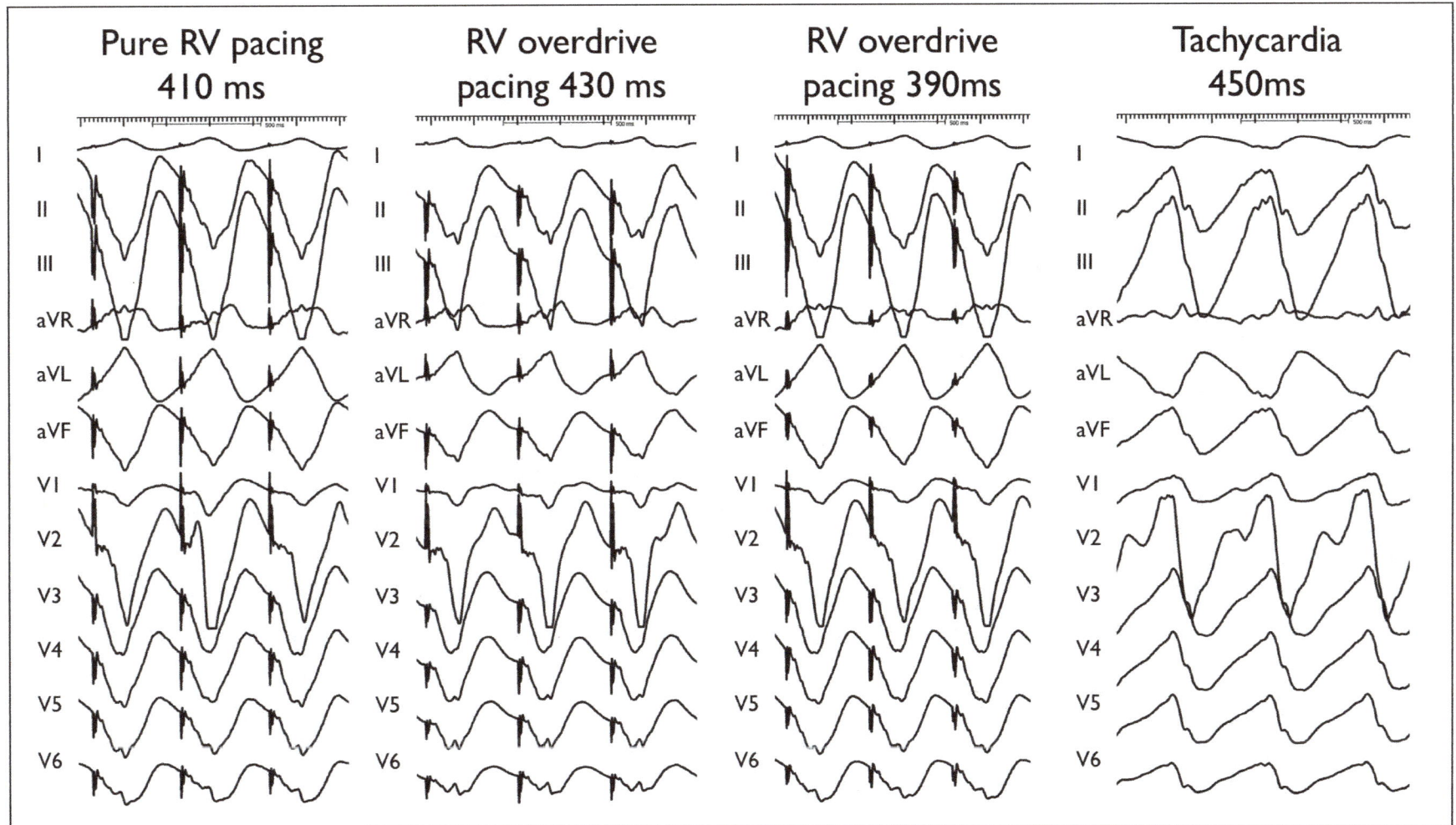

Pure RV pacing 410 ms | RV overdrive pacing 430 ms | RV overdrive pacing 390ms | Tachycardia 450ms

Answer

The correct answer is **D**. Overdrive pacing results in a QRS that appears identical to the ventricular tachycardia. The postpacing interval is within 30 ms of the tachycardia cycle length and the stimulus–QRS interval is similar to the EGM–QRS interval.

However, this maneuver does not prove the mechanism of tachycardia, as an automatic focus can be overdriven from a site close to the site of origin. Classical entrainment requires the fulfillment of at least one of three criteria to prove reentry: 1) constant fusion beats during rapid pacing at a constant rate except for the last captured beat; 2) progressive fusion with different degrees of fusion at the different rate; and 3) interruption of the tachycardia by rapid pacing associated with localized conduction block to a site followed by activation of that site from a different direction and with a shorter conduction time by the next pacing impulse.

Overdrive pacing during tachycardia is performed from the RV apex and activation mapping is performed after substrate mapping.

Figure 4.K.3

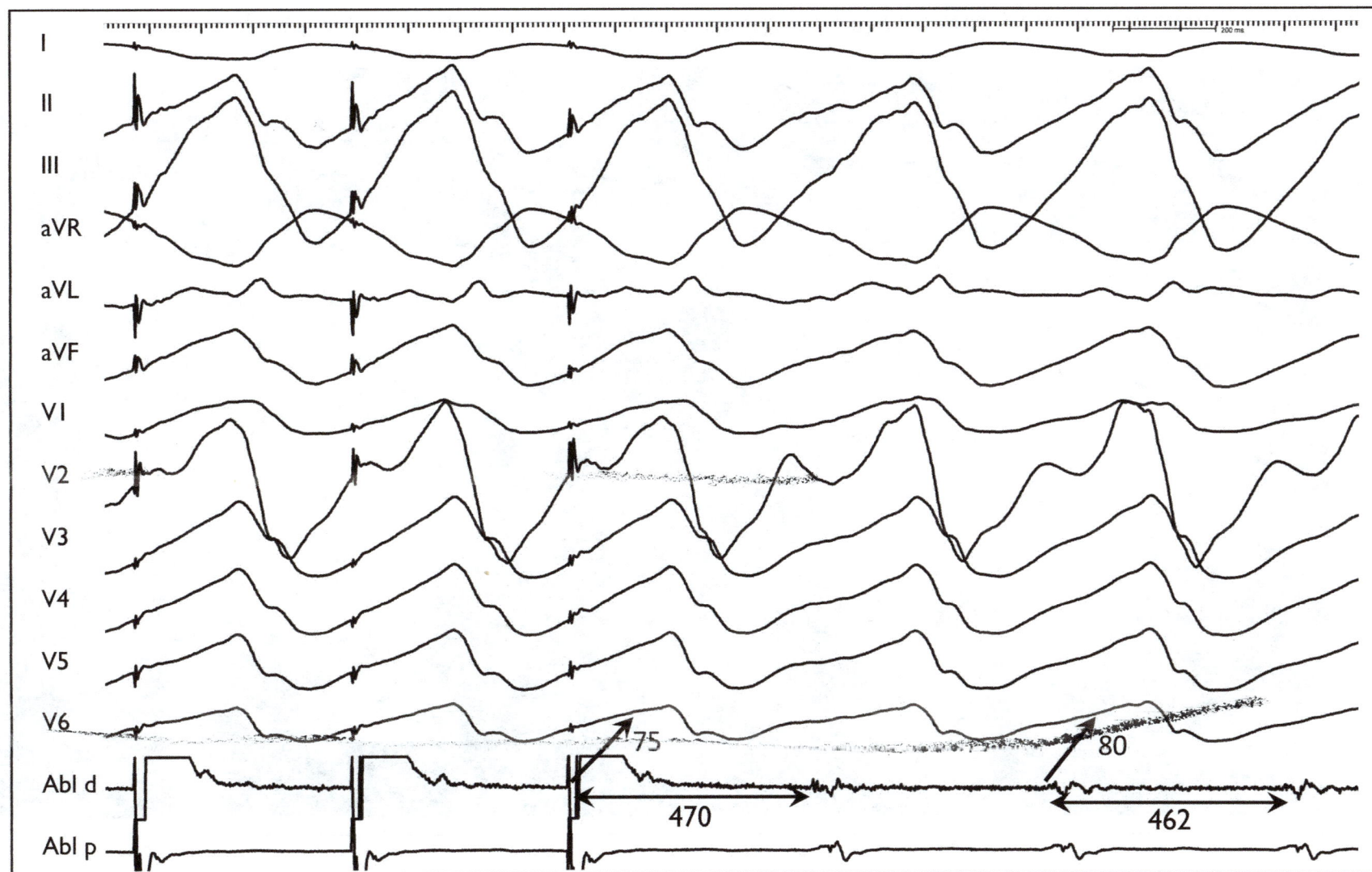

Figure 4.K.4

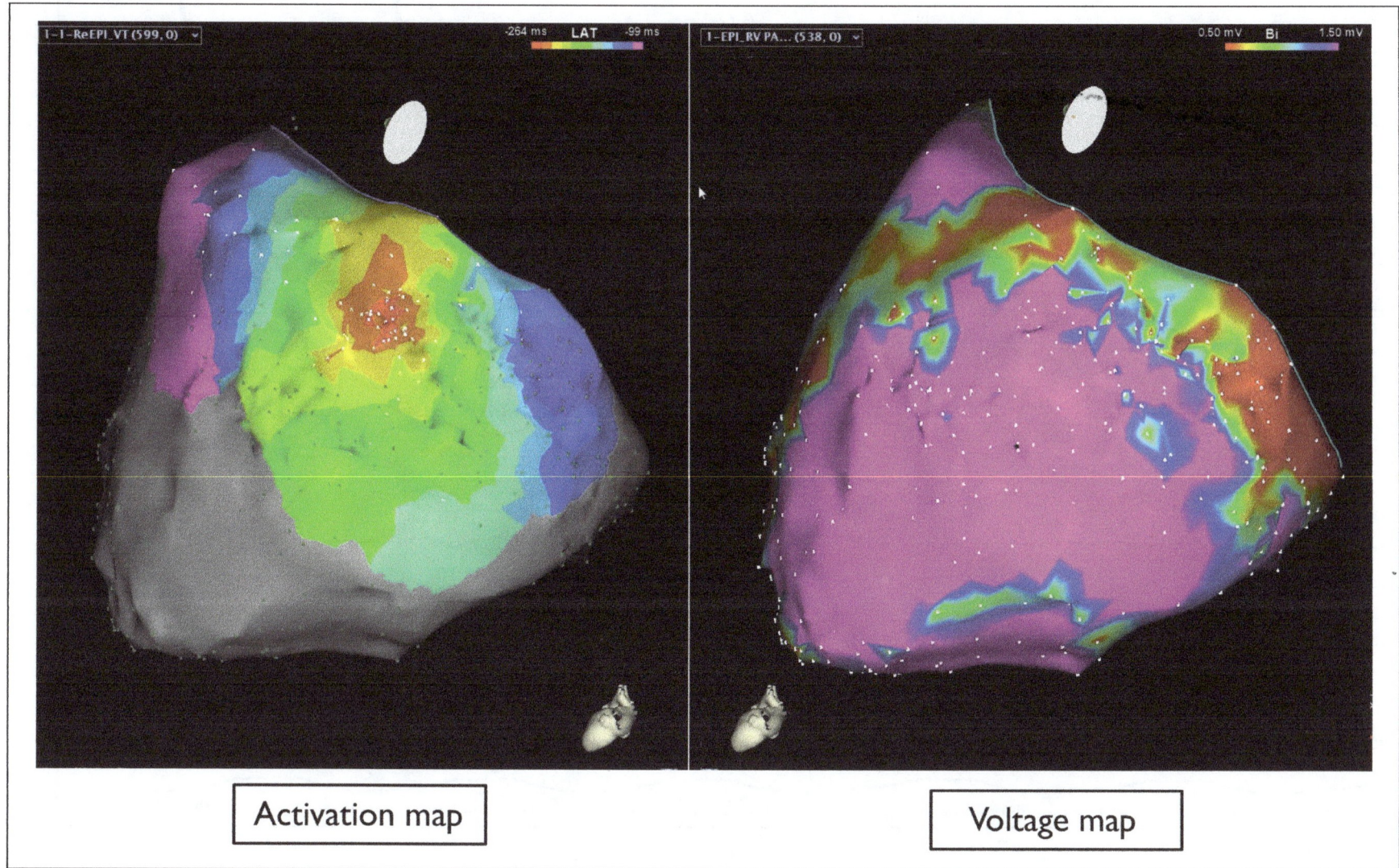

Activation map

Voltage map

References

1. Waldo AL, Henthorn RW, Plumb VJ, MacLean WAH. Demonstration of the mechanism of transient entrainment and interruption of ventricular tachycardia with rapid atrial pacing. *J Am Coll Cardiol.* 1984;3:422–430.

2. Brugada P, Wellens HJJ. Entrainment as an electrophysiologic phenomenon. *J Am Coll Cardiol.* 1984;3:451–454.

3. Anderson KP, Swerdlow CD, Mason JW. Entrainment of ventricular tachycardia. *Am J Cardiol.* 1984;53:335–340.

4. Josephson ME, Horowitz LN, Farshidi A, Spielman SR, Michelson EL, Greenspan AM. Sustained ventricular tachycardia: evidence for protected localized reentry. *Am J Cardiol.* 1978;42:416–424.

5. Das MK, Scott LR, Miller JM. Focal mechanism of ventricular tachycardia in coronary artery disease. *Heart Rhythm.* 2010;7:305–311.

6. Ellis E, Shvilkin A, Josephson ME. Nonreentrant ventricular arrhythmias in patients with structural heart disease unrelated to abnormal myocardial substrate. *Heart Rhythm.* 2014;11(6):946–952.

Case 4.L

Question

A 46-year-old woman who had suffered an acute inferior myocardial infarction 5 months earlier underwent electrophysiologic study for recurrent, symptomatic narrow QRS complex tachycardia.

Based on the information, what is the most likely diagnosis?

A) AVNRT with upper common final pathway block

B) Orthodromic reentrant tachycardia using a nodofascicular accessory pathway

C) Automatic junctional tachycardia

D) Ventricular tachycardia

Figure 4.L.1

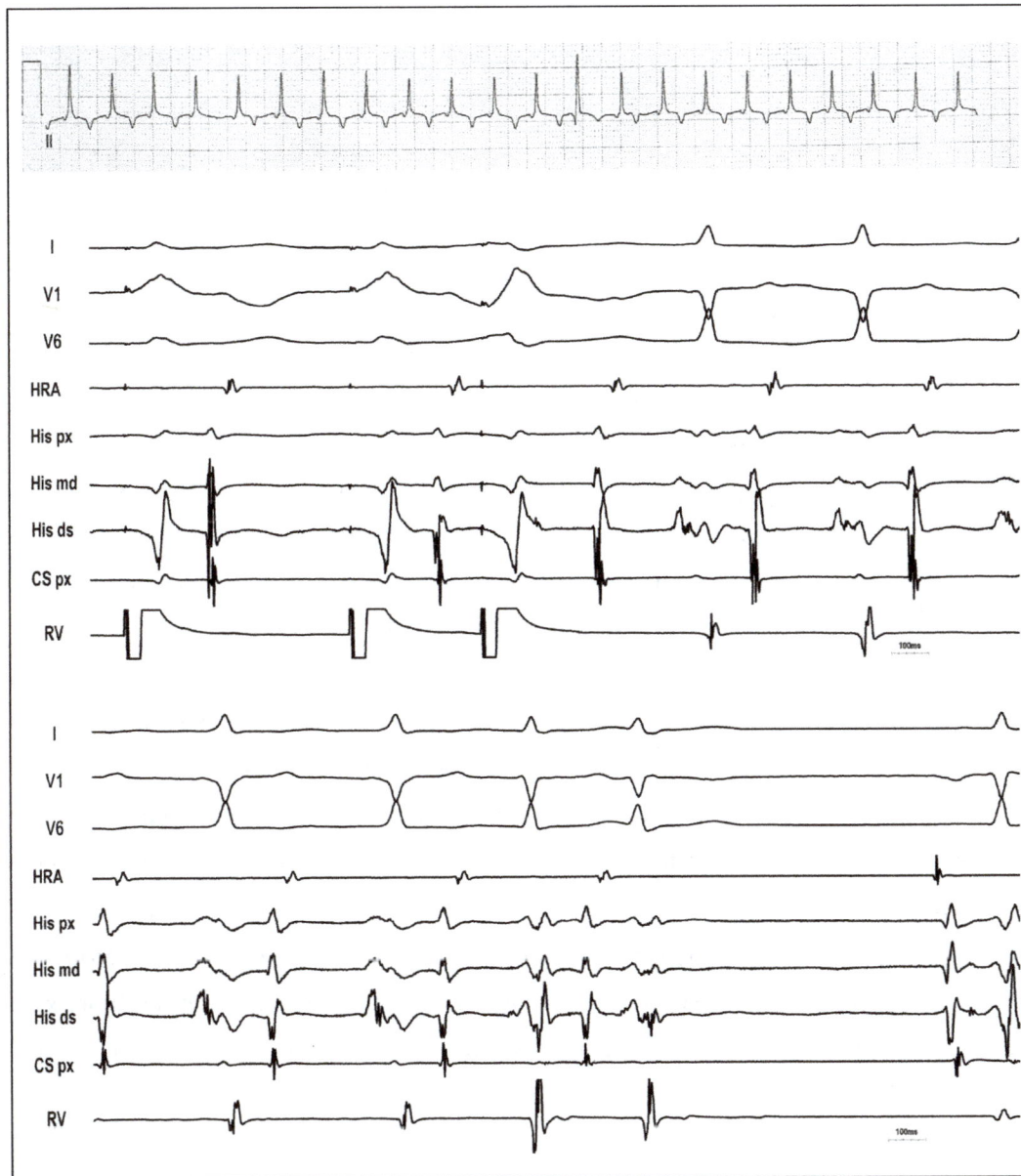

Answer

The correct answer is **D**. A single extrastimulus induces a narrow complex tachycardia with a concentric atrial activation pattern. A His bundle potential (rH) occurs after the extrastimulus ("VH jump") and upon termination of tachycardia, indicating that the His bundle catheter is in good position. During tachycardia, however, His bundle electrograms are absent before each QRS complex, indicating a nonsupraventricular origin. All narrow complex supraventricular tachycardias (AVNRT, ORT, JT) have His bundle potentials preceding each QRS complex. Narrow complex (≤ 120 ms) VT is rare and tends to be associated with inferior myocardial infarctions. The II–lead ECG strip shows VT with VA Wenckebach. The single supraventricular QRS complex (★) follows the longest RP interval on the tracing and is an atypical AV nodal echo. Note that its QRS morphology is slightly narrower and different from tachycardia. VT is interrupted by two short-coupled His bundle extrasystoles (the first of which has a supraventricular QRS morphology, while the second shows incomplete RBBB— but both have short HV intervals (14–20 ms)).

References

1. Sakamoto T, Fujiki A, Nakatani Y, Sakabe M, Mizumaki K, Inoue H. Narrow QRS ventricular tachycardia from the posterior mitral annulus without involvement of the His-Purkinje system in a patient with prior inferior myocardial infarction. *Heart Vessels*. 2010;25:170–173.

2. Bogun F, Good E, Reich S, et al. Role of Purkinje fibers in post-infarction ventricular tachycardia. *J Am Coll Cardiol*. 2006;48: 2500–2507.

Figure 4.L.2

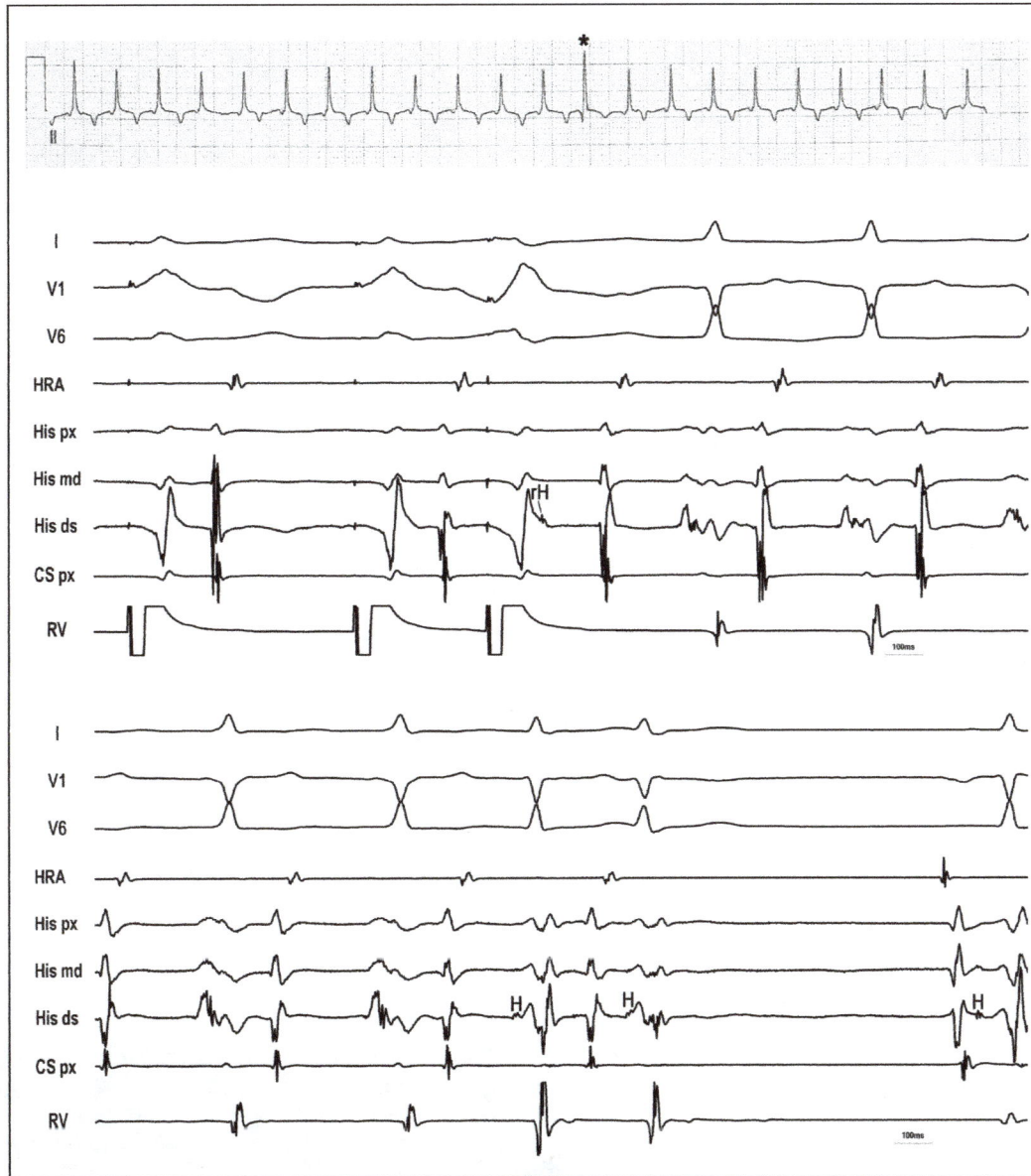

Question

Entrainment mapping is attempted in a 36-year-old patient with arrhythmogenic right ventricular cardiomyopathy.

Why is classical entrainment not demonstrated?

A) Concealed fusion is not consistent

B) The postpacing interval is shorter than the TCL

C) The VT cycle length oscillates

D) All of the above

E) None of the above

Figure 4.M.1

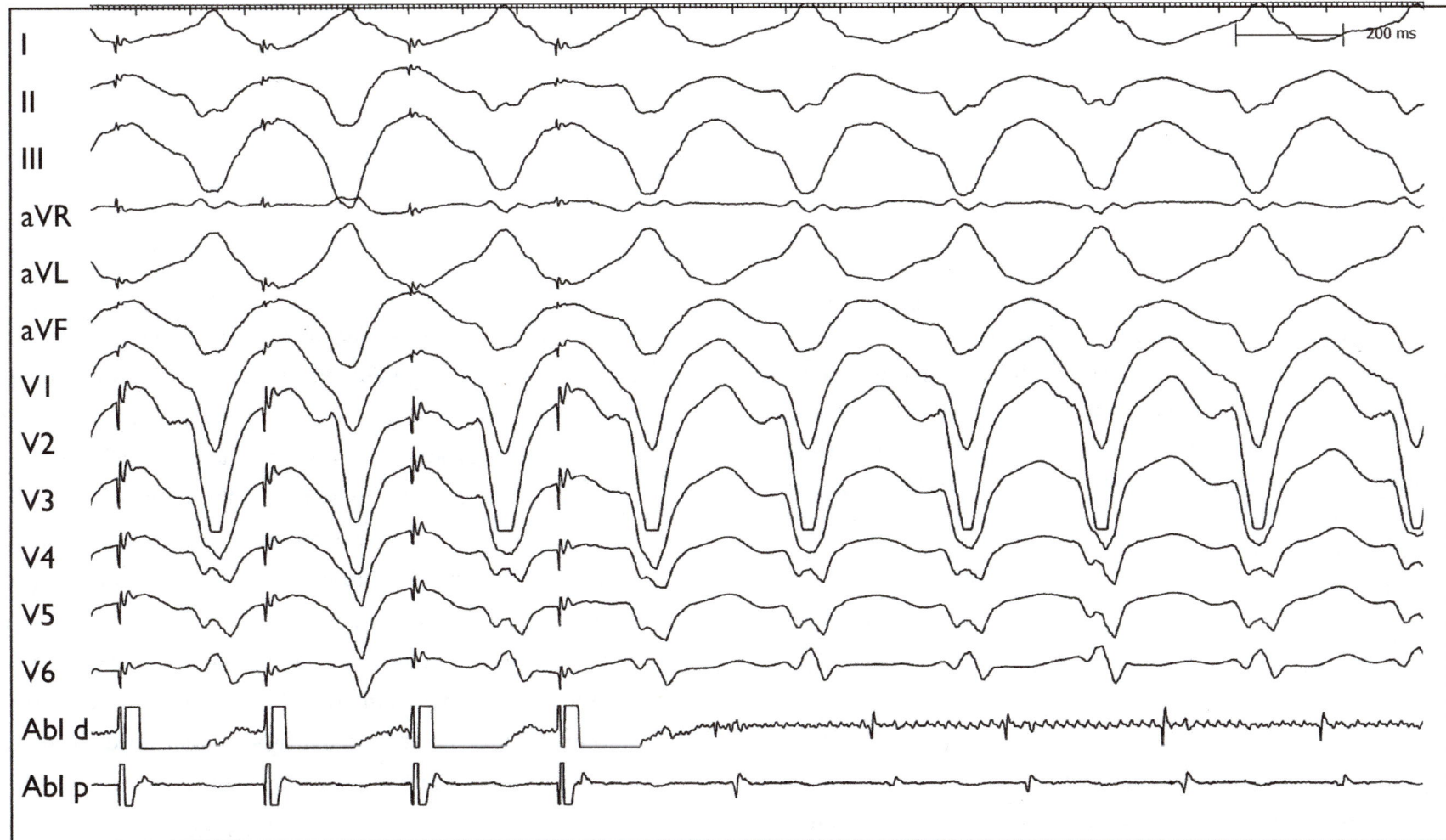

*A*nswer

The correct answer is **D**. All of the above are correct. Classical entrainment criteria for proof of an isthmus requires concealed fusion during pacing and a postpacing interval within 30 ms of the tachycardia cycle length. During entrainment, the second beat and last beat of pacing demonstrate overt fusion, most evident in leads II, III, and V_6. However, the first and third beats are an exact match for the VT, demonstrating concealed fusion. Although not typically seen, multiple exit site morphologies from a common isthmus can be seen with pacemapping as well as during entrainment.

The postpacing interval of 280 ms is shorter than the tachycardia cycle length (295 ms). However, significant oscillation is noted after entrainment with shortening of the cycle length to 250 ms. Variations in tachycardia cycle length are likely due to functional slowing with recovery in the circuit and limits the interpretation of entrainment. A short PPI may also result from far field capture more remote from the pacing electrode, which shortens the distance that the circuit needs to complete when returning to the pacing site.

References

1. Stevenson WG, Khan H, Sager P, Saxon LA, Middlekauf HR, Natterson PD, Wiener I. Identification of reentry circuit sites during catheter mapping and radiofrequency ablation of ventricular tachycardia late after myocardial infarction. *Circulation*. 1993;88:1647–1670.
2. Tung R, Shivkumar K. Unusual response to entrainment of ventricular tachycardia: In or out? *Heart Rhythm*. 2014;11(4):725–727.
3. Kaneko Y1, Nakajima T, Irie T, Ota M, Iijima T, Tamura M, et al. Mechanism of shorter postpacing interval than the tachycardia cycle after high-output entrainment pacing of atrial flutter. *J Cardiovasc Electrophysiol*. 2013;24(8):936–938.

Figure 4.M.2

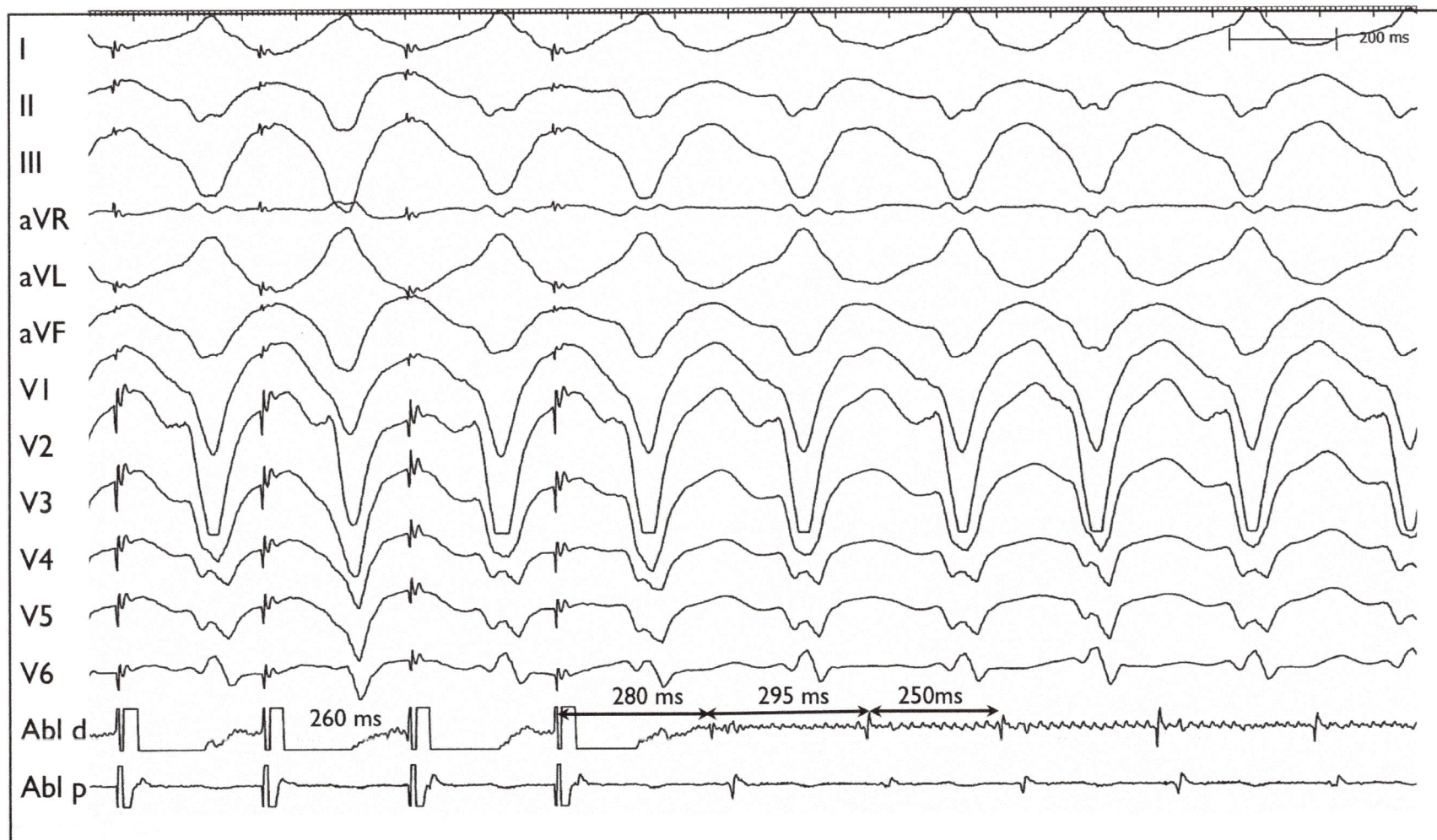

Question

What is the most likely mechanism of the wide complex tachycardia observed during the second rhythm strip?

A) Supraventricular tachycardia with aberrancy

B) Antidromic atrioventricular reentrant tachycardia

C) AV nodal reentrant tachycardia with bystander ventricular preexcitation

D) Ventricular tachycardia

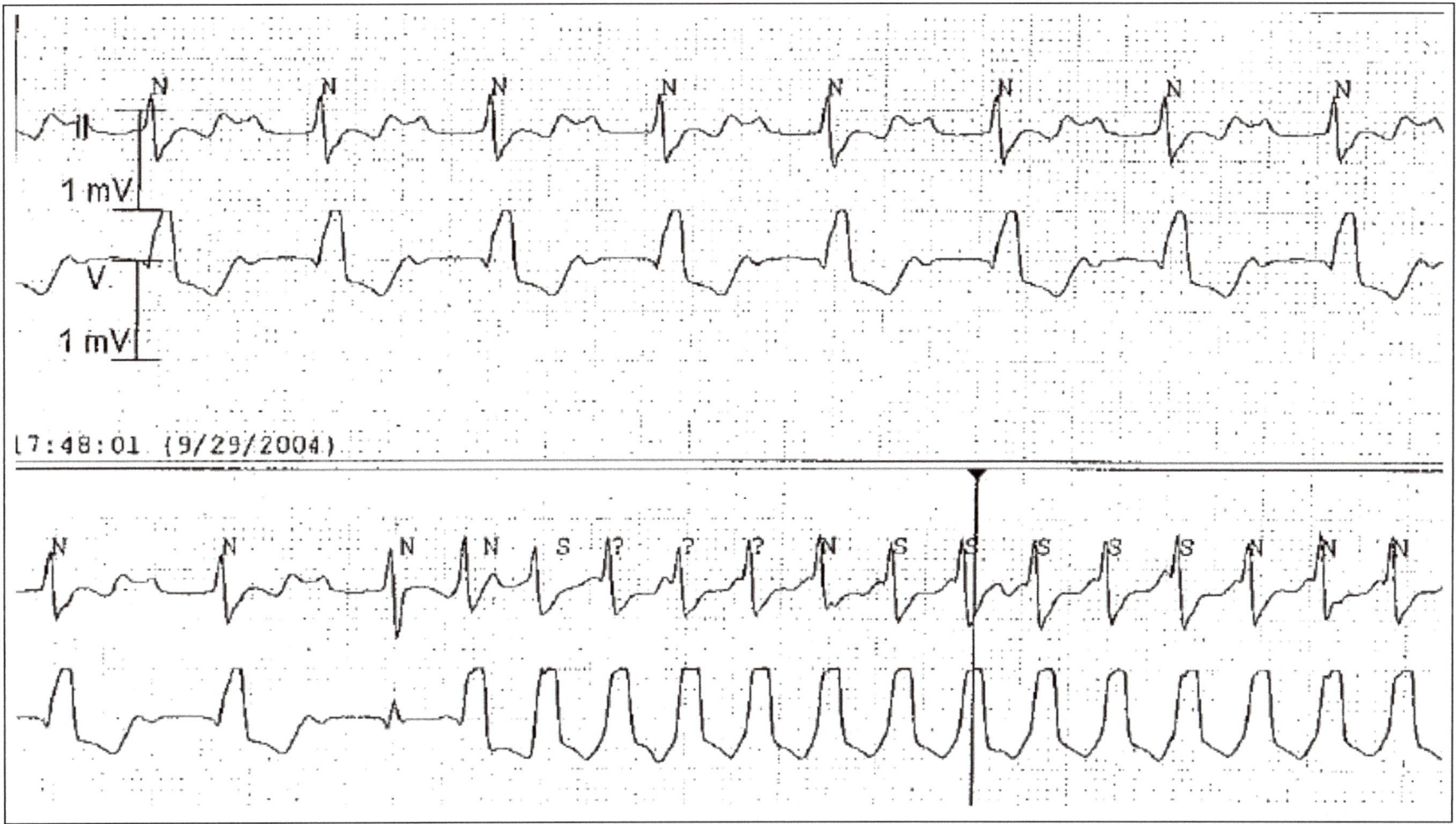

Figure 4.N.1

Answer

The correct answer is **D**. The initial portion of the tracing demonstrates sinus rhythm with first-degree AV bock and right bundle branch block. Next, a wide complex tachycardia initiates, with QRS morphology similar to native conduction. However, **AV dissociation is clearly present, establishing the diagnosis of ventricular tachycardia with certainty**. The sinus P waves (annotated with ⋆) march through the rhythm strip uninterrupted. Note the first beat of VT (arrow) is fused with native conduction, resulting in a narrower QRS complex than either native conduction or VT. Choices A, B, and C all have a 1:1 AV relationship.

Reference

1. Brugada P, Brugada J, Mont L, Smeets J, Andries EW. A new approach to the differential diagnosis of a regular tachycardia with a wide QRS complex. *Circulation*. 1991;83(5):1649–1659.

Figure 4.N.2

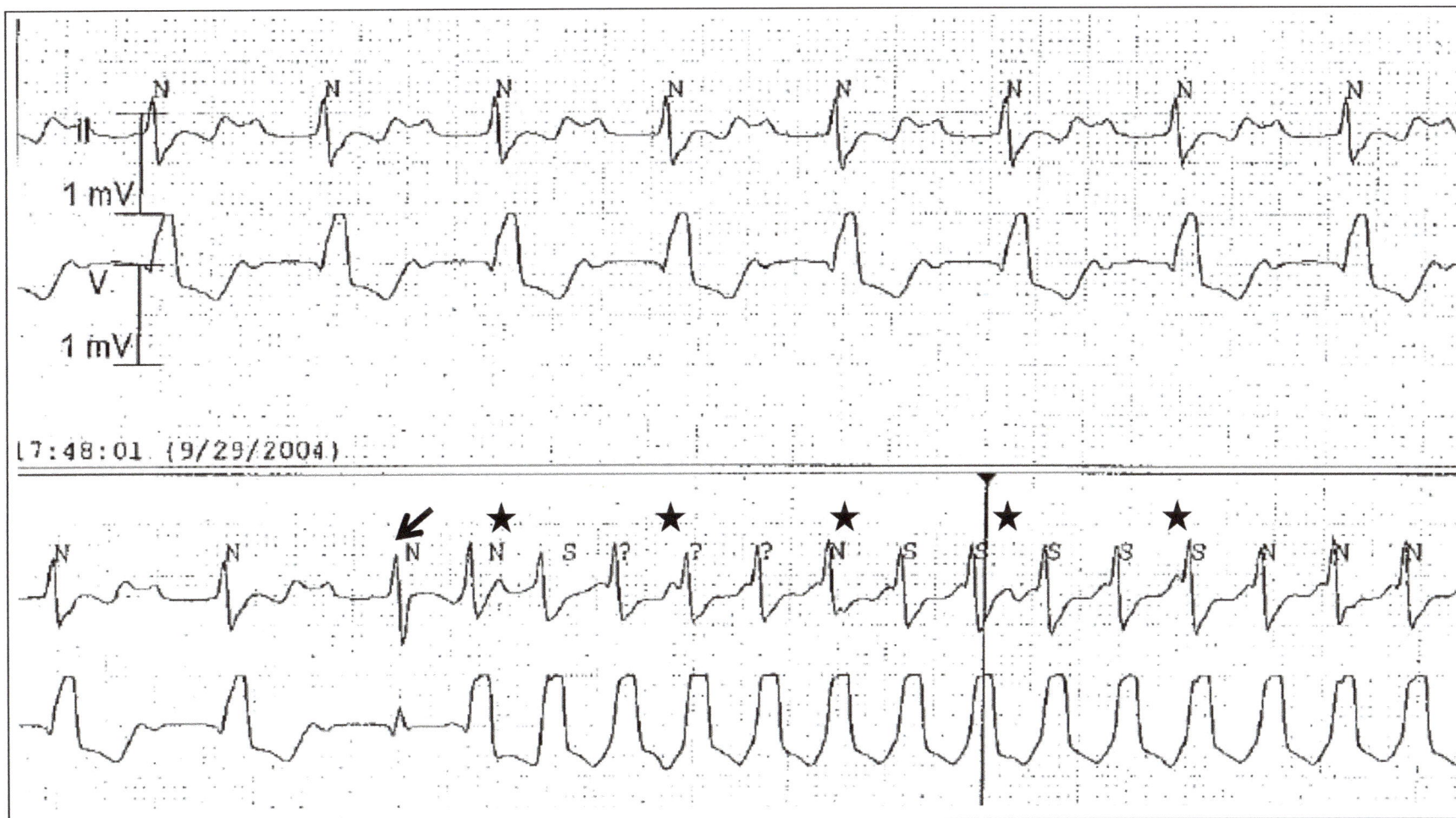

Question

The following phenomenon is seen during pacemapping within scar.

What should be the next step?

A) Pacemap in a different region

B) Map for diastolic signal

C) Ablate at this site

D) Ablate if entrainment criteria are fulfilled

Figure 4.O.1

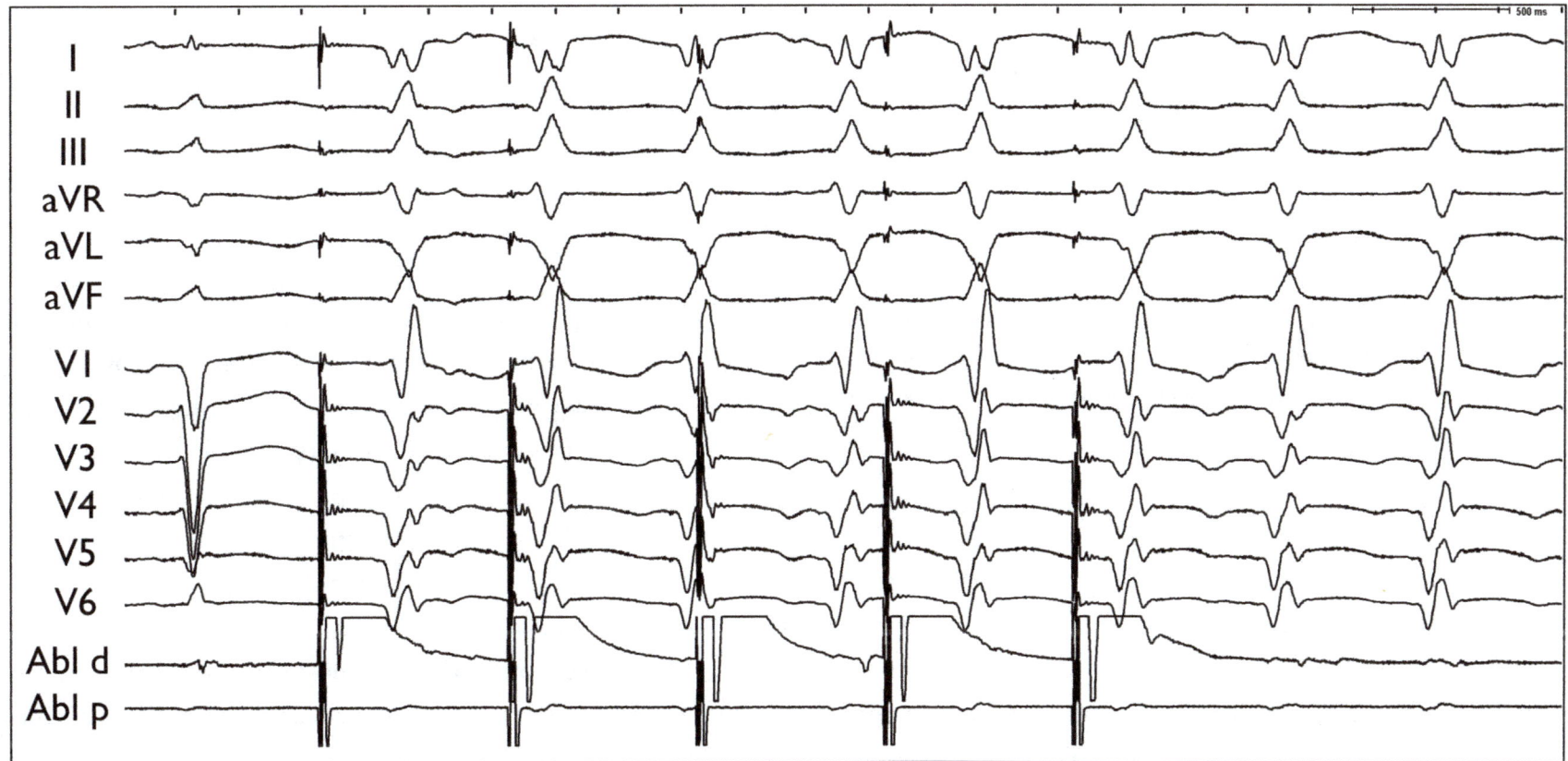

Figure 4.O.1

*A*nswer

The correct answer is **C**. Ablation at this site is likely to be successful.

The unintended induction of ventricular tachycardia during pacemapping at a relatively slow drive cycle (600 ms) has been termed a **pacemapped induction**. This phenomenon occurs without the need for an extrastimulus to initiate reentry and occurs more frequently during pacing from within the reentrant path. Decremental conduction with unidirectional block with a pacing drive is specific for the isthmus and results in termination of VT in >90% of cases. An exact pacemap match is not a requirement, as isthmus sites may have multiple exit sites.

In this case, the first beat of pacing is captured with a long stimulus–QRS interval. The second pacing spike is unlikely to capture, as there is effectively no stimulus latency. VT is initiated, and the morphology is a close match to the first pacemap beat. Note that the VT has subtle morphology changes with alternans most apparent in V_2. Despite the lack of overt diastolic activity, rapid termination of VT was achieved at this site. Although entrainment can be attempted, termination of VT, transition to a different morphology, or failure to capture may result.

Reference

1. Tung R, Mathuria N, Michowitz Y, Yu R, Buch E, Bradfield J, et al. Functional pace-mapping responses for identification of targets for catheter ablation of scar-mediated ventricular tachycardia. *Circ Arrhythm Electrophysiol.* 2012;5(2):264–272.

Figure 4.O.2

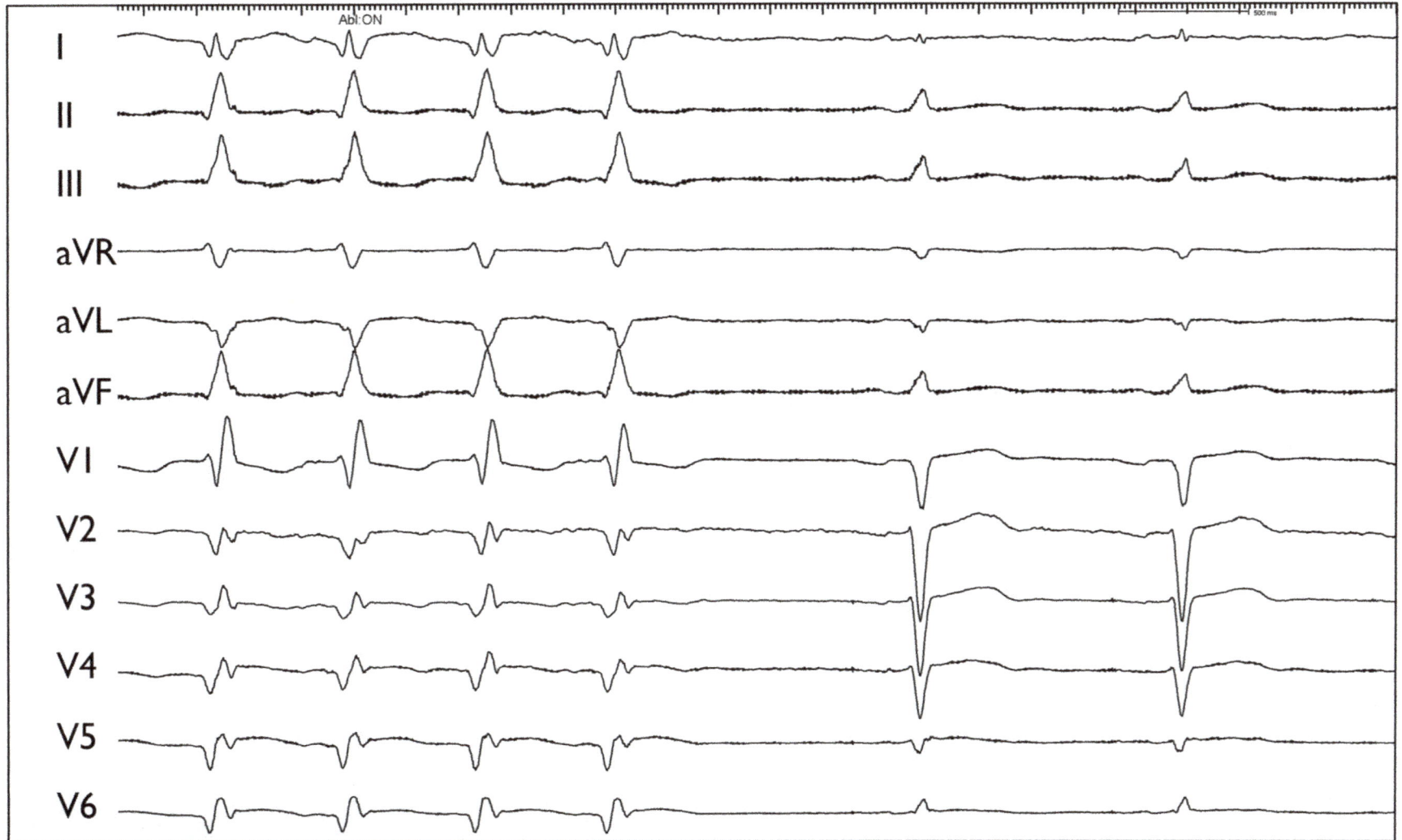

Question

What is the most likely substrate in this patient with three ventricular tachycardia morphologies?

A) Arrhythmogenic right ventricular cardiomyopathy

B) Anterior myocardial infarction

C) Idiopathic

D) Nonischemic left ventricular cardiomyopathy with basal lateral predominance

E) Nonischemic left ventricular cardiomyopathy with septal predominance

Figure 4.P.1

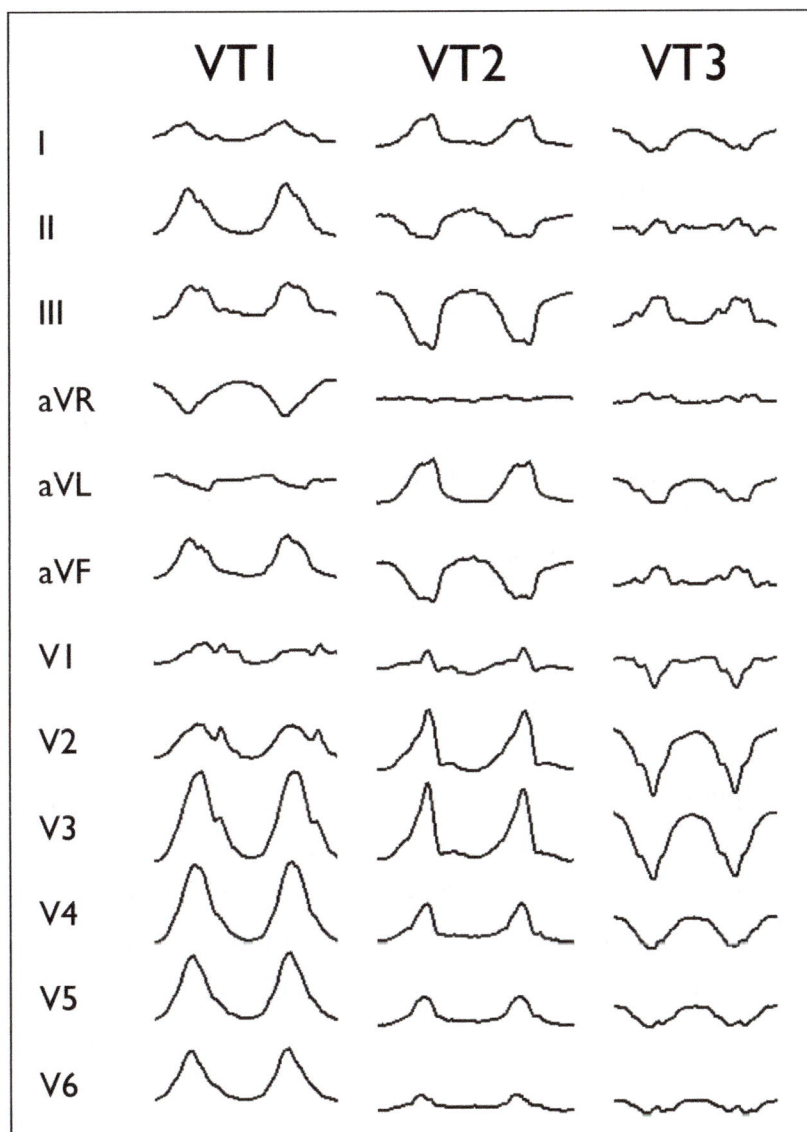

Answer

The correct answer is **E**. The first and second VTs have a right bundle configuration in lead V_1 and are positive throughout the precordium, consistent with exit sites in the basal left ventricle. Both are positive in lead 1, indicating exit sites on the septum. The first VT is inferiorly directed, while the second VT is superiorly directed. Thus the first VT is exiting at the top of the basal LV septum and the second at the bottom of the basal LV septum. The third VT has a left bundle configuration in lead V_1 with late precordial transition, consistent with an exit more apically along the LV septum.

When multiple VT morphologies are observed exiting along various septal sites, a septal nonischemic substrate should be suspected. Septal scarring is frequently midmyocardial, and thus bipolar voltage can be normal along both sides of the septum, as was the case in this patient. However, unipolar voltage is more sensitive for deeper substrate, and large areas of unipolar LV and RV voltage abnormality were detected in this patient.

Unipolar abnormality is most commonly defined as < 8.3 mV in the LV and < 5.5 mV in the RV. Cardiac MRI prior to ablation is useful for identifying septal scar, which is often challenging to ablate.

References

1. Haqqani HM, Tschabrunn CM, Tzou WS, et al. Isolated septal substrate for ventricular tachycardia in nonischemic dilated cardiomyopathy: incidence, characterization, and implications. *Heart Rhythm.* 2011;8:1169–1176.

2. Hutchinson MD, Gerstenfeld EP, Desjardins B, et al. Endocardial unipolar voltage mapping to detect epicardial ventricular tachycardia substrate in patients with nonischemic left ventricular cardiomyopathy. *Circ Arrhythm Electrophysiol.* 2011;4:49–55.

3. Polin GM, Haqqani H, Tzou W, et al. Endocardial unipolar voltage mapping to identify epicardial substrate in arrhythmogenic right ventricular cardiomyopathy/dysplasia. *Heart Rhythm.* 2011;8:76-83.

Figure 4.P.2

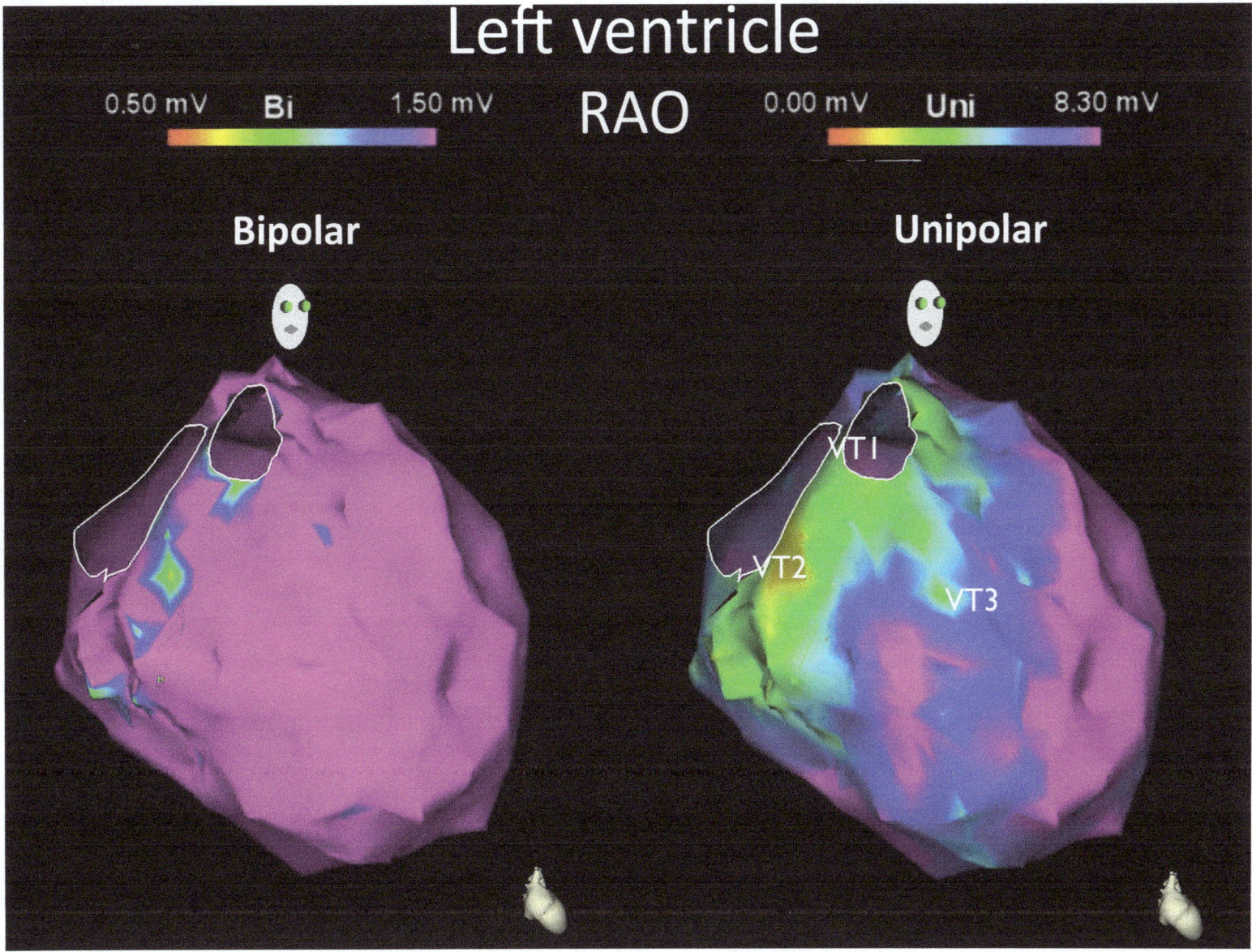

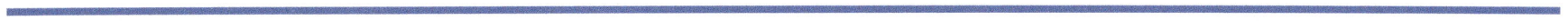

Figure 4.P.3

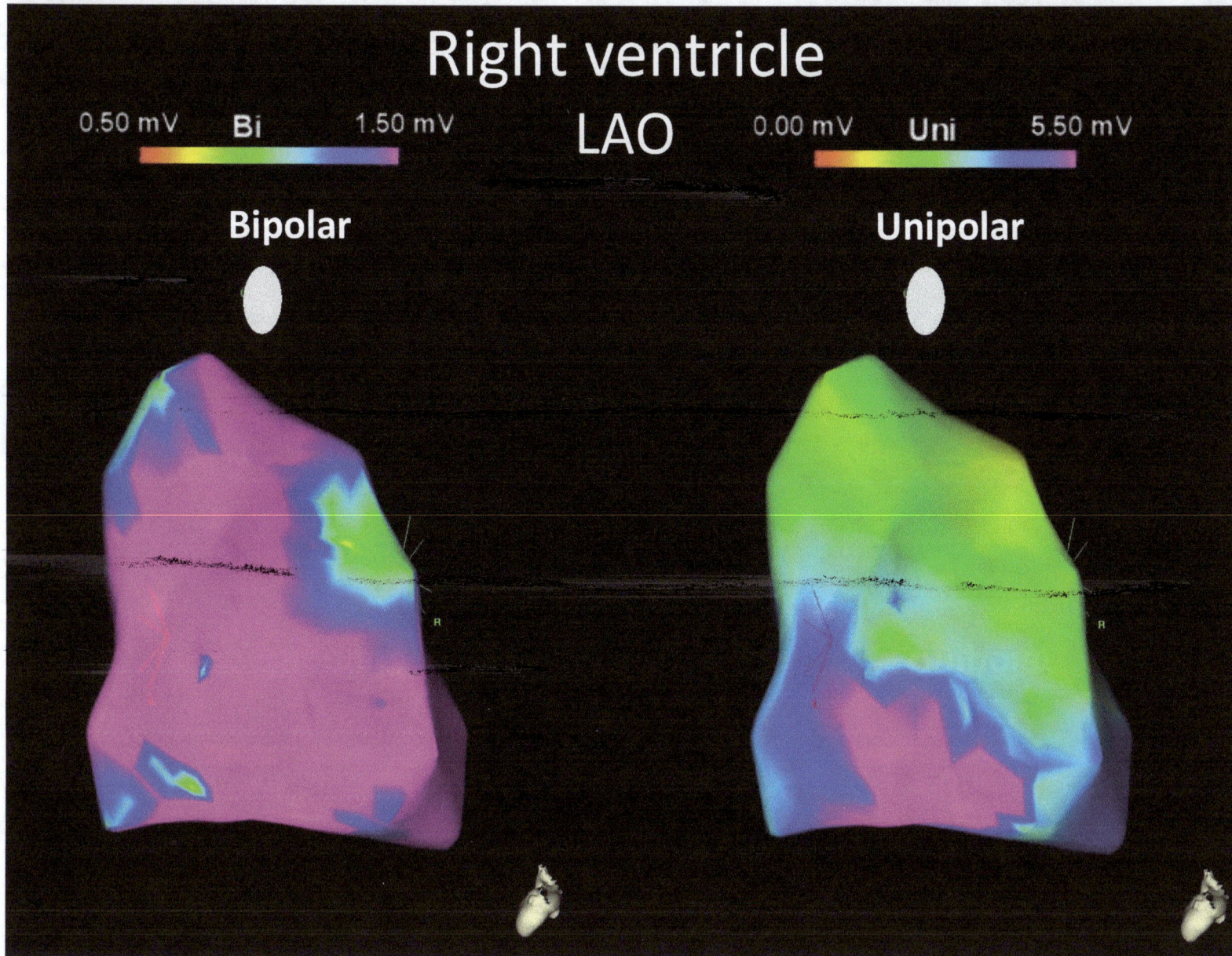

Question

A 61-year-old man with dilated cardiomyopathy under–goes endocardial mapping of ventricular tachycardia. Which site is demonstrated with entrainment?

A) Isthmus

B) Outer loop

C) Adjacent bystander

D) Electrogram not captured

Figure 4.Q.1

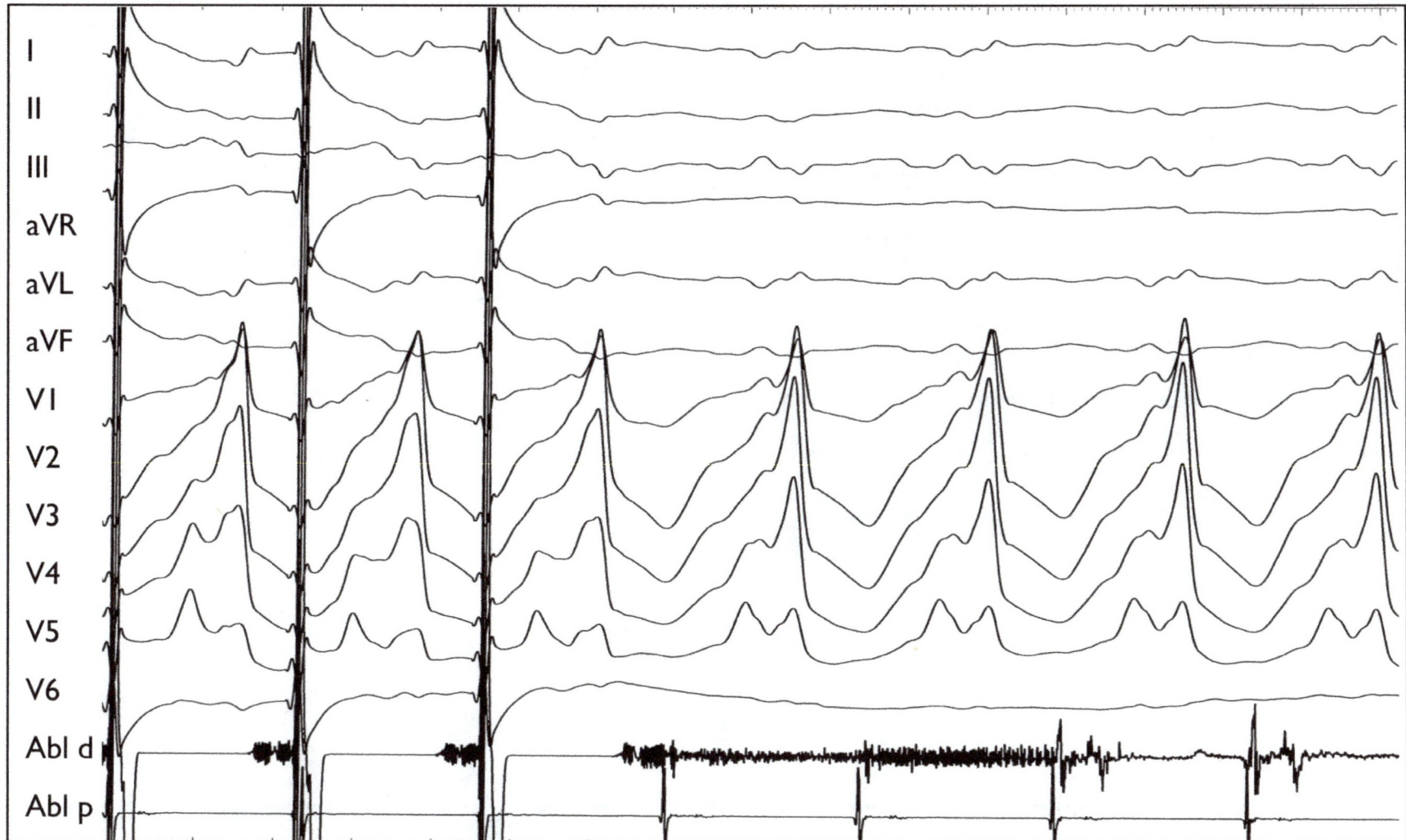

Figure 4.Q.2

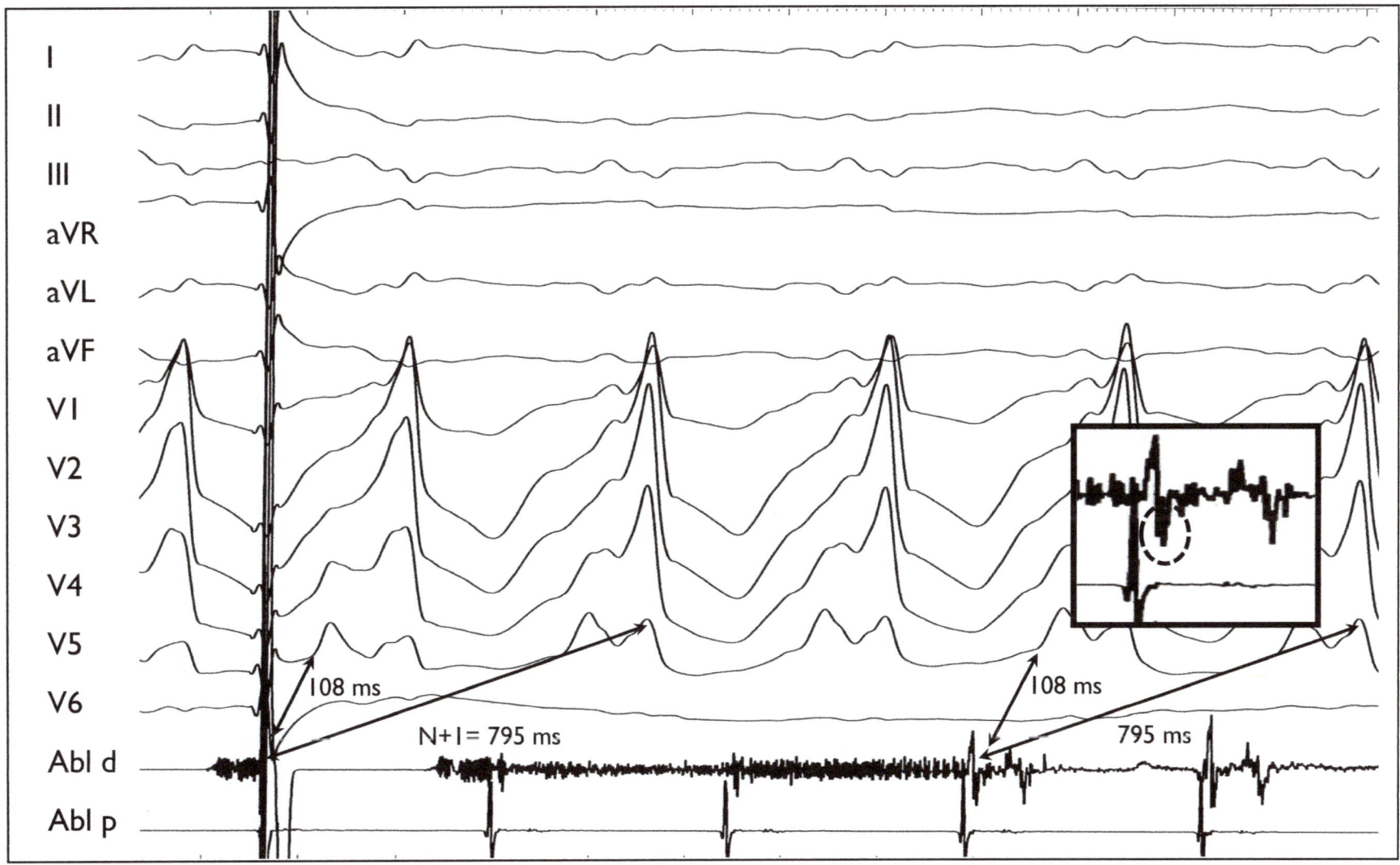

Answer

The correct answer is **B. Entrainment from an outer loop site** is shown.

Significant artifact from saturation in the pacing channel of the distal ablation electrode is seen after entrainment. This commonly obscures the return electrogram, which makes measurement of the postpacing interval a challenge. The N+1 technique can be implemented, where measurement from the last pacing stimulus to a fiducial point on the following QRS serves as a PPI surrogate. Measuring to the second R-wave peak in V_5 yields an N+1 interval of 795 ms, which is an exact match when measuring back from the last QRS complex at the same peak after the artifact has resolved.

Importantly, the actual electrogram component captured is the small negative component (dashed circle) that has an EGM-QRS interval of 108 ms, which matches the S-QRS interval. Measuring to the onset of the tallest positive electrogram component is 120 ms. Capture is present as overt fusion is seen. Due to the presence of slight fusion, most apparent in V_3 and V_4, an isthmus site is not proven. Outer loop sites exhibit overt fusion, as the antidromic wavefront is not bound within a protected isthmus. However, as they are within the circuit, the postpacing interval is within 30 ms of the tachycardia cycle length.

Adjacent bystander sites demonstrated concealed entrainment with a long S-QRS interval. The response to entrainment in various parts of the reentrant circuit are summarized in the Figure 4.Q.4.

Figure 4.Q.3

- At an outer loop site, the antidromic wavefront is not bound within the scar channel, resulting in myocardial capture spatially distinct from the circuit exit site. The PPI is within 30 ms of the TCL, indicating that it is in the circuit.

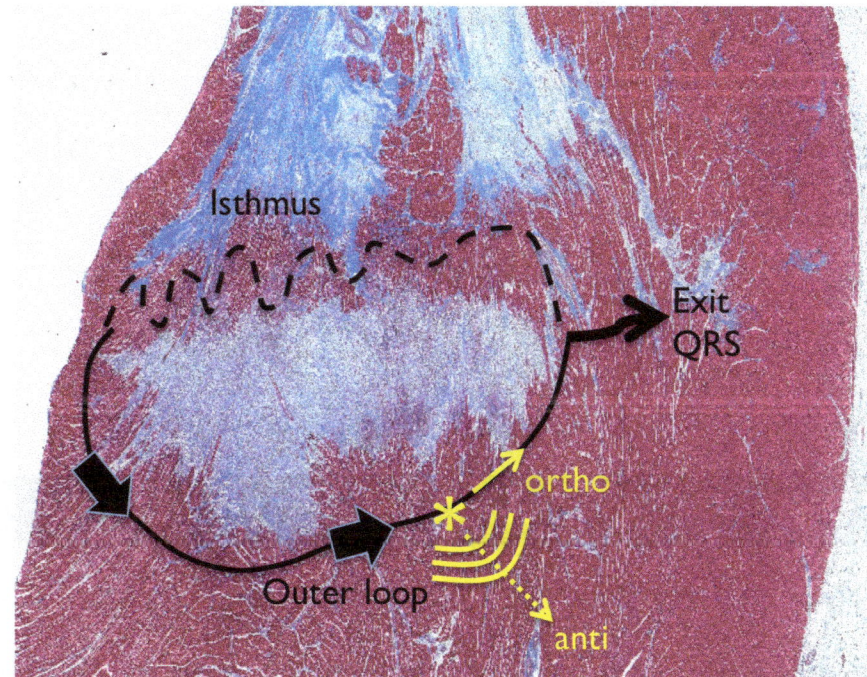

Figure 4.Q.4

Circuit location	Fusion	PPI	EGM-QRS
Remote bystander	overt	>TCL	variable
Outer loop	overt	=TCL±30ms	variable
Inner loop	concealed	=TCL±30ms	>70%
Isthmus (Central)	concealed	=TCL±30ms	30-70% TCL
Distal Isthmus (Exit)	concealed	=TCL±30ms	<30% TCL
Proximal isthmus (Entrance)	concealed	=TCL±30ms	70-100% TCL
Adjacent bystander	concealed	>TCL	<S-QRS

References

1. Stevenson WG, Khan H, Sager P, Saxon LA, Middlekauf HR, Natterson PD, Wiener I. Identification of reentry circuit sites during catheter mapping and radiofrequency ablation of ventricular tachycardia late after myocardial infarction. *Circulation.* 1993;88:1647–1670.

2. Soejima K, Stevenson WG, Maisel WH, Delacretaz E, Brunckhorst CB, Ellison KE, Friedman PL. The N + 1 difference: a new measure for entrainment mapping. *J Am Coll Cardiol.* 2001;37(5):1386–1394.

3. Derejko P, Szumowski ŁJ, Sanders P, et al. Clinical validation and comparison of alternative methods for evaluation of entrainment mapping. *J Cardiovasc Electrophysiol.* 2009;20(7):741–748.

Question

Entrainment mapping is performed in a 61-year-old man with dilated cardiomyopathy.

The following response demonstrates:

A) Isthmus

B) Outer loop

C) Adjacent bystander

D) Remote bystander

E) None of the above

Figure 4.R.1

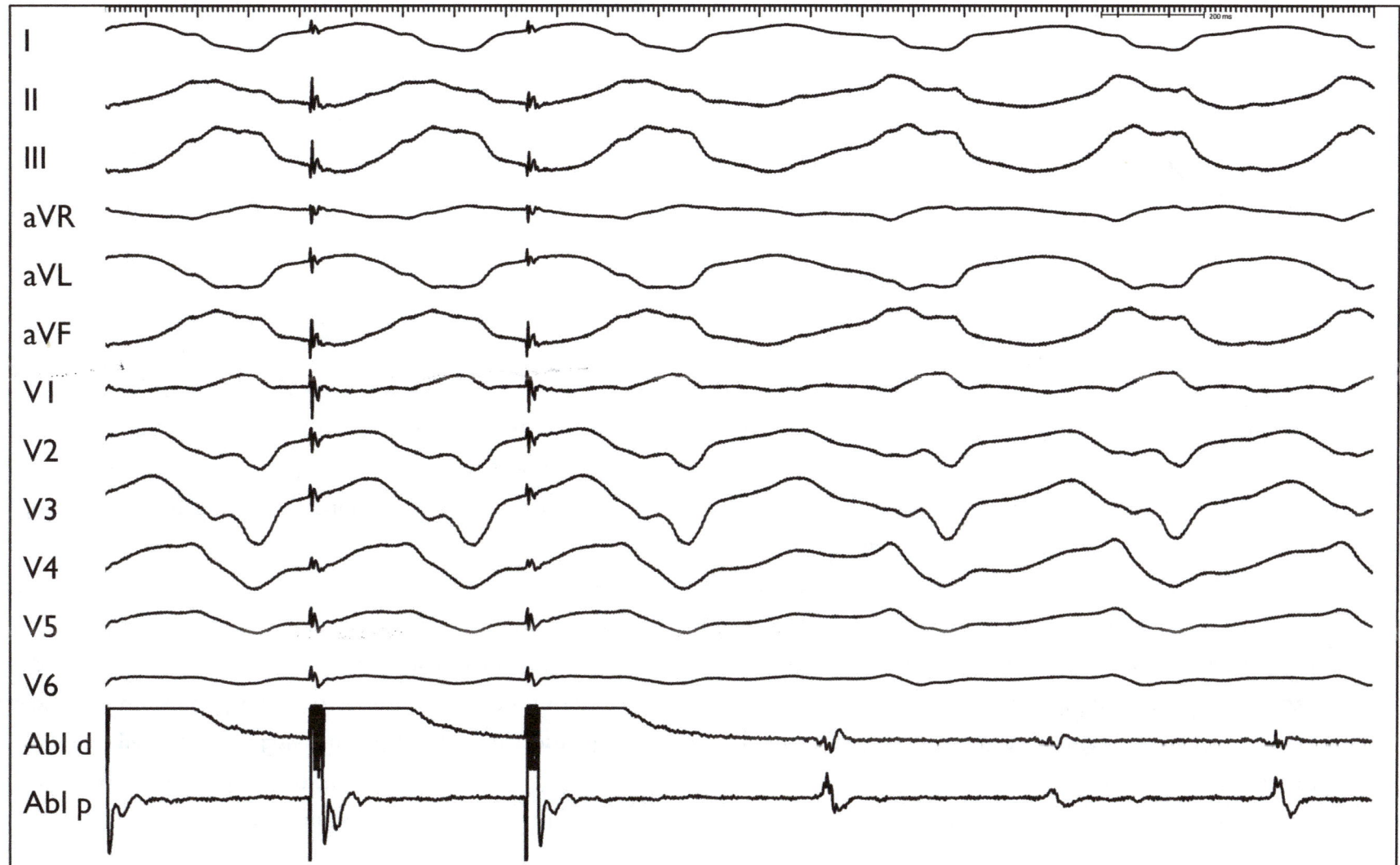

Answer

The correct answer is **E**. The entrainment response is not characteristic of any of the preceding answers.

Overdrive pacing 25 ms faster than the TCL is performed with capture of the local electogram. Concealed fusion is seen during pacing. Note the T wave fuses into the QRS onset during faster pacing, which commonly confounds analysis of morphologic match. Overt fusion should be seen at remote bystander and outer loop sites.

Closer analysis suggests the possibility of subtle fusion in the inferior leads, but this is not conclusive. Importantly, the postpacing interval (555 ms) is 100 ms longer than the TCL (445 ms), which excludes an isthmus site or an outer loop site.

Proof of an adjacent bystander or "blind loop" attached to an isthmus requires that the PPI-TCL difference (110 ms) is the same as the S-QRS-EGM-QRS difference (26 ms). This is not the case, which suggests several possibilities: 1) the electrogram captured may not be seen on the distal ablation catheter, 2) anodal capture was present, or 3) decremental conduction occurred due to entrainment, resulting in a longer postpacing interval.

Despite the absence of classical entrainment response for any circuit location, prompt termination occurred at this site during ablation.

This case highlights some of the limitations of entrainment mapping.

Figure 4.R.2

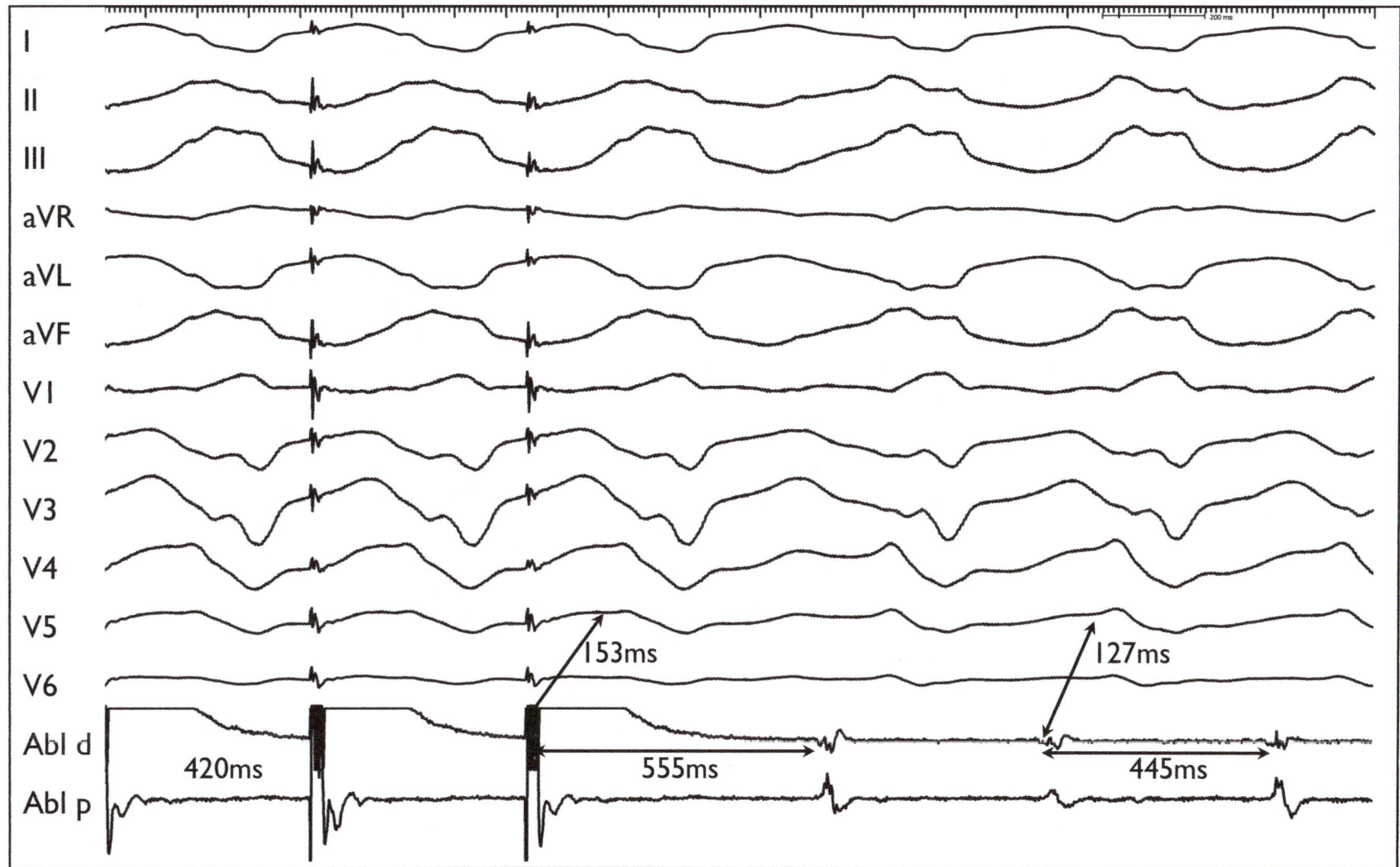

Figure 4.R.3

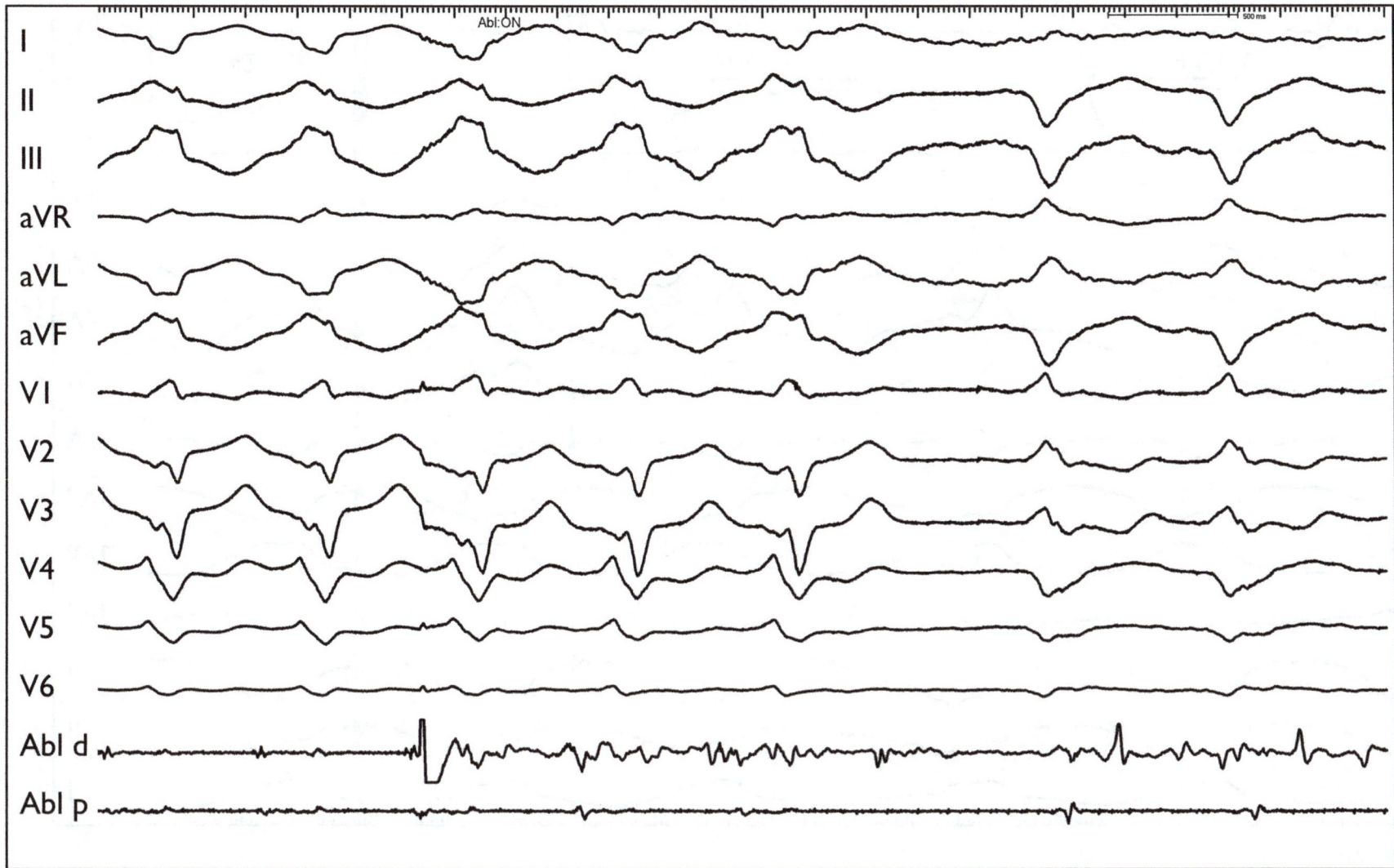

Figure 4.R.4

Limitations of Entrainment Mapping

1. Failure to capture—pacing too slow, too low of an output, or tissue is inexcitable

2. Assuming a macroreentrant mechanism—focal can be overdriven

3. Decremental conduction—pacing too fast yields long postpacing interval

4. Far-field capture—pacing at high output can result in shorter PPI

5. Inability to distinguish near field electrogram components

6. Pacing artifact obscures local electrogram making it difficult to assess return interval—use N+1 technique

7. Termination of tachycardia

8. Acceleration of tachycardia or transition to a different tachycardia

Figure 4.R.5

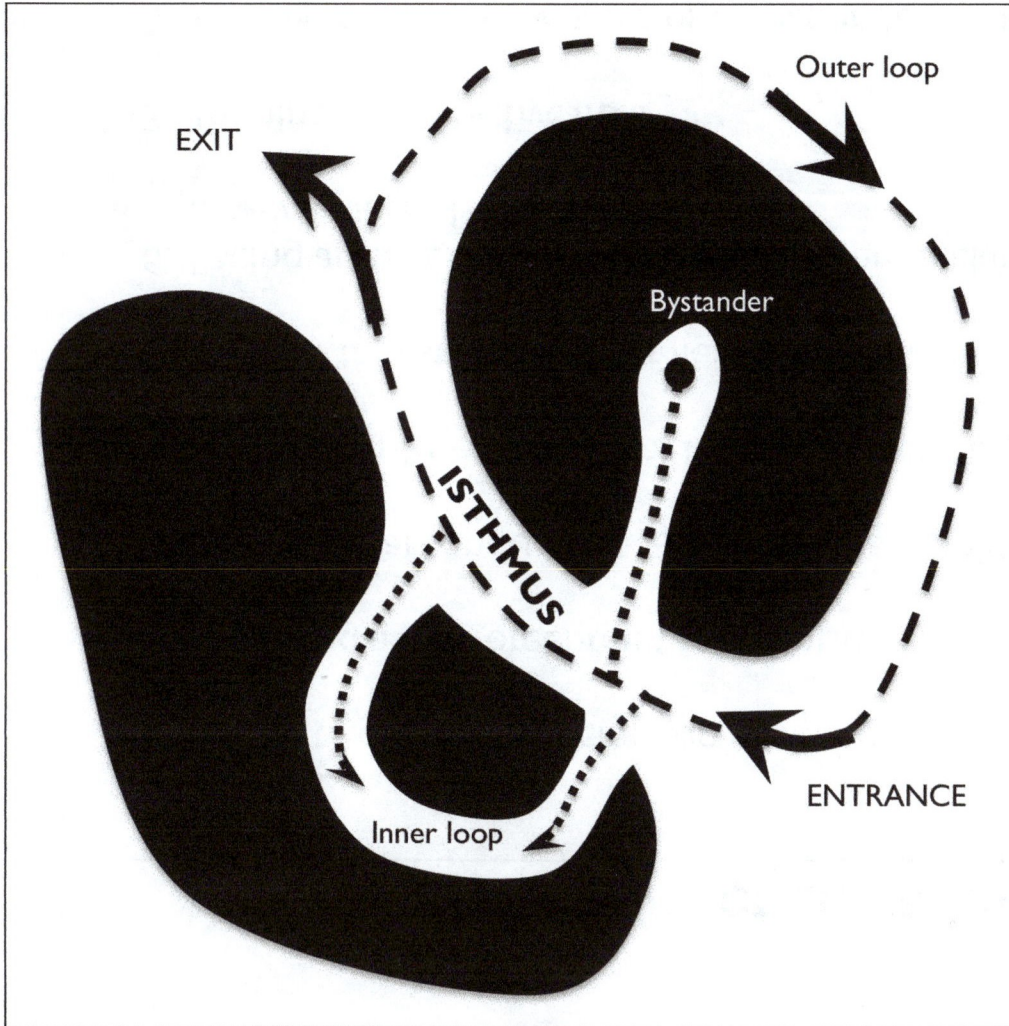

Reference

1. Josephson ME. *Clinical Cardiac Electrophysiology: Techniques and Interpretations*, 4th ed. Philadelphia: Lippincott Williams & Wilkins; 2008.

*Q*uestion

A 62-year-old man with history of remote anterior myocardial infarction presented with ventricular tachycardia. Catheter ablation was performed. Pacing was delivered from the ablation catheter.

The ablation catheter is most likely positioned in:

A) Entrance site

B) Isthmus site

C) Exit site

D) Outer loop

E) Remote bystander

Figure 4.S.1

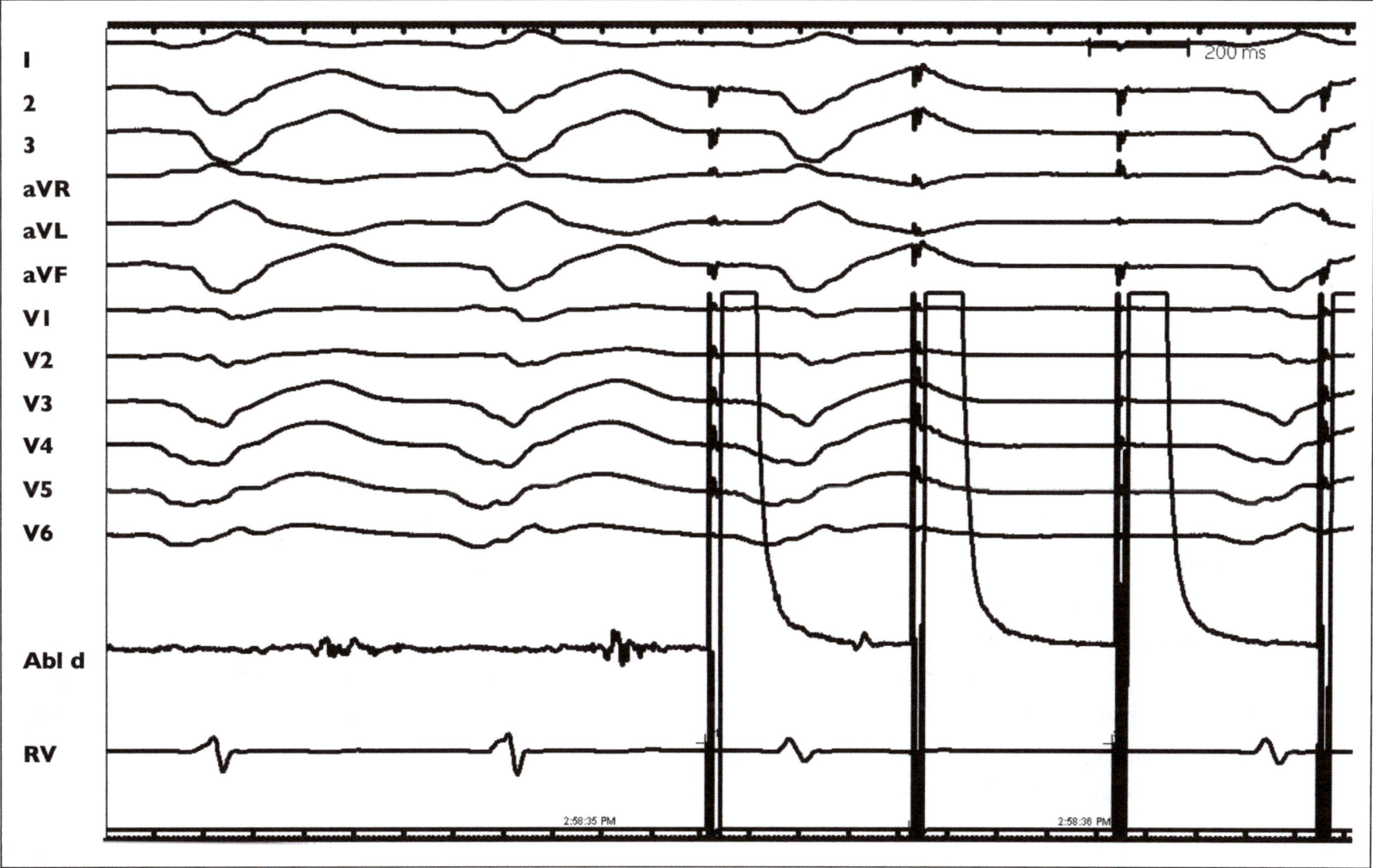

Figure 4.S.1

Answer

The correct answer is **B**. The ventricular tachycardia cycle length is 590 ms. There is a long, mid-diastolic potential recorded by the ablation catheter (annotated with ⋆). The first pacing stimulus does not affect the tachycardia. The second pacing stimulus terminates VT without generating a QRS complex (nonpropagated extrastimulus). The third pacing stimulus produces a perfect pacemap for the VT, with a long stimulus to QRS. **A nonpropagated extrastimulus occurs when pacing inside a narrow, protected isthmus of the tachycardia circuit**. The paced wavefront collides with the refractory tail of the VT wavefront in the orthodromic direction,

and with the head of the VT wavefront in the antidromic direction, thereby extinguishing the tachycardia. It is highly predictive of a successful ablation site. In this case, VT was reinduced and then promptly terminated with ablation in this location.

The stimulus to QRS interval on the paced beat is 240 ms, which is 41% of the tachycardia cycle length. Pacing at an entrance or exit site would result in a stimulus to QRS interval $>70\%$ or $<30\%$ of the tachycardia cycle length, respectively. Pacing at an outer loop or remote bystander site would generate a QRS complex of different morphology than the ventricular tachycardia.

Figure 4.S.2

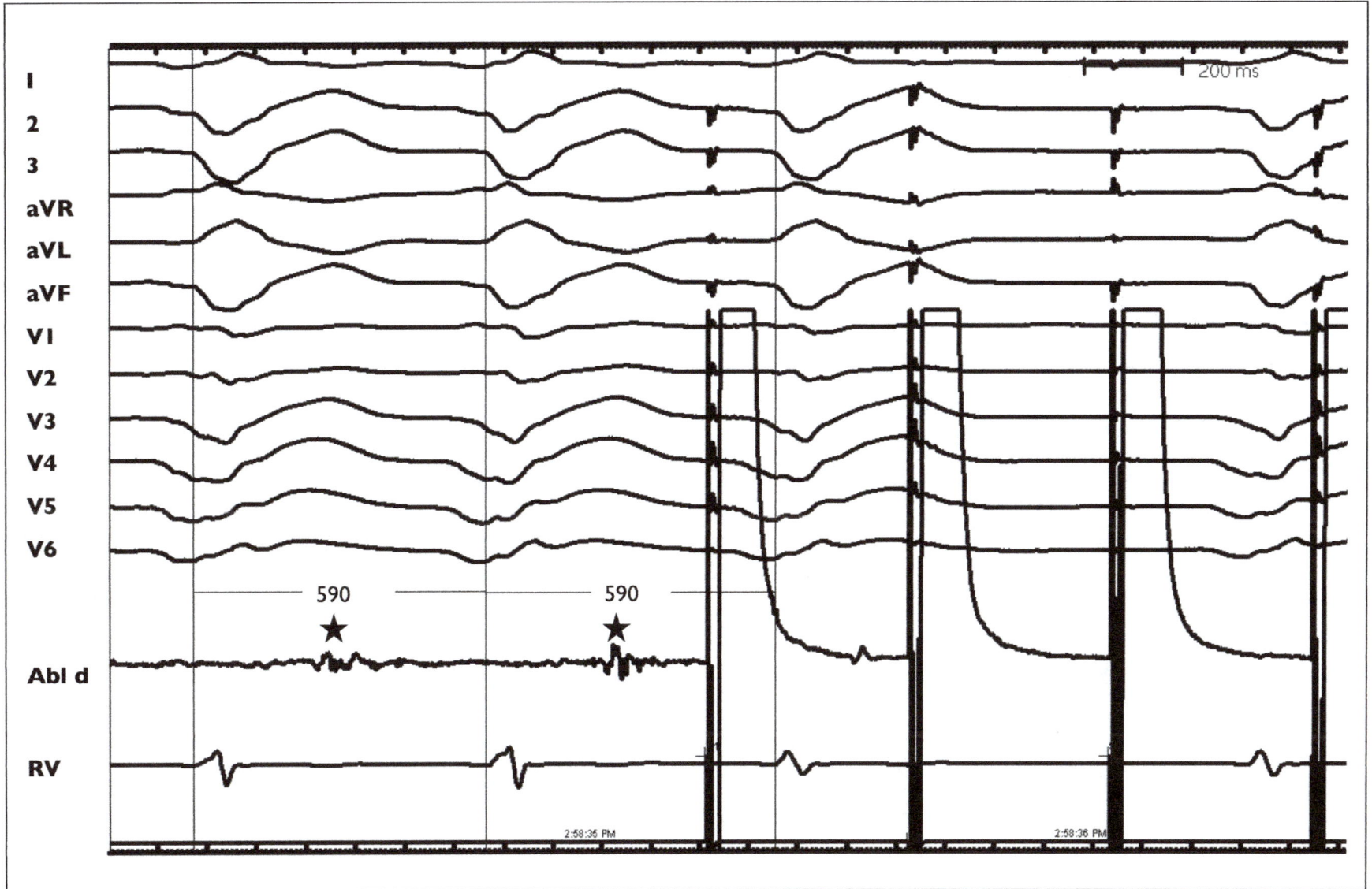

References

1. Altemose GT, Miller JM. Termination of ventricular tachycardia by a nonpropagated extrastimulus. *J Cardiovasc Electrophysiol*. 2000;11:125.

2. Stevenson WG, Khan H, Sager P, et al. Identification of reentry circuit sites during catheter mapping and radiofrequency ablation of ventricular tachycardia late after myocardial infarction. *Circulation*. 1993;88:1647–1670.

Appendix A

Spoiler alert! Because the case titles are by diagnosis, they may suggest an answer to the case question. Therefore, they are presented as an appendix, rather than as a table of contents.

Appendix B

www.ingramcontent.com/pod-product-compliance
Lightning Source LLC
Chambersburg PA
CBHW080920220326
41598CB00034B/5627

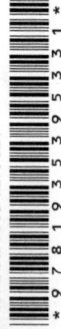